QM Library

KU-627-423

23 1370011 2

Research Methods for Clinical Therapists

WITHDRAWN
FROM STOCK
QMUL LIBRARY

For Peter, Tom and Laura and in memory of my parents – with my love and thanks

Commissioning Editor: Mairi McCubbin
Development Editor: Sheila Black
Project Manager: Morven Dean/Sruthi Viswam
Designer: George Ajayi
Illustrator: Chartwell/Cactus

Research Methods for Clinical Therapists

Applied Project Design and Analysis

Carolyn M. Hicks BA MA PhD PGCE CPsychol

Professor of Health Care Psychology
College of Medical and Dental Sciences
University of Birmingham, UK

FIFTH EDITION

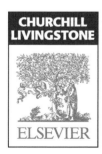

EDINBURGH LONDON NEW YORK OXFORD PHILADELPHIA ST LOUIS SYDNEY TORONTO 2009

CHURCHILL
LIVINGSTONE
ELSEVIER

An imprint of Elsevier Limited

© Harcourt Brace and Company Limited 1999
© Harcourt Publishers Limited 2000
© Elsevier Limited 2004
© 2009, Elsevier Limited. All rights reserved

No part of this publication may be reproduced or transmitted in any form or by any means, electronic or mechanical, including photocopying, recording, or any information storage and retrieval system, without permission in writing from the publisher. Permissions may be sought directly from Elsevier's Rights Department: phone: (+1) 215 239 3804 (US) or (+44) 1865 843830 (UK); fax: (+44) 1865 853333; e-mail: healthpermissions@elsevier.com. You may also complete your request on-line via the Elsevier website at http://www.elsevier.com/permissions.

First published 1988
Second edition 1995
Third edition 1999
    Reprinted 2000
Fourth edition 2004
Fifth edition 2009

ISBN: 978-0-7020-2998-1

British Library Cataloguing in Publication Data
A catalogue record for this book is available from the British Library

Library of Congress Cataloging in Publication Data
A catalog record for this book is available from the Library of Congress

Notice
Neither the Publisher nor the Author assumes any responsibility for any loss or injury and/or damage to persons or property arising out of or related to any use of the material contained in this book. It is the responsibility of the treating practitioner, relying on independent expertise and knowledge of the patient, to determine the best treatment and method of application for the patient.
The Publisher

Printed and bound by CPI Group (UK) Ltd, Croydon, CR0 4YY

Transferred to Digital Print 2012

The
publisher's
policy is to use
**paper manufactured
from sustainable forests**

QM LIBRARY (WHITECHAPEL)

Contents

Preface

It is now 20 years since the first edition of this text and the demand for top quality, cost-effective healthcare has never been greater. Increased access to information technology, international advances in healthcare knowledge and technology, and the empowerment of patients have all contributed to the expectation that healthcare delivery will be based not on hunch and ritual, but on leading-edge science. This means that the evidence-based healthcare culture, with its focus on scientific rigour and objective evidence, is now centre stage in the drive towards best care at best prices. As a result, healthcare professionals have an imperative to ensure that their clinical decisions can be justified on empirical grounds and that they can withstand fiscal and clinical scrutiny. Added to this is the rise in healthcare litigation, which means that, increasingly, health professionals must be fully accountable for their practice and able to defend treatment interventions in the light of available research evidence. The case for evidence-based healthcare would seem to be unassailable. Yet, while few would attempt to mount any counter argument, good quality research studies that address fundamental issues in care provision have not been as plentiful as is either desirable or necessary. Without published research, there is no facility for healthcarers to collate and evaluate the necessary information that could radically alter and improve their traditional practices. It is a truism that for healthcare practice to be evidence based, there must be evidence on which to base it. There is, then,

responsibility on the healthcare professions to ensure that there is a constant output of well-conducted research studies that have the power and potential to inform and modify outdated practices. A fertile research culture must be a key means by which patient care can be enhanced, without squandering limited resources. That this research nirvana has not yet been achieved has been the focus of considerable research interest in itself. While the causes of low research output and low research uptake have been debated at length elsewhere, of particular relevance to the present text is the issue of essential competences. Clearly, one reason why many healthcare professionals avoid the concept and practice of evidence-based care derives from the fact that many feel they lack the necessary knowledge and skills either to conduct research or to evaluate published research findings. The pre- and post-qualifying courses that have been introduced over the last few years have been quick to address this problem, by making research methodology modules a core and compulsory aspect of the curriculum. Yet those healthcarers who qualified before the introduction of these changes have not been exposed to research as a fundamental and integrated feature of their training, and as a result may feel themselves to be disadvantaged in the brave new world of evidence-based healthcare. One aim of this book is to guide this group through the building block processes of research design and data analysis; therefore, many examples and illustrations have been included which target management and educational problems that senior professionals may encounter in the course of their work. This, of course, is not to ignore current students of the clinical therapies who may be required to produce a research-based assignment in part fulfilment of their pre-registration education. The book is intended to support their projects too.

Allied to the issue of education and training is the fact that healthcare courses reside firmly within the domain of academia. Changes in basic funding provision for the university sector were introduced in the 1980s, with money now being dependent in part upon research productivity. This has created a near obsession with research in many institutions, with the result that there is enormous pressure on academic staff to increase both the quality and quantity of their research output. Whatever the merits of this situation, there is little doubt that research will continue to be a major focus of activity throughout the tertiary education sector. The knock-on effect of this means that university-based departments of clinical therapy are subject to this research pressure. The pincers are unavoidable, then. Healthcare professionals of all types and strata must ensure that they are research-informed, research-aware and research-active if they are to meet the twin demands of health strategy and tertiary education.

This book is one attempt to facilitate this process. As a partial response to changing healthcare provision, there has been a surge in the publication of research texts for various professional groups, yet there is little doubt that the subject area remains a dry and boring one for many people. Many research methods and statistics books are stuffed full of complex, esoteric and incomprehensible words and symbols, and their message, inevitably, will remain inaccessible to all but the most intrepid and determined of readers. I hope that this text will not fall into the same trap. I am not a statistician but rather a psychologist who often has a mental block when confronted with new statistical formulae and concepts. This, I trust, will mean that I am perhaps more aware of the anxieties and problems many new researchers and non-statisticians experience when confronted with numbers; as a result I have attempted, as far as possible, to demystify the text and remove the jargon. Similarly, if indi-

viduals are to be enticed into the research arena, it is important that the essential, but turgid concepts of research methodologies are made meaningful to them. Consequently, a text on clinical therapy research should translate the theoretical ideas into situations and terms which make sense to a clinical therapist. I have, over the years, taught numerous research methods courses to a wide range of healthcare professionals, and all my experience suggests that the most effective way of engaging the participants' interest and enhancing their understanding is to 'customise' the essential concepts, using examples relevant to their own experience. This text attempts to do that.

The emphasis in this text is primarily on experimental research in clinical therapy. A full explanation of what this means in practice will be given later, but it is important to justify, at this point, why this particular research approach has been chosen. Experimental research is important for all the healthcare professionals because it allows them to compare procedures, treatments and patient groups. In the context of clinical therapy, this means that the relative effectiveness of different interventions for a given medical problem can be evaluated, allowing therapists to rationalise their practices; it allows the comparison of different patient groups, so that it can be ascertained whether one type of person is more likely to benefit from a given procedure than another, and it allows the evaluation of the efficiency or reliability of various makes and types of equipment. In short, the experimental approach is critical in the development of the clinical therapies as research-based professions. It should be noted, however, that it is not the only valid approach to research and nor is it the most valid, but it is a particularly worthwhile way of investigating many problems which arise in clinical therapy practice. While other methodologies will be referred to in the text, it is the experimental approach and the statistical analyses which go with it that will receive most attention.

In these ways, this edition is similar to the previous one. However, there is some new material which has been incorporated, largely on the recommendations of many of the therapists who were kind enough to provide feedback on the previous editions. There are numerous minor changes and updatings (for example, on information sources and ethics procedures), which will, I hope, serve to clarify the essential points. However, the most significant modifications to this edition have been the inclusion of additional material.

The book is still divided into three main sections (the basic principles of research design, a range of statistical analyses and some applications to practice) and its target audience remains a range of manual and clinical therapists. However, this edition has some additional features. Firstly, there is an expanded section on calculating the size of samples required for various research projects. The meteoric rise in health research as the principal means of informing clinical interventions has brought with it demands for greater stringency in its conduct. Clearly, if patient care is to be delivered in line with leading-edge research findings, then those findings must be properly and scientifically obtained. This is not to suggest that, hitherto, health research was either mediocre in quality or sloppy in its execution, but rather that the criteria that guide research activity are now more clearly articulated. This is evident in the research governance framework, laid down by the UK Department of Health and operationalised through the ethics committees. One issue that has received attention is that of obtaining a sample of adequate size from which to draw sound and valid conclusions. While for a whole range of practical reasons, many researchers just starting out cannot possibly obtain vast numbers of study participants, it is still important to know the basis on which suitable sample sizes are calculated.

A second new feature of this edition is a small section on preparing posters for presentation. Increasingly used as a method of assessing students' work, posters are also an excellent way of getting research findings disseminated in a relatively informal setting. Less intimidating than a conference paper, the poster has become a preferred method for researchers wanting to test the publication water.

But it is the final 'Applications' section of the text that has seen the addition of most new material. Here, there are four new chapters. The first – Receiver Operating Characteristics – is an invaluable approach to developing and validating diagnostic and screening tests. With the expansion of clinical therapists' roles, there is a commensurate demand for diagnostic skills and risk assessments; to check therapists' clinical decision-making in these areas against accepted gold-standards, and to develop new criteria for referral and treatments, a recognised protocol is required. The Receiver Operating Characteristics technique is therefore central to these activities. The second new chapter describes a long-established method – the Thurstone Paired Comparison Technique – as a means by which the user voice can be captured. Government policy has been clear on the role of the consumer, or user, of healthcare as a source of information by which service planning and improvements can be made. Focus and local interest groups have been commonly used in this regard, but the Thurstone approach enables the researcher to reach a wider population, through the use of a forced-choice questionnaire. The third new chapter focuses on inter-rater agreements – an area familiar to many clinical therapists. Where it is necessary to double-check instrument readings, or clinical decisions, or to verify measurements of any sort, the therapist may well seek independent assessments to ensure that the measurements are accurate. Interclass correlations are the accepted method of undertaking this; I have also included a technique of graphical representation to supplement the method, as this is now increasingly being seen as an essential part of the process. And finally, there is a chapter on conducting systematic reviews. Seen as a rigorous and objective approach to analysing and synthesising large numbers of research studies, the systematic review is central to the application of evidence-based healthcare; it is also increasingly being used as an alternative to the research dissertation at pre- and post-registration level, in order to avoid the problems students so frequently encounter with ethics applications and patient access.

I really hope this text will be a help to those clinical therapists who want to conduct research at whatever level and for whatever purpose.

Finally, I would like to acknowledge the many people who helped and supported me in writing this book.

I am indebted to my research students and to the many healthcare practitioners who have participated in my research methods courses, all of whom have furnished me with numerous examples and insights into their own practice. If inaccurate statements about clinical therapy remain in the text, it is because I misused their advice. Dr Fred Barwell, as ever, has been the personification of patience and a continuous fount of knowledge on all matters statistical. And I am inordinately grateful both to my husband, Professor Peter Spurgeon, who has (several times) read and constructively commented on the various drafts of the new material, and to my children, Tom and Laura, for their unerring ability to help me keep things in proportion. My sincere thanks to them all.

Birmingham, 2008 CH

Acknowledgements

I am indebted to the following sources for granting permission to reproduce the statistical tables in Appendix 2 of this book:

Tables A2.1, A2.5 and A2.6 from Lindley DV, Scott WF 1995 New Cambridge Statistical Tables, 2nd edn. Cambridge University Press, Cambridge

Table A2.2 from Wilcoxon F, Wilcox RA 1949 Some rapid approximate statistical procedures. American Cyanamid Company. Reproduced with the permission of the American Cyanamid Company

Table A2.3 from Friedman M 1937 The use of ranks to avoid the assumptions of normality implicit in the analysis of variance. Reprinted with permission from the Journal of the American Statistical Association. Copyright (1937) by the American Statistical Association. All rights reserved

Table A2.4 from Page EE 1963 Reprinted with permission from the Journal of the American Statistical Association. Copyright (1963) by the American Statistical Association. All rights reserved

Table A2.7 from Runyon RP, Haber A 1991 Fundamentals of Behavioral Statistics, 7th edn. McGraw-Hill, New York

Table A2.8 from Kruskal WH, Wallis WA 1952 The use of ranks in one-criterion variance analysis. Reprinted with permission from the Journal of the American Statistical Association. Copyright (1952) by the American Statistical Association. All rights reserved

Table A2.9 from Jonckheere AR 1954 A distribution-free k-sample test against ordered alternatives. Biometrika 41 (Biometrika Trustees)

Table A2.10 from Olds EG 1949 The 5% significance levels for sums of squares of rank differences and a correction. Annals of Mathematical Statistics 20 (The Institute of Mathematical Statistics)

Table A2.11 from Table VII (p. 63) of Fisher RA, Yates F 1974 Statistical Tables for Biological, Agricultural and Medical Research, Longman Group Ltd, London (previously published by Oliver and Boyd Ltd, Edinburgh). I am grateful to the Literary Executor of the late Sir Ronald Fisher FRS, to Dr Frank Yates and to Longman Group Ltd, London, for permission to reprint Table VII from their book, Statistical Tables for Biological, Agriculture and Medical Research, 6th edn. 1974

Table A2.12 adapted from Friedman M 1940 A comparison of alternative tests of significance for the problem of m rankings. Annals of Mathematical Statistics 11. (The Institute of Mathematical Statistics)

SECTION 1

Basic principles of research

SECTION CONTENTS

Chapter 1

Introduction

THE NEED FOR RESEARCH IN CLINICAL THERAPY

Why carry out research in clinical therapy? Surely the professions are sufficiently well established to make such activities irrelevant – after all, many of the therapeutic techniques currently in practice have been developed over the years and consequently are tried and tested. Moreover, many of these professions owe a great deal of their clinical effectiveness to issues that defy quantification, such as the relationship that builds up between the therapist and the patient. Is there really any need to start introducing experiments and statistical analysis?

I have heard these arguments on a number of occasions and accept their value. There is no doubt in my mind that good patient outcomes are as much dependent upon art as on science, and upon the therapeutic relationship, as well as on well-researched clinical interventions. In this sense, then, there is room for both qualitative and quantitative methodologies in clinical therapy research; neither of these approaches should be seen as superior to the other, but rather as complementary techniques, each with the power and potential to inform the other. It follows from this, then, that there are some research topics, particularly those that cannot be reduced to number crunching and bean counting, that are better investigated using qualitative techniques. By the same token, there are many research questions that routinely emerge in clinical practice that are more appropriately answered using experimental methods and formal scientific designs. For a whole host of reasons that have been debated at length elsewhere, experimental research has a relatively recent history in the professions allied to medicine and yet, in an era of evidence-based health care, its importance to the professions and the care they deliver has never been greater. Perhaps it may be relevant here to revisit some of the arguments that are supporting the emergence of scientific research in health care.

The first argument is a general one. There is an increasing movement towards enhanced professionalisation of the allied health care occupations. Two key criteria of a profession are, first, that there should be a body of specific knowledge that is directly relevant to, and developed by, the profession's members, and, second, that the essential training should be education based rather than apprenticeship based. In pursuit of greater professional status, the allied health care professions are moving towards all-graduate membership, with preregistration education now grounded in academia. As an essential feature of these courses, students are expected to complete broad-spectrum research methodology modules, which typically cover both qualitative and quantitative approaches. Where the course is assessed by completion of a research project, not only will the students be better equipped to undertake independent research, but the empirical skills and evidence that are amassed in the process will have the capacity to inform clinical practice. Consequently, the allegiance with higher education has provided more opportunities to develop the occupation-specific body of knowledge that will help to define each of the clinical therapies as professions. The necessary inclusion of a wide range of research skills training in the existing degree courses means that, alongside the qualitative approaches, scientific research methodology and statistics also occupy an essential part of the preregistration training. Such a component lends breadth, depth and credibility, not only academically, but professionally.

A second point relates to the need for clinical therapists to understand research methods and statistics in order to evaluate other professionals' research activities and reports. In a climate of increasing accountability, particularly in the public service sector, it is becoming imperative for professionals to justify their clinical decisions and actions and to increase their effectiveness and efficiency. Clearly, one way to achieve these aims is to ensure that clinical practice is fully informed by proper empirical evidence rather than simply being based on more traditional or ritualistic modes of operating. As a result, health-care professionals are turning increasingly to published research, in order to inform their practice, and thus to rationalise and streamline their own service delivery. Consequently, it is essential that health carers are able to understand and evaluate the quality of published research that is germane to their own interest, prior to any decision to implement the conclusions in their own practice. Therefore, an additional, equally important reason for clinical therapists to develop their research competencies is the need to be able to make properly informed judgements concerning published research. Without this, it is highly likely that patients' wellbeing, both physical and psychological, might be adversely affected in a direct or indirect way, through the implementation of unchallenged findings from poorly conducted research. Of course, it should be noted that there are a number of sophisticated sources of healthcare guidance, based on the analysis and synthesis of high quality research, for example:

- The Cochrane Collaboration: an independent, international, not-for-profit centre that conducts systematic reviews of high quality research on a variety of topics, with the aim of improving health care decisions.
- The Centre for Reviews and Dissemination: reviews research about treatment effectiveness in a range of health and social care areas and provides an enquiry service. The Centre also provides databases of structured abstracts of research reviews, which have been independently evaluated, an NHS Economic Evaluation database and a Health Technology Assessment database, all of which can be accessed via the website cited at the end of this chapter
- National Institute for Health and Clinical Excellence (NICE): an independent organisation that synthesises research and expert

opinion to provide health guidance on a range of diseases and conditions.

- National Service Frameworks: evaluates research with the aim of providing guidance and long-term strategies for managing a wide range of health care problems.
- *BMJ Clinical Evidence*: provides updated reviews on a variety of clinical conditions

While these organisations provide an invaluable source of independent information, their coverage is by no means exhaustive, further emphasising the need for the health care professional to be able to make informed assessments of relevant research studies. If there are no readily available systematic reviews in your area of interest, you may need to conduct your own evaluation of relevant available research. Chapter 25 of this text provides a framework for undertaking this, but there are many other dedicated sources of help, such as the Public Health Resource Unit, which provides appraisal tools for assessing research studies that use a range of different methodologies.

The third argument in favour of research in the clinical therapies relates to much more specific problem-driven issues. There are many clinical therapists who, at the risk of disagreement from their colleagues, would admit that many of the therapeutic procedures they use are selected on the basis of intuition, personal preference and familiarity, rather than on the basis of empirically established information. To illustrate this point, consider the following problems:

1. You are about to treat a recent injury where pain is the predominant symptom. Do you select ice or ultrasound? Why? When I asked these questions of a group of highly trained physiotherapists, their opinions were divided. While this could suggest that both methods are equally effective, in this instance I do not think this was the case. Every member of the group put forward an argument for one treatment or the other, based on his/her own experience and not on any research evidence. In other words, their views were divided because treatment selection was a matter of opinion and not of hard factual evidence deriving from scientific research. Research in any of the clinical therapies might compare the outcomes of different types of treatment, thus removing the subjective element and making the decision process clearer, less ambiguous and hopefully more effective.

2. The uniform/no uniform issue continues to be contentious in some quarters of the paramedical professions. There are sound arguments on both sides, with the pro-uniform lobby claiming that the uniform inspires greater confidence and trust in the patient, while the anti-uniform contingent argues that it decreases rapport. So how can the issue be resolved? The answer lies in the use of experimental method and statistical analysis: if the effects of wearing uniform versus wearing 'civvies' are measured and analysed using scientific techniques, the debate can be settled.

3. You are informed about a new manual technique for dealing with a musculoskeletal problem. Do you try it on the first patient who comes along and then, if the outcome appears to be favourable, try it on everyone else who presents with the same problem? Or do you set up a controlled experiment whereby you systematically compare the effectiveness of the new technique with that of the standard treatment procedure? If you opt for the latter you will need a sound knowledge of scientific methodology and data analysis.

I hope that you can see from these examples of problem-driven issues that experimentation and statistical analysis are essential if clinical therapy procedures are to be appropriately and effectively used.

In the current era of increasing pressure on resources, hit-and-miss policies of treatment, based on opinion and preference rather than hard evidence, are too wasteful of time and money to be justified. Moreover, the growing realisation of the importance of complementary therapies means that practitioners must be able to confirm the value of their interventions through systematic evaluation if they are to withstand the scepticism of conventional medicine. Establishing clinical practices on a firm professional foundation by demonstrating their efficiency, cost-effectiveness and success is a crucial defence against the imperialists and the cynics. And to do this, a knowledge of experimental design, research methods and statistical analysis is essential.

APPROACHES TO RESEARCH

The main emphasis of this book is on experimental research. This doesn't mean that clinical therapists are expected to sit in laboratories surrounded by chemicals and Bunsen burners, but rather that they apply the basic principles of experimental methods to their own clinical practice. In this context, an experiment simply means that different groups of people – patients, colleagues or whoever – are treated in certain ways, to see if there are any differences in the groups' outcomes which could be attributed to the intervention they received. In this way, treatments can be compared for effectiveness, along objective scientific lines, in order to try to optimise procedures. The whole issue of designing an experiment will be dealt with in more detail in the course of the book.

However, the experimental approach is not the only way of conducting health care research, and nor is it necessarily the most valid. It should be remembered that research is about asking questions and finding answers to those questions in a systematic and logical way. There are many ways of asking and answering questions and these variations constitute the different methodologies in research. Experimental research techniques deal with research problems in a way which has enormous value to the clinical therapies, as I hope you will discover as you read this text. However, there are alternative approaches that are more appropriate under certain circumstances. Moreover, there is a strong argument to be made for the use of multiple methodologies to investigate a research question, since this may provide a more comprehensive answer. To include all the possible variations on the research theme would be impossible in a single text, but it may be useful to refer to some of them briefly here.

SINGLE-CASE DESIGNS

Like all person-oriented professions, the clinical therapies are involved in treating individuals, with their own particular medical problems, personality, motivations, etc. Consequently, it may be appropriate on occasions, not to establish whether groups of patients do better on a given intervention than another group, but rather to ask whether a single individual patient is benefiting from the treatment given. This has given rise to a research approach known as the single-case design.

Let us imagine you are dealing with a 73-year-old woman who has just had a stroke and has lost the use of her left arm which now has very weak muscle contraction. You decide to try to increase the strength of contraction by the use of sensory facilitation. After five treatments, you check her movement control and note that it has improved. This would appear to confirm your choice of treatment for her. (Other clinical therapists could also think of an intervention specific to their own practice that would aid arm movement, and which they could use here by way of illustration.)

The phases in such a procedure are given labels. The period prior to beginning treatment is called the baseline phase or A. The period during which the patient received the facilitation is called the treatment phase or B. Hence this design is known as an AB design.

However, the approach is not quite as conclusive as might appear at first, since it is possible that the patient's movement control would have improved over time anyway, just as a result of the natural recovery process. The AB design, then, by itself, cannot prove definitively that an improvement occurred as a function of treatment, because that improvement might have happened irrespective of any therapy. One way of getting over this problem is the ABAB design.

In this single-case ABAB approach, our patient would have the sensory facilitation treatment stopped, and consequently would enter another no-treatment phase (a second A stage). If the facilitation had been responsible for the improvement previously observed, we would anticipate that during the second A phase there would be some deterioration in movement control. Then another treatment phase (the second B phase) would be introduced into the study, to find out whether movement control improved again, as a

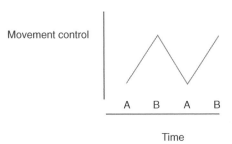

Figure 1.1 Graph of patient's movement control whilst being treated by sensory facilitation on an ABAB design.

result of sensory facilitation. These phases are outlined in Figure 1.1

Whilst this design might be useful for looking at individual case histories, it is clearly inappropriate in some situations. For example, it is quite likely that the improvement in movement control noted during the first treatment phase is irreversible and would not, therefore, deteriorate. There are also serious ethical objections, too, in terms of withholding treatment and this must, of necessity, be a cause for deliberation prior to the use of an ABAB design. Finally, these single-case designs have little predictive power for other comparable situations. Our stroke patient in this study might have improved, but we have no basis for expecting other stroke patients to derive benefit from the same treatment. Where quick decisions have to be made, it is often more useful to be able to rely on findings derived from groups of people rather than from individuals.

QUALITATIVE RESEARCH

All research involves the collection of facts about an individual or a group of people. Where this information is numerical in nature (such as percentage range of movement, distance walked, degree of spine curvature, a score on a self-help questionnaire, blood pressure and temperature readings, etc.), the research is classified as quantitative. However, how do you quantify a patient's feelings about their condition, or their thoughts on their progress? While numbers can be used to measure many fairly objective events, a person's thoughts, feelings and beliefs cannot adequately be subjected to this type of numerical assessment. What is often more appropriate in

these circumstances is a description, such as a verbal or pictorial recording, of the individual's responses. Information collection that avoids numerical approaches is called qualitative research, and is a means by which the researcher can gain insights into another person's views, opinions, feelings and beliefs, within their own natural settings, usually using techniques such as interviews.

Techniques of qualitative research rely heavily on accurate reporting in a natural environment, without control or restriction being imposed by the investigator. Moreover, unlike quantitative research where small aspects of an individual's behaviour are selected for study, in qualitative research, the individual as a whole and in relation to their social setting is described. Thus, qualitative research can be thought of as holistic. Furthermore, qualitative approaches usually focus on specific individuals, rather than on groups, or types, of individuals, although focus groups are becoming increasingly popular as a source of qualitative data.

Another important aspect of qualitative research is the role of the investigator who, rather than being detached and objective as in quantitative research, must become enmeshed and integral with the people being studied. This subjectivity, while bringing bias to the research environment, allows for a measure of sensitivity and intuition in the assessment and this can have a considerable benefit in some subject areas. Nonetheless, it should be pointed out that unless the information collection process in qualitative approaches is carefully structured, there is enormous potential for researcher bias. Furthermore, analysis of interview transcripts, video recordings and the like, is very labour intensive and may be difficult to distil to the core issues. This problem is made worse by the involvement the investigator typically has with the people being studied, since when people know they are being watched or monitored their behaviour changes, often in quite fundamental ways.

Such qualitative approaches can be of great importance to paramedical research. It should be pointed out, though, that academic and professional regard for quantitative techniques, rather unjustifiably, tends to be higher, which may mean that qualitative research is disregarded and trivialised. The current overwhelming interest in the randomised controlled trial in medical/health care research (known as the gold-standard) testifies to the high prestige attributed to scientific methodologies and number crunching. Yet it is often criticised for being reductionist and losing sight of the whole person or the real nature of the clinical condition. Qualitative techniques, on the other hand, because of their more holistic approach, can be very usefully employed to describe phenomena such as hospital or health centre cultures, or patient experiences, particularly where these are likely to be unusual. My own feeling is that qualitative and quantitative research should be seen not in superior/inferior terms, but rather as complementary techniques, each bringing their own insights to a given problem. Indeed, I am increasingly of the opinion that multi-methods approaches provide a much more valuable and informed picture and therefore, I would recommend that qualitative and quantitative techniques should be used in tandem where feasible.

One technique to which I have recently been introduced (and about which I am now behaving like a proselytising zealot!) is Q-methodology. Because it relies on computer analysis of the data, it cannot be included in this text, but the technique combines the statistical rigour of the quantitative approach, with the rich subjective data of the qualitative. It is particularly useful for looking at patients' experiences of treatment, illness, and rehabilitation, or carers' experiences of the treatment journey – indeed, anywhere that the individual experiential account is of interest. The technique then groups respondents' accounts according to the similarity of the stories they tell. For example, if you were interested in the carers' experiences of looking after a physically disabled child, you might use Q-methodology with 20 or 30 carers to see what their particular problems, concerns etc were, and the Q analysis procedure would then group these viewpoints according to their resemblance to one another. In this way, you might end up with four or five different stories which each told a story about how the carers perceived the journey of caring for their disabled children. If you are interested in pursuing this technique further, there are references at the end of this chapter.

OBSERVATIONAL TECHNIQUES

One research technique that is inherent to both qualitative and quantitative approaches is observation. Observation in research simply means that a researcher can collect information on a given topic through direct recording and perception of the relevant events.

Observational techniques may involve self- or other-evaluations. Self-evaluations are simply reports of subjective responses to certain situations. Pain measurement is a classic example of self-observation, where a patient is required to make a subjective evaluation, of either a numerical or qualitative kind, of how much pain they are experiencing. Other-evaluation involves the use of a third party to observe and record events. Many clinical assessments of students rely on observations of aspects of their clinical expertise, such as the ability to establish rapport with the patient and, as such, these assessments constitute an observational technique.

Observations may be carried out either in natural settings, such as clinics, or in more controlled environments, such as laboratories. Both have advantages and disadvantages; for example, while a natural setting cannot be adequately controlled in terms of external or biasing influences, it does have the advantage of realism, so that events can be observed in the way in which they normally occur. Laboratory settings, on the other hand, can control extraneous influences, but the results so obtained may not translate into more natural surroundings.

Inevitably there are problems with observational techniques, just as there are with all research methodologies. The reliability of an observation may be a problem, and, consequently, some research topics may require a number of different independent observers, or the use of video monitoring systems. Nonetheless, observational information gathering can be an invaluable approach, either on its own or in conjunction with other data collection techniques.

These topics are covered in more detail in Robson (2002), Polit & Hungler (2002), Bowling (2002) and Polgar & Thomas (2007), and the reader is referred to these books for a fuller explanation of the range of approaches to research.

SURVEYS, QUESTIONNAIRES AND OTHER DESCRIPTIVE TECHNIQUES

These approaches to research are essential tools for the health care researcher and will be covered separately in Chapter 3. The techniques are useful for establishing an overview or picture of a given problem within a specified group of people. For example, the researcher might wish to follow up a group of spinal injury patients to establish whether or not they have had any further physical problems, such as residual pain or restricted movement; whether or not they have complied with their exercise plan; attended their outpatients' appointment, or whatever. The survey technique, using a specially devised questionnaire, would be a highly appropriate way of conducting such a study. An introduction to these approaches will be described in more detail in Chapter 3.

ACTION RESEARCH

The term 'action research' is increasingly used to describe a cycle of events that is intended to help the practitioner evaluate and modify practice. There are several models of action research and the reader is referred to Hart & Bond (1995) for a review. In essence, however, the action research process is problem-driven, in that a practice-based problem is identified, the practitioner and researcher design a research programme to investigate it; they develop a package of change based on the results and then evaluate the impact of the change package. For example, a problem may be identified that is concerned with enabling stroke patients to perform the activities of daily living. The researcher together with the community physiotherapists and occupational therapists would collectively design an intervention which would facilitate the patient group in bathing and toileting. The package would be implemented and evaluated. Any potentially valuable modifications might be identified and included in a revised care package which would

then be tested and evaluated and so on in an iterative cycle. While this may appear to be very similar to the sorts of research issues that are the focus of this text, action research particularly emphasises the collaborative involvement between practitioner and researcher, the practical nature of the research problem, a change in practice intervention based on the research findings and the development of a theoretical framework into which the entire dynamic cycle of practice–informing research–informing practice–informing research sits. Because the research is not conducted solely by a researcher in a clinical setting, but rather in co-operation with the practitioners in that setting, action research has the capacity to empower practitioners and to integrate research with practice, thereby overcoming the well-known practice/research divide. The research methods used may be qualitative or quantitative.

GROUNDED THEORY

This is another research variant that may be particularly useful in an era of clinical audit. The term refers to hypotheses or theories that emerge from existing data. So, rather than generating hypotheses and then collecting data to establish whether or not the hypothesis has been supported, grounded theory starts off with the information from which hypotheses and theories emerge. For example, an epidemiologist might systematically collect data about the incidence of multiple sclerosis and find that clusters of the disease occur in cold climates, in younger people and in social classes 2 and 3. This constitutes the data base from which hypotheses and theories might emerge to explain the pattern of distribution. With the advent of clinical audit, large data bases are now routinely collected which could be interpreted using grounded theory methods. For more information, a seminal text is Glaser & Strauss (1999).

USING STATISTICS

Statistics are a crucial part of quantitative research. Whenever someone carries out an experiment it is essential that the results are analysed and presented in a way that can be understood by other interested parties. Statistics are one means by which this is achieved. For example, if an experiment had been carried out to compare two different treatment procedures for arthritic toe joints, it is insufficient just to present a table of figures showing the range of movement and pain levels for each patient following treatment and expect the reader to make sense of it. The data have to be analysed, described and interpreted using statistical methods, so that an objective conclusion can be reached about the study's outcomes.

The main type of data analysis covered in this book is a technique known as inferential statistics, which is the most common way of analysing results derived from experiments. The concepts and procedures relating to this approach are described in Chapters 6–9 and 13–18.

However, data can also be analysed using techniques of descriptive statistics. This method allows the researcher to describe the findings in terms of their most interesting features. Descriptive statistics are often used to analyse survey data and for this reason will be referred to in more detail in Chapters 3–5.

Unfortunately, many people are put off research because of the statistical procedures that are required. They see a page of formulae and figures, panic and slam the book shut. This suggests the first and most important rule of statistics – don't panic! Inability to understand statistics is usually an emotional problem, and anyone who feels diffident in the face of figures should remember this. As long as you approach the statistical analysis systematically and in a step-by-step manner, there should be few problems.

Another point should be raised here. Do not imagine that the object of statistical analysis is to test your long multiplication and division – it isn't. Statistics are no more than a tool for analysing data. So, always use a calculator, or a computer, as they are faster and usually more reliable than even the quickest mind. This text provides a guide to calculating by hand some of the most commonly used tests. This obviously will involve the researcher in a lot of mathematical activity. There are, of course, a number of software packages that are commonly available and which will do the statistical analyses in a matter of seconds, once the data have been entered. These packages are readily available; one of the easiest to access and use is SPSS (Statistical Package for the Social Sciences). This offers a wide range of statistical tests and is reasonably user friendly. In my experience, once the data have been entered, the rest is relatively easy, although the package does generate a huge amount of output, much of which is not always directly relevant, especially to the beginning researcher. I would recommend two texts that are enormously helpful in guiding the beginning researcher through SPSS:

- Julie Pallant (2007) SPSS survival guide. Open University Press, Milton Keynes (a very readable, non-threatening book that is an invaluable aid to data inputting, using the commands and menu options and interpreting the print-out).
- Denis Anthony (1999) Understanding advanced statistics. Churchill Livingstone, Edinburgh (another step-by-step approach to statistics and SPSS analysis of data, but deals more specifically with health care research).

Of course, once the researcher has set up the SPSS database, this can be explored and expanded with great ease. Nonetheless, it should be pointed out that unless your organisation has a site licence, this is an expensive package (and one which takes up a lot of computer memory). Where the research is small scale, and the researcher unfamiliar with computer analysis, manual calculations are often quicker and therefore preferable. It is also the case that working out your statistical calculations by hand, at least in the first instance, is very useful for showing how statistical tests 'work'; the vast majority of my students have commented that, despite their initial anxieties, working through a database with only a pen, paper and calculator has been very informative and helpful to their overall understanding of a range of fundamental concepts. It is hoped that this book will be useful in these situations.

Lastly, remember that you don't need to memorise the statistical formulae presented in this book; as long as you know where to look them up and how to use them, there is no need to commit them to memory. Further, at the risk of being hammered by the purists, I would also add that there is no need to understand how the formulae were derived from statistical theory. While many statisticians would vehemently disagree with that rather bald statement, I would liken statistical analysis to any other tool or piece of apparatus; you don't need to understand the workings of a car or television in order to use it. If that were the case, only garage mechanics would be allowed to drive cars. Many would argue, of course, that if you do understand the mechanism, then you are able to put it right if the apparatus goes wrong. However, if you know when, why and how to use a statistical method, and if you follow the procedure step-by-step, then the statistical tool will not break down. It is the when, why and how of statistics that this book aims to explain.

STRUCTURE OF THE BOOK

The book has been divided into three sections, the first of which is devoted to the design of research projects, the second to statistical procedures and the third to some research applications. I would recommend that anyone who feels unsure of themselves mathematically should read Appendix 1 (pp. 337–340). The rest of you may only want to refresh your memories on some basic rules of mathematics. These are presented briefly in the next section. Once you have read as far as Chapter 10 you should have a sound idea of how to design research studies and which analysis to use on any data resulting from them. In Section 2, the chapters are devoted to outlining the procedures involved in particular statistical tests. You should read the relevant chapter as and when required. For this reason, these chapters are relatively independent of each other and so may contain common material. I make no apologies for this repetition, since I find nothing more irritating than to open a statistics book at the appropriate chapter only to discover that certain essential elements have been covered earlier, necessitating the reading of additional chapters in which I have little immediate interest. For this reason, the chapters on statistical tests are virtually self-contained. Section 3 provides

seven examples of applied research techniques that use some of the statistical procedures covered in the second section.

Throughout the book, too, there are exercises to test your understanding of a particular principle. If you decide to do these, you will find the answers at the back of the book. Also, within each chapter, at appropriate intervals, there are 'Key Concepts' boxes, which summarise the most important points. These can be used to refresh your memory without having to plough through several pages to find what you want. And at the end of each chapter there is a list of recommended further readings. These relate to books and articles that I and my students have found useful, but there are many others available, the style of which may suit you better. There is a particularly extensive list at the end of this chapter, which I hope won't be too daunting. As a number of concepts have been briefly covered here, it seems important to provide a range of reading in order to enable any interested reader to pursue any aspect of interest; many of these readings will also appear at the end of other chapters in this book.

Finally, there aren't a lot of laughs in statistics. Because many students find the topic dry I've tried to make the style as chatty as possible. Nonetheless, jokes are hard to come by, but do persevere – statistics are an essential part of clinical therapy and research life.

So, I hope you will find that this book equips you with the basic elements you need for your research. Happy experimenting!

P.S. All the experiments and data in the book are entirely fictitious!

P.P.S. Please note that all the calculations in the examples and activities have been worked to three decimal places throughout.

P.P.P.S. A final caveat: I am not a clinical therapist, a point which will undoubtedly become clear to you as you read this book. As a result, I have a tendency to make up health care as I go along, so if there are examples which strike you as ludicrous, naive or just impossible, please forgive me.

And a final word from a student: 'If I had only one day to live, I would spend it in my statistics class. It would seem so much longer.' (Sanders et al 1985).

SOME BASIC MATHS

Most of us have forgotten many of the basic mathematical concepts we learnt for 'O'-level or GCSE, simply because we don't use them very often. Even though you are advised to use a calculator for the statistical tests in this book, it is still essential that you are familiar with the basic mathematical principles, for two main reasons. First, even though a calculator will do all the most complex multiplying, dividing and square-rooting for you, you will need to know the order in which these processes are carried out, because, as you will no doubt remember, some types of computation must be done before others. This will be clarified later. Second, even though you will be using a calculator, it is still quite possible to come up with some odd results, either because some information has been entered wrongly, or simply because, on occasions, calculators have been known to go haywire. So you need to be able to 'eyeball' the results of your calculations to see if they look right. If you have any doubts or reservations about any of this, read on.

This section is just a brief reminder of some of the basic principles you will need. These principles are discussed in greater detail in Appendix 1, so if you are unsure of any of them, turn to page 337.

BASIC RULES

1. If the formula contains brackets, you must carry out all the calculations inside them first.
2. If the formula contains brackets within brackets, you must do the calculations in the innermost brackets first.
3. If the formula contains only additions and subtractions, or multiplications and divisions, work from left to right.
4. Adding two negative numbers results in a negative answer.
5. Adding a plus number to a minus number is the same as taking the minus number from the plus number.
6. Multiplying two positive numbers gives a positive answer.
7. Multiplying a positive number and a negative number together gives a negative answer.
8. Multiplying two negative numbers gives a positive answer.
9. Dividing a positive number by a negative number (or vice versa) gives a negative answer.
10. Dividing two negative numbers gives a positive answer.
11. The square of a number is that number multiplied by itself. It is expressed as ^{2}.
12. The square root of a given number is a number which when multiplied by itself gives the number you already have. It is expressed as $\sqrt{\ }$.
13. To round up decimal points, start at the extreme right-hand number. If it is 5 or more, increase the number to its left by 1. If it is less than 5, the number to its left remains the same.
14. If there is no mathematical symbol contained within a formula, a multiplication sign is assumed; e.g. $5(4 + 8)$ means $5 \times (4 + 8)$.

Activity 1.1 (Answers on p. 359)

Calculate the following:

1. $14 + 8 + 27 - 3$
2. $14 + 8 - (27 - 3)$
3. $17 + (30 - 4)$
4. $11(19 + 4)$
5. $74 - [(19 \times 3) + 8]$
6. $12 + (14 \times 3) - 5$
7. $6[(4 + 8) - 3]$
8. $15 - 4 - 4 + 12$
9. $(49 - 1) + (7 \times 8)$
10. $36 - (12 - 6) + 17$
11. $-18 + 22 - 10$
12. $-24 + 16$
13. $-12 \times +4$
14. $-18 - 26$
15. 14×-3
16. $- 51 + 3$
17. $51 - (+3 \times + 2)$
18. $+17 - 4 - 26$
19. $-19 + 11 + 15$
20. $-5(4 \times 12)$

One easy mnemonic that may help with the basic order of calculation is <u>B</u>less <u>M</u>y <u>D</u>ear <u>A</u>unt <u>S</u>ue (<u>B</u>rackets <u>M</u>ultiplication <u>D</u>ivision <u>A</u>ddition <u>S</u>ubtraction).

You might like to do the exercises in Activity 1.1 just to satisfy yourself that you're happy with these rules.

SYMBOLS IN STATISTICS

You will find the following symbols appearing in formulae throughout the book. Although they will be explained when they appear, this page can serve as a quick reference point.

Σ = sum or total of all the calculations to the right of the symbol, e.g.

$$\Sigma 3^2 + 6^2 + 4^2 = 61$$

x = an individual score
$\bar{x}$ = the average score
$\sqrt{}$ = the square root of a figure or calculations, e.g.

$$\sqrt{89} = 9.434$$

$$\sqrt{17 + 15 + 86} = 10.863$$

$$\sqrt{51 \times 3} + 4 = 12.369 + 4 = 16.369$$

N = the total number of scores in an experiment
n^2 = the number times itself, e.g.

$$8^2 = 8 \times 8$$
$$= 64$$

$<$ = less than, e.g.
$5 < 7$ (5 is less than 7)
$>$ = more than, e.g.
$10 > 2$ (10 is more than 2)
C = the number of conditions in the experiment
n = the number of scores in a subgroup or condition.

FURTHER READING

General research texts

Bowling A 2002 Research methods in health, 2nd edition. Open University Press, Buckingham

Brown B, Crawford P, Hicks C 2003. Evidence-based research: dilemmas and debates in health care. Open University Press, Maidenhead

Bryman A 2001 Social research methods. Oxford University Press, Oxford

Coolican H 2004 Research methods and statistics in psychology, 4th edition. Hodder and Stoughton, London

Glaser B, Strauss A 1999 The discovery of grounded theory. Chicago, Aldine

Hart E, Bond M 1995 Action research for health and social care: a guide to practice. Buckingham, Open University Press, Buckingham

Polgar S, Thomas S 2007 Introduction to research in the health sciences. Edinburgh, Churchill Livingstone.

Polit DE, Beck CT 2006 Essentials of nursing research: methods, appraisal and utilization, 4th edition. Lippincott, Philadelphia

Polit DE, Hungler B 2002 Nursing research: principles and methods, 6th edition. JP Lippincott and Co, Philadelphia

Rees C 2005 An introduction to research for midwives, 2nd edition. Elsevier Science, London

Robson C 2000 Small scale evaluation: principles and practice. Sage Publications, London

Robson C 2002 Real world research: a resource for social scientists and practitioner-researchers. Blackwell Publishing, Oxford

Saks M, Allsop J 2007 Researching health: qualitative, quantitative and mixed methods. Sage Publishing, London

Sanders DH, Eng RJ, Murph AF 1985 Statistics: a fresh approach. McGraw Hill, New York

Sim J, Wright C 2002 Research in health care: concepts, designs and methods. Nelson Thornes, Cheltenham

Smith K 2005 Understanding grounded theory principles and evaluation. Online. Available: http://nurseresearcher.rcnpublishing.co.uk/resources/archive/GetArticleById.asp?ArticleId=5870

Watson,R, McKenna H, Cowman S, Keady J 2008 Nursing research: designs and methods. Edinburgh, Churchill Livingstone

Qualitative research

Cavanagh S 2005 Content analysis: concepts, methods and applications. Online. Available: http://nurseresearcher.rcnpublishing.co.uk/resources/archive/GetArticleById.asp?ArticleId=5869

Conneeley AL 2002 Methodological issues in qualitative research for the researcher/practitioner. British Journal of Occupational Therapy 65(4):185–190

Fielding N 2005 Varieties of research interviews. Online. Available: http://nurseresearcher.rcnpublishing.co.uk/resources/archive/GetArticleById.asp?ArticleId=6292

Greenhalgh T, Taylor R 1997 How to read a paper: papers that go beyond numbers (qualitative research). BMJ 315:740–743

Hammell KW, Carpenter C, Dyck I 2000 Using qualitative research: a practical introduction for occupational and physical therapists. Churchill Livingstone, Edinburgh

Hammell KW, Carpenter C 2004 Qualitative research in evidence-based rehabilitation. Churchill Livingstone, Edinburgh

http://www.qualitaveresearch.uga.edu/QualPage/ 10 December 2008

Lane P 2005 Focus group methodology. Online. Available: http://nurseresearcher.rcnpublishing.co.uk/resources/archive/GetArticleById.asp?ArticleId=6157

Mays N, Pope C 1995 Qualitative research: rigour and qualitative research. BMJ 311:109–112

Mays N, Pope C 2000 Qualitative research in health care: assessing quality in in qualitative research. BMJ 320:50–52

Pope C, Mays N 1995 Qualitative research; reaching the parts other methods cannot reach: an introduction to qualitative analysis in health and health services research. BMJ 311: 42–45

Pope C, Mays N 2000 Qualitative research in health care: analysing qualitative data. BMJ 320: 114–116

Pope C, Mays N 2006 Qualitative research in health care, 3rd edition. BMJ Publishing, London

Morse J 1992 Qualitative health research. Sage Publications, California

Morse J, Field P 1995 Nursing research: the application of qualitative approaches. Chapman & Hall, London

Roberts P 2005 Planning and running a focus group. Online. Available: http://nurseresearcher.rcnpublishing.co.uk/resources/archive/GetArticleById.asp?ArticleId=6067

Rose K 2005 Unstructured and semi-structured interviewing. Online. Available: http://nurseresearcher.rcnpublishing.co.uk/resources/archive/GetArticleById.asp?ArticleId=6294

Stevenson C 2005 Theoretical and methodological approaches in discourse analysis. Online. Available: http://nurseresearcher.rcnpublishing.co.uk/resources/archive/GetArticleById.asp?ArticleId=5936

Wainwright SR 2005 Analysing data using grounded theory. Online. Available: http://nurseresearcher.rcnpublishing.co.uk/resources/archive/GetArticleById.asp?ArticleId=6296

There are a number of online journals specialising in qualitative methods, two useful examples of which are:

The Qualitative Report. Online. Available http://www.nova.edu/ssss/QR December 10 2008

Qualitative Research. Online. Available http://qrj.sagepub.com/ December 10 2008

The *BMJ* and *Nurse Researcher* are also online

Evidence–based healthcare

BMJ Clinical Evidence. Online. Available http://clinicalevidence.bmj.com/ceweb/index.jsp December 10 2008

Bury T, Mead J 2002 Evidence-based healthcare; a practical guide for therapists, 2nd edition. Butterworth Heinemann, Edinburgh

Carnwell R 2005 Essential differences between research and evidence-based practice. Online. Available: http://nurseresearcher.rcnpublishing.co.uk/resources/archive/GetArticleById.asp?ArticleId=6150

Centre for Reviews and Dissemination. Online. Available http://www.york.ac.uk/inst/crd and http://www.york.ac.uk/inst/crd/crddatabases.htm for the economic and health technology evaluations December 10 2008

Cochrane Collaboration. Online. Available http://www.cochrane.org December 10 2008

Evans D 2003 Hierarchy of evidence: a framework for ranking evidence evaluating healthcare interventions. Journal of Clinical Nursing 12:77–84

Goding L, Edwards K 2005 Evidence-based practice. Online. Available: http://nurseresearcher.rcnpublishing.co.uk/resources/archive/GetArticleById.asp?ArticleId=6197

Gray M 2001 Evidence based healthcare, 2nd edition. Churchill Livingstone, Edinburgh

Hamer S, Collinson G 2005 Achieving evidence-based practice; a handbook for practitioners. Bailliere-Tindall, Edinburgh

http://www.patient.co.uk/printer.asp?doc=40002064

National Institute for Clinical Excellence. http://www.nice.org.uk December 10 2008

National Service Frameworks. Online. Available http://www.dh.gov.uk/en/Policyandguidance/healthandsocialcaretopics/DH_4070951 December 10 2008

Physiotherapy Evidence Database (PEDro). Online. Available http://www.pedro.fhs.usyd.edu.au/links.html December 10 2008

Public Health Research Unit. Online. Available http://www.phru.nhs.uk/Pages/PHD/resources.htm December 10 2008

Sackett D, Haynes B 1995 On the need for evidence-based medicine. Evidence Based Medicine 1: 4–5

Sackett D, Rosenberg WMC, Gray JAM, Haynes RB, Richardson WS 1996 Evidence-based medicine: what it is and what it isn't. BMJ 312:71–72

Taylor MC 2007 Evidence-based practice for occupational therapists, 2nd edition. Blackwell Science, Oxford

The quantitative/qualitative debate and some methodological approaches

Bryman A 1988 Quantity and quality in social research. Routledge, London

Carr L 1994 The strengths and weaknesses of quantitative and qualitative research: what method for nursing? Journal of Advanced Nursing 20: 716–721

Clark AM 1998 The qualitative–quantitative debate: moving from positivism and confrontation to post-positivism and reconciliation. Journal of Advanced Nursing 27(6):1242–1249

Creswell JW 2003 Research design: qualitative, quantitative and mixed methods approaches, 2nd edition. Sage Publications, London

Hammersley M 1991 Deconstructing the qualitative–quantitative divide. In Hammersley M (ed) What's wrong with ethnography? Routledge, London

Kelly B, Long A 2005 Quantity or quality. Online. Available: http://nurseresearcher.rcnpublishing.co.uk/resources/archive/GetArticleById.asp?ArticleId=6151

Newell R 2005 Single case experimental design: controlling the study. Online. Available: http://nurseresearcher. rcnpublishing.co.uk/resources/archive/GetArticleById. asp?ArticleId=6071

Rose S 1976 The conscious brain. Penguin, Harmondsworth.

Williamson GR 2005 Illustrating triangulation in mixed-methods nursing research. Online. Available: http://nurseresearcher.rcnpublishing.co.uk/resources/archive/GetArticleById.asp?ArticleId=5955

Q-methodology

Cordingly L 2005. Q methodology. http://nurseresearcher. rcnpublishing.co.uk/resources/archive/GetArticleById. asp?ArticleId=5871

Herron-Marx S, Williams A, Hicks C 2007 A Q methodology study of women's experiences of enduring post-natal perineal and pelvic floor morbidity. Midwifery 23(3):322–334. Online. Available http://www.ncbi.nlm.nih.gov/sites/entrez?db=pubmed&uid=17126457&cmd=showdetailview&indexed=google December 10 2008

Statistics and computer software

Pallant J 2007 SPSS survival manual, 3rd edition. Open University Press, Buckingham

Anthony D 1999 Understanding advanced statistics. Churchill Livingstone, Edinburgh

Chapter 2

Research design and statistics: some basic concepts

When you engage in research, you will almost always end up collecting information, or measuring something: muscle tone, recovery rate, vital capacity, patient satisfaction, numbers of patients, pain levels, competence with activities of daily living, etc. This information is called data. In order for the research to have some value, the meaning of these data has to be presented in ways that other research workers can understand. For example, there is no point in carrying out a well-designed experiment to compare the effectiveness of reflexology versus remedial massage for promoting leg movement in multiple sclerosis sufferers if the data on this are left as a jumbled mass of figures. In other words, the researcher has to make sense of the results.

There are various ways of making sense of the results, but for the clinical therapist two methods are of major importance. The first approach is called descriptive statistics, where the researcher collects a set of data, usually from a form of survey, and then describes it in terms of its most important features (e.g. average scores, range of scores, etc.). The second approach is called inferential statistics, in which the data, which have usually been collected from an experiment, are subjected to statistical analysis, using tests which allow the researcher to make inferences beyond the actual data in front of him/her. The differences between these approaches will be discussed briefly now, and then in more detail in later chapters.

DESCRIPTIVE STATISTICS

As has already been mentioned, descriptive statistics are often used in conjunction with survey methods. A survey is a research approach that involves collecting information from a large number of people using interviews or questionnaires, in order that an overall picture of that group can be described in terms of any characteristics that are of interest to the researcher. It may be worth noting that a lot of audit data that are routinely collected now as part of the UK government's target-setting agenda could easily be analysed using techniques of descriptive statistics. Examples are take-up of community podiatry services or breast screening, satisfaction with osteopathy treatment, Did Not Attend rates for an out-patient physiotherapy clinic, use of antenatal clinics, vaccination rates, etc. The information that is collected in this way can be analysed using techniques of descriptive statistics in order to highlight some of the most interesting findings. Indeed, at the time of writing, the UK government is proposing to introduce a mass screening programme to identify people at risk from key illnesses, such as diabetes and coronary heart disease. Following implementation, a survey would be useful, to assess the uptake of the screening, which areas and which groups show the lowest and highest uptakes, the public's reactions and perceptions, the longer-term health impact of early screening, cost-effectiveness, etc. Many of the results from a survey of this kind would be analysed using techniques of descriptive statistics.

The way in which a survey is carried out will be described in more detail in the next chapter. However, some general introductory points about survey methods and descriptive statistics will be described here so that the reader can get an overview of how descriptive and inferential statistics differ.

Let's take an example. Supposing you are interested in the general topic of community podiatry. You could easily gather a vast quantity of data on this topic; for example:

1. The number of community podiatrists currently employed in a particular district, and their specialities.

2. The average number of calls made per podiatrist per week within the district over the last year.
3. The types of patients seen (their ages, medical condition, ethnic origin, social class, sex, etc.) over the last year.
4. The average amount of time spent treating a particular category of patient.
5. Any changes in the delivery of community podiatry over the previous 10-year period could be noted (e.g. any increase in provision to a particular patient group).

From all this survey data, you could gain the following sorts of information:

- what is going on in a particular area (type and extent of community podiatry service provision)
- identification of areas of existing or potential problems (e.g. less provision in some geographical areas or for some categories of patient)
- measurement of the extent of these problems
- the generation of possible explanations for them.

In addition to all this, the survey could identify past trends and so could be used to predict future patterns. (For example, with the population growth in the over-75 age group and the increasing trend towards community-based care, the need for greater provision of community podiatrists with a special interest in the problems of the older person might be highlighted.)

The outcome of such surveys can radically influence major, as well as minor, policy decisions. And if such policy changes are implemented, survey techniques may be used to evaluate the impact these changes have. It might be useful at this point to look at some of the ways in which descriptive statistics might be useful to the clinical therapist, by means of a more specific illustration.

DESCRIPTIVE STATISTICS: AN EXAMPLE

Suppose that you are the head of a school of osteopathy. Obviously, in this role you will be concerned about the standards of student per-

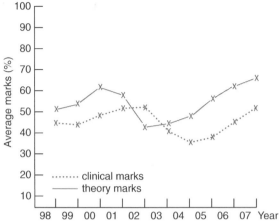

Figure 2.1   Average clinical and theory marks over the past 10 years in a school of osteopathy.

Table 2.1   Average exam marks from all the other schools of osteopathy in 2007

School	Average theory mark (%)	Average clinical mark (%)
A	63	58
B	45	55
C	48	59
D	57	45
E	70	50
F	52	60
G	54	61
H	67	66

formance, both clinical and theoretical, in your school. In particular, you may want to find out: (a) whether these standards are dropping or rising from year to year, and (b) how they compare with other schools throughout the country. To do this you need to employ some common mathematical techniques in order to highlight certain features of the data, in other words, descriptive statistics. Let's take the first example. To find out whether the standards are changing from year to year, you could take the average mark in both final theory and clinical exams over, say, the last 10 years. From this you can draw a graph to get the general picture of the standards of performance. You might end up with something like Figure 2.1.

From such a graph of average marks, you can get the general picture of the trend of perform-ance and also the comparative performance on clinical and theory exams.

To solve your second problem of how your school compares with others, you can collect the average marks from all the other schools for 2007, and then compare your marks with these. You might obtain the data in Table 2.1.

Your own averages for 2007 (66% for theory, 52% for clinical; see Figure 2.1) can be compared with those of other schools to find out how well your own school is doing. It can be seen, then, from this information that your school comes third in the theory exams, but only seventh in the clinical exams. From this information, too, you can see that, although school E has the best marks

on theory, they have the biggest discrepancy between theory and practice, while school H appears to be the most consistent. In other words, you can glean a considerable amount of informa-tion from such data.

It should be pointed out that there are many ways of describing your data besides the methods illustrated above. However, the three most com-monly used forms of descriptive statistics are: graphs; measures of central tendency, which present data in terms of the most typical scores and results; and measures of dispersion, which present data in terms of the variation in the scores. Each of these will be discussed in Chapter 5, 'Techniques of descriptive statistics'.

Descriptive statistics, then, are used when the researcher has collected a large quantity of data, usually from a survey of some sort, and wishes to extract certain sorts of information from it in order to provide a description of the data.

It is important to recognise that descriptive statistics allow you to make statements about features of your data that are of interest, but they do not allow you to infer anything beyond the results you have in front of you. In other words, if you were measuring the muscle power of a group of 20 muscular dystrophy patients, you could use descriptive statistics to make state-ments about the muscle power data of that par-ticular group of patients in terms of average power, range of power measurements, speed of contractions, etc. What you could not do would be to infer anything about the muscle power of muscular dystrophy patients as a whole, simply on the basis of the data from your particular group. To be able to do that you have to use the techniques of inferential statistics.

INFERENTIAL STATISTICS

Prior to every election, we are bombarded with the results of opinion polls which tell us how well one political party is likely to do compared with the others. In order to obtain this sort of information, a sample of the general public is questioned, since it would be impossible to ask the opinions of every member of the electorate. In any case, collecting the views from the entire population would constitute the general election itself. From the responses given by this sample, the attitudes of the rest of the voters are predicted, or inferred. However, we all know that these opinion polls may be quite incorrect. For example, if the opinion pollsters only went to a polo match in Surrey and asked the views of the spectators, they would be likely to get a very different picture of the prevailing political opinion than if they only went to a football match in an inner city area. In other words, if the opinion poll is to have any value in predicting the outcome of an election, the sample selected for the poll must be representative of the population as a whole and not representative of just one section of it.

The usual method of selecting a sample that is representative of the population from which it is drawn is a technique called random sampling. For a sample to be random, it must have been selected in such a way that every member of the relevant population had an equal chance of being chosen. For example, if six playing cards are to be randomly selected from a pack, the pack is first shuffled and any six cards are chosen. Assuming the dealer did not hide any or keep his thumb on some, then these six cards will be a random sample because every one of the 52 cards had an equal chance of selection.

Now, there are two important points here. First, if these cards are not replaced and a second random sample is drawn from the same population, it will not be the same; so, if another set of six cards is selected from the pack, they will be different from the first set because there is only one ace of clubs, seven of hearts, etc., in a pack. Similarly, any two groups of hysterectomy patients, if randomly drawn from a population of hysterectomy patients, will not be identical in their characteristics (age, height, fitness, etc.). Second, the larger the random sample drawn, the more likely it is that it will be reasonably representative of the population from which it comes. So, a random sample of three hysterectomy patients out of a total population of 60 will stand less chance of being representative than a random sample of 35. More information about the ways in which the researcher can select a random sample in practice and other ways of selecting a sample are provided in Chapter 3.

Returning to the opinion poll, even if the sample is representative of the whole population, there will still be an element of error in the predictions about the election (because some voters subsequently change their views, fail to vote, or misunderstand the questions, etc.).

Nonetheless, if the voters selected for the poll have been chosen randomly, according to certain statistical principles, then this degree of error can be calculated using a branch of statistics known as inferential statistics. Essentially, what this approach enables the researcher to do is to select a small sample of people for study, and from the results of that study to make inferences about the larger group from which that sample was drawn. In other words, techniques of inferential statistics allow the researcher to move from what they know to be the case, as indicated by the data they have collected, to what they predict will be the case in other similar situations.

In case this sounds a rather complex procedure, it should be stated that these inferential techniques are used by everyone on a daily basis. For example, your children, for as long as you can remember, have had cereal for breakfast. These are your data, the facts that you know to be true. On this basis, then, you anticipate that this morning they will again want cereal so you put the packets out for them on the assumption that this is what they will want. This is your inference, based on the information collected from previous mornings and generalised to another similar situation. There are doubtless numerous examples that you can think of where your knowledge about one situation leads you to make assumptions about other comparable situations. The actual techniques of inferential statistics are rather more complex than this, but the basic idea is the same.

The proper scientific procedure for making these inferences involves formulating an hypothesis, setting up an experiment to test the hypothesis and using inferential statistics to analyse the results of your experiment to see if your hypothesis has been supported. Thus, inferential statistics are used in testing hypotheses. It should be pointed out at this stage, that there are two main types of research design which are used to test hypotheses: experimental designs and correlational designs. These will be described in detail in Chapter 6.

USING INFERENTIAL STATISTICS: AN EXAMPLE

A classic way in which the clinical therapist might use this approach is in the comparison of different treatment techniques with patients. Let's suppose you were interested in trying to improve hip movement, using conservative techniques, in a group of elderly patients awaiting a total hip replacement operation. You have two techniques, A and B, and you want to find out which is more effective.

For a host of practical reasons, you cannot test every patient awaiting a total hip replacement, and so you select a random sample of, say, 60 patients and randomly assign half of them to treatment A and the other half to treatment B. Both groups are managed in exactly the same way except for the nature of their treatment, and at the end of a given period you compare the groups in terms of their range of movement.

Suppose you find that the range of movement is greater (i.e. improved) for the treatment A group than for the treatment B group. Now you would expect that there would be some differences between the groups anyway, simply because of chance factors, like the mood swings of the patients, personality factors, current state of health, fatigue, etc., but the question is whether the difference between the two groups in terms of range of movement can be accounted for by these chance factors, or whether the difference is due to the relative effectiveness of the treatments.

If the experiment has been carried out properly and in accordance with certain prerequisite conditions (see Chapters 7 and 8 for details on this), then statistical tests can be used to analyse the data and to conclude whether or not the difference between the groups is, in fact, attributable to the type of treatment. If it is found to be due to the treatment procedure, then you would conclude that treatment A is more effective with this group. If you have selected your sample of patients randomly from the whole group of patients waiting for total hip replacements, then you could reasonably infer that treatment A is likely to be more effective than treatment B with other similar patients, and hence you would recommend it to other clinical therapists.

In other words, you have selected a small sample for study and from the results of this study you can make inferences about the whole population from which the sample was drawn. This is the basis of inferential statistics.

Key Concepts

Data from research must be presented in a way that can be understood by the reader. There are two main ways of doing this:

- Descriptive statistics, which summarise the main features of the results from a survey by describing the average scores, etc.
- Inferential statistics, which are used to test hypotheses, and which involve selecting a small sample of people for study. The results of the study allow the researcher to make inferences about the population from which the sample was drawn.

In other words, descriptive statistics allow the researcher to make statements only about the results obtained, but do not permit any assumptions to be made beyond the data collected, whereas inferential statistics allow the researcher to make assumptions beyond the set of data in front of her/him.

FURTHER READING

Boynton P 2005 The research companion: a practical guide for the social and health sciences. Psychology Press, Hove

Cohen L, Holliday M 1996 Practical statistics for students. London, Paul Chapman Publishing

Coolican H 2004 Research methods and statistics in psychology, 4th edition. London, Hodder Arnold

QM LIBRARY (WHITECHAPEL)

Coolican H 2006 Introduction to research methods in psychology, 3rd edition. London, Hodder Arnold

Field A, Hole G 2004 How to design and report experiments. London, Sage

Parahoo K 2006 Nursing research: principles, process and issues, 2nd edition. Macmillan, London

Polgar S, Thomas S 2007 Introduction to research in the health sciences. Churchill Livingstone, Edinburgh

Robson C 2004 Real world research, 2nd edition. Blackwell Publishing, Oxford.

Robson C 1999 Experiment, design and statistics in psychology. Penguin Psychology, Harmondsworth

Scott I, Mazhindu D 2005 Statistics for health care professionals. Sage Publications, London

Watson R, McKenna H, Cowman S, Keady J 2008 Nursing research: designs and methods. Edinburgh, Churchill Livingstone

Chapter 3

Questionnaires, surveys and sampling

It was noted in the previous chapter that surveys often use questionnaires as a means of collecting information about a group of people. However, while questionnaires are commonly used in this way, they can also be used in experimental or single-case designs, and as such are an invaluable method of data collection. This chapter will look at the basic principles of questionnaire design, as well as providing more details on carrying out surveys. Chapter 19 will look in more detail at a specific form of questionnaire – attitude measures.

QUESTIONNAIRE DESIGN

Designing a good questionnaire is a skilled business and does not involve simply jotting a few questions down on paper. The design and use of a good questionnaire should follow six steps:

1. Identifying the general topics to be covered by the questionnaire, which will reflect the objectives the researcher has in mind.
2. Initial draft of the questions covering all these topics.
3. Piloting the questionnaire; i.e. giving out the questionnaire to a number of people (who do not necessarily come from the population at whom the questionnaire is targeted) in order to collect feedback on unclear or insensitive questions, ambiguous instructions, etc.

4. Modification of the questionnaire using the information collected from the pilot trial.
5. A second pilot trial to establish whether or not the earlier problems have been ironed out.
6. Final administration of the questionnaire in the actual study or survey. The completed questionnaire can then be analysed in a variety of different ways.

It is important that the questions are properly informed and do not just arise from what the researcher believes to be relevant. This means that a thorough review of the literature should be undertaken first to identify the main themes. From each of these themes, a set of questions can be constructed. This thematic review of the literature provides some degree of validity (see Chapter 19) for the questionnaire, which is essential if the tool is to measure what it is intended to measure. If you are writing your work up as an assignment or for publication, it is also important to justify the themes (and by implication the questions) by citing the associated research work. For example, if you are developing a questionnaire that is concerned with patients' evaluations of an early discharge programme following total joint replacement, a literature search may generate, say, 5 commonly emerging issues, which would form the foundation for a set of questions that address each theme. This might be reported in the following way:

- Theme 1: pressure on informal carers (Smith 2006; Jones 2007; Bloggs 2007; Brown 2008)
- Theme 2: familiarity of home surroundings (Andrews 2005; Blake 2006; Clark 2007; Davies 2007)
- Theme 3: clinically related anxieties (Evans 2004; Freeman 2006; Gold 2007; Harris 2008), etc.

This research-based support for the questions demonstrates that the researcher is familiar with the core issues, and also adds justification for the inclusion of the items in the questionnaire. However, the available literature is not the only source of knowledge that can be used in the development of your questionnaire – running focus groups or conducting informal interviews with relevant people can embellish and corroborate the findings from the literature search. For

example, in the above illustration, you could interview some early and standard discharge patients, as well as hospital and community health care professionals, to get their views on what the issues are surrounding early discharge.

ASKING THE QUESTIONS

Questions come in two main forms: open-ended and closed. Open-ended questions are those that allow respondents free range when supplying their answers. They are questions that do not provide boundaries or constraints on the answers. Closed questions, on the other hand, do just that: they allow the respondent only a limited choice of how to answer the question.

To illustrate the difference between the two, let us take a simple enquiry that any clinical therapist might make about a patient's health. He/she might ask the patient:

'How do you feel today?'

or, alternatively

'Are you feeling any better today?'

The first is an open-ended question since the patient is being given the opportunity to make statements about their pain levels, appetite, anxiety level or whatever. The second example is a closed question, since the patient can really only answer 'yes' or 'no'. This example is a simplistic one, but it does illustrate the different ways in which questions can be used to elicit information.

As with every other aspect of research, both types of question have their pros and cons. Open-ended questions allow the respondent more flexibility and consequently much more information can be derived, often of a type the researcher had not thought of. On the debit side, though, such answers are difficult to analyse objectively, which means that it can be difficult to compare one person's answer with that of another, and it may also be very labour-intensive. Really, in order to analyse open responses properly, a detailed and systematic content analysis is required; the reader is referred to any of the texts listed under 'Qualitative Research' at the end of Chapter 1 and to Attride-Stirling's excellent (2001) paper on thematic analysis of qualitative data. (It may be worth pointing out that there are software packages available for analysing this sort of qualitative data, but these still require a lot of time to input the responses. A particularly popular package is NVivo.) In addition, open-ended questions are more time-consuming for the respondent to complete, and without answer guidelines many participants may miss the point completely, give only a very superficial answer or provide responses that are neither relevant nor useful.

Closed questions overcome many of these difficulties, since the structured response format means that answers can be completed quickly, analysed easily and direct comparisons between people can be made. However, the analysis will inevitably be restricted by the response categories offered by each question and so some richness of data may be lost. (This point will be discussed in more detail later in this chapter as well as in Chapter 4.) The value of such questions is largely governed by the skill of the question-setter, who needs both to ask sound questions, devoid of ambiguities and bias and to provide a comprehensive and appropriate answer structure. Too often respondents get irritated by answer formats that do not meet their needs and consequently they refuse to reply.

These points raise two particularly important issues in questionnaire design: how to word the questions and how to structure a response format for closed questions.

WORDING THE QUESTIONS

Asking the right questions is a skilled science and is not a topic that can be covered adequately here. I would therefore refer the reader to Oppenheim's (1992) seminal text 'Questionnaire design and attitude measurement' which remains a leader in the field.

However, some guidelines can be given here, as a start. Good question design is dictated by a list of dos and don'ts, each of which will be illustrated in turn:

1. Don't use complex sentence structures.
Do keep your sentences clear and simple. For example, ask:

'Do you think that cystic fibrosis merits top priority for Government funding for genetic engineering?'

and not:

'Do you think that cystic fibrosis, which is a life-threatening and frightening disease and one which causes untold anxiety, misery and pain to sufferers and families alike, should be given top priority in terms of Government funding for genetic engineering projects?'

2. Don't use medical or professional jargon.
Do use words and phrases that the respondents will understand. For example, ask:

'When did you have your gallbladder operation?'

and not:

'When did you have your cholecystectomy?'

3. Don't confuse the respondent by asking about more than one thing at a time.
Do keep to one idea per sentence. For example, ask:

'Do you experience any pain after eating?'

and

'Do you experience any pain after walking?'

and not:

'Do you experience any pain after eating or walking?'

4. Don't assume everyone will know what you mean.
Do keep your questions unambiguous. For example, ask:

'Do you do your exercises for at least 20 minutes every day?'

and not:

'Do you do your exercises regularly?'

5. Don't use double negatives.
Do ask questions positively. For example, ask:

'Have you ever wanted anything to eat after doing your exercises?'

and not:

'Have you ever not wanted to have nothing to eat after doing your exercises?'

6. Don't ask leading questions.

Do ask questions in an unbiased, unemotional way. For example, ask:

> 'Do you think that smokers should be debarred from treatment for smoking-related diseases?

and not:

> 'Do you agree that smokers should not be entitled to any treatment for their self-inflicted smoking diseases?

Instructions on how to complete the questionnaire should also be clear and unambiguous. In addition, it may be necessary to enclose a definition of what the essential terms are, to avoid misunderstanding; for example:

> 'Doing your exercises' should be taken to mean 'Doing all the exercises you have been shown in the way they were demonstrated and for the time suggested'.

Remember that piloting a questionnaire is an essential stage in the research process, since it provides an opportunity to identify and iron out potential problems.

RESPONSE FORMATS FOR CLOSED-ENDED QUESTIONS

The way in which the response options are structured is important in questionnaire design, since it can dictate how honestly the respondent answers, as well as the value and amount of information that can be derived from the questionnaire. These response formats can be thought of as ways of measuring a person's reply to your question and the measurements range from simple through to sophisticated scales. The whole area of scales or levels of measurement is a crucial one in all sorts of research and is dealt with in Chapter 4 in much more detail. However, a brief introduction will be given here.

Let's imagine you have been treating a group of prostatectomy patients for postoperative incontinence, and you wish to send them a follow-up questionnaire, 6 months after the operation, to find out how they are progressing. One question you want to ask is: Do you still suffer any incontinence?

You can structure the possible answers to this in a number of ways, for example:

(a) Do you still suffer any incontinence?

  Yes ☐   No ☐

(b) Do you still suffer any incontinence?

1	2	3	4	5
Never	Infrequently	Often	Very often	All the time

(c) Do you still suffer any incontinence?

  Never   ☐
  Once a day   ☐
  Twice a day   ☐
  Three times a day   ☐
  Four times a day   ☐
  Five times a day   ☐

The first response format is a simple one and gives us only basic information. For instance, a respondent who ticks the 'Yes' box might suffer urinary incontinence once a month or once an hour, but this sort of answer format doesn't provide that level of detail.

The second answer format is somewhat more sophisticated, since it allows us to collect a range of information on the overall frequency of incontinence. However, the descriptions 'infrequently', 'often', etc. are open to subjective interpretation, and while they provide more information about the patient's level of incontinence than the previous format, are still lacking in objectivity and precision.

The last response format is the most sophisticated of the three, since it gives us detailed and accurate information about how often the patient is incontinent, in absolute terms.

These different types of response need different techniques to analyse them and this point is referred to in some detail later. As a rule of thumb, it is better, where possible, to use the most sophisticated and objective response formats as they supply a lot more information about the respondents.

It is also important to note, too, that respondents are not always honest in their answers, not necessarily because they deliberately wish to deceive the researcher, but simply because they want to present themselves in the best possible light. This tendency is known as a social-desirability response set and topics which are sensitive or emotive are particularly vulnerable to this type of bias. The researcher should be cognisant of this when analysing the data.

Finally, do treat your respondents with respect. Don't ask embarrassing or intrusive questions, don't use their replies to compromise them, don't mislead them in any way and if you tell them their responses are anonymous or confidential, mean it. For further guidance on this issue, the section on ethics in Chapter 6 provides a more detailed discussion.

ADVANTAGES AND DISADVANTAGES OF QUESTIONNAIRES

The main advantage of questionnaires is that they can be designed and customised for any purpose or group of people.

In addition, because a questionnaire does not have to be administered by the researcher in person, it means that a large sample of people can be included in the study by posting the questionnaire to them. This has added advantages. First, posting a questionnaire is considerably cheaper than the time and travel expenses that would be incurred either by transporting the individual participants into the project centre, or by the researcher travelling to meet the participants. Second, if questionnaires are to be posted, the possibility of the researcher influencing the respondent's answers either unwittingly or deliberately is reduced considerably.

However, questionnaires also have their disadvantages. If the questionnaires are sent by post there is a very high chance that a lot of recipients will not return them. While this non-return rate can be reduced somewhat by the inclusion of stamped addressed envelopes, it does, nonetheless, mean that the researcher usually has to send out considerably more questionnaires than are actually needed in order to compensate for the non-returners, and this, of course, adds to the cost. However, sending out reminders to respondents can increase the response rate. It should be remembered too, that the non-responders may have very different views to the the responders and consequently the results from a low return rate may not be representative.

For postal questionnaires, a return of about 40% is considered adequate.

Furthermore, whether a questionnaire is administered in person or by post there is still a high probability that some questions will be ignored, or incorrectly completed, instructions may be misinterpreted and some answers will be inadequately detailed.

Also, while it seems an unbelievably obvious thing to say, it is still a point which is commonly overlooked by a lot of researchers: the respondent should be able to read the questions. This means that issues of visual impairment, non-English speakers and illiteracy must be considered. And, of course, because of their ease and efficiency as a data-gathering tool, questionnaires are very widely used, which means that your target group may be suffering questionnaire fatigue.

This having been said, questionnaires are still a very popular and very useful technique of data collection within the health care area.

Key Concepts

- Questionnaires are a very useful way of collecting data in the health care area.
- Asking the appropriate questions is a very skilled task and requires consideration of a number of issues.
- Questions can be open-ended or closed-ended, both of which have advantages and disadvantages.
- Closed-ended questions require structured answers, and the way in which the questioner sets out the answer structures is an important consideration.

SURVEYS

In the previous chapter a survey was described as a research technique which involves collecting data from a large number of people, so that a general overview of the group can be obtained. Surveys usually use questionnaires or interviews as a means by which information is gathered, but, since a key characteristic of the survey is the large number of people who take part, it is often quicker and much cheaper to use questionnaires rather than interviews. Indeed, so costly is it to interview hundreds of people that it is often outside the scope of most researchers. Consequently, issues concerning interviews will not be covered here. If you would like to find more about interview techniques, Polgar & Thomas (2007) and Robson (2002) provide useful overviews.

GENERAL PRINCIPLES OF SURVEYS

The first stage in designing a survey is to establish its aims. In other words, what questions do you want answered? So, for example, you may want to audit the services of a back pain clinic, and consequently might want to ask:

1. How many people use it in the course of a year?
2. Where do they come from?
3. How many men use the clinic?
4. How many women use the clinic?
5. What are the ethnic origins of the users?
6. What are the ages of the users?
7. What are the occupations of the users?
8. What were the presenting medical problems?
9. For how long do users come to the clinic per session?
10. How do the users rate the quality of care they receive at the clinic? etc.

You then have to decide the best ways of finding answers to these questions; in other words, you have to design your survey.

THE DESIGN OF THE SURVEY

Two commonly used survey designs are prospective designs and retrospective designs.

Prospective designs involve identifying the group of people you want to study and then collecting the information you require when they use the particular service. So, for example, you might want to focus on patients using a back pain clinic who have had no known injury to the back. As soon as such patients enter the clinic the researcher would collect the relevant information from them. While this approach allows the researcher to select participants according to clearly defined criteria, it can obviously be a very

time-consuming process to access an adequate number of suitable participants.

However, a commonly used survey approach is the retrospective design, which focuses particularly on past events. For example, you might identify, from the medical records department in the back pain clinic, patients who presented with back pain but who had no known injury. You would then contact these patients to collect the information you require, such as their subsequent problems, perceptions of care, etc. The main problem with this approach is the fact that when people are asked to recall events their memory may be selective and, consequently, this might bias the data you collect.

Once you have decided on the design, you then have to identify the people who will take part in your survey.

SELECTING THE PEOPLE TO TAKE PART

Finding the appropriate number and type of people to take part in your study is called sampling. This is an essential part of good research design of any sort, whether it be surveys or experimental approaches. While some reference has already been made to sampling in the earlier section on inferential statistics (Ch. 2), it is sufficiently important to merit a section on its own.

Sampling

When you carry out a piece of research it is impossible to involve every person who might be of interest to you, both for practical and financial reasons. For example, you might want to conduct some research on women with osteoporosis, but as there must be many thousands of these women within the UK it would be completely impossible to study them all. Consequently, you would select just some of them to take part in your study. These women would be your sample.

However, if the data collected from the sample are to be of any value, the sample must be representative of female osteoporosis sufferers as a whole. This entire group of all the osteoporosis patients is called the population. The population can be defined as all those people (or even events) who possess the characteristic(s) in which the researcher is interested. This parent population is sometimes called the sampling frame. Thus, the sample of osteoporosis sufferers is a subset of the population of osteoporosis sufferers as a whole. To take another example, you may wish to look at the treatment procedures for asthma patients in a regional health authority. All the asthma patients in that authority would constitute the population and you might select a sample of 500 of them for your study.

However, if you are to collect any useful information from your sample, you have got to try to ensure that the sample is pretty well representative of the population from which they are drawn. If it is not, then the conclusions you reach from your study cannot readily be generalised to the rest of the population and might lead you to make invalid assumptions about that population. In other words, when selecting a sample, the sample mean (or average) for any given characteristic should be the same as the population mean, because, in this way, any results from the sample can more confidently be assumed to apply to the population from which it was drawn. However, in reality, there will always be a difference between the sample mean and the population mean and this difference is called the sampling error. In general, the larger the sample and the more rigorous the sampling methods used, the smaller the sampling error.

Let's illustrate this idea with an example. Supposing you wanted to conduct a survey looking at the incidence of asthma in the under-fives, perhaps with a view to planning future clinical therapy provision more carefully. You devise your questionnaire and send it out to every family within two postal districts. When you get the returns and analyse the data, you find to your amazement that 70% of the respondents' under-five children suffer from asthma. You then assume that 70% of all under-fives in your region have asthma and you set about recruiting four specialist therapists to meet the anticipated demand for services. Two years later, you find that two of these specially recruited therapists have insufficient work to do and you have to terminate their contracts. What could have gone wrong with your planning?

One possible reason might be the way in which you selected your survey sample. When you go back to check this, you realise that the two

postal areas you chose were both inner city areas lying close to a network of motorway junctions. Consequently, atmospheric pollution was likely to be extremely high in the areas. Moreover, you then read a new report which claims that smoking is more prevalent in inner city areas. Therefore, the children in your sample were also likely to have been subjected to high levels of atmospheric pollution in their home as well. Small wonder, then, that your survey results suggested an incredibly high incidence of early childhood asthma. It also becomes clear why your specialist therapists were underemployed – your resource planning was based on findings from a very biased sample which could not be generalised to the rest of the region's population.

Consequently, it is imperative that the sampling techniques employed in any study, be it survey or experimental, must be sound if you are to draw valid conclusions from your data. The most commonly used sampling methods in scientific and health research are incidental sampling and random sampling.

Incidental sampling

Incidental sampling is a generic term which involves selecting the most easily accessible people from your population; consequently, it is relatively easy to do. However, it is a non-probability method of collecting a sample and therefore, because the process isn't random, should not, strictly speaking, be used in experimental research (although it often is). Let's imagine you're interested in conducting a questionnaire survey of the counselling needs of quadriplegic patients presenting for treatment. You ask a friend who's a clinical therapist in your local hospital to give your questionnaire to all the relevant patients s/he sees in the unit.

This is undoubtedly an easy way of accessing a sample but it may not give you a representative selection of patients. For example, because of workload allocations, the clinical therapist may only see those patients who have recently become quadriplegic, or alternatively he or she may only see the patients whose condition is progressive. Since the parent population of quadriplegic patients is not necessarily suffering only from progressive diseases, nor are they all newly paralysed, this incidental sample is unlikely to be representative. Moreover, because it is conceivable that newly diagnosed quadriplegic patients, or those with progressive conditions, might have more counselling support needs because of the newness or the degenerative nature of their condition, the results from your survey would probably not reflect the support needs of quadriplegic patients as a whole. But, unless you had a lot more information about the population of quadriplegic patients, you wouldn't know whether the sample was biased or representative, and, consequently, whether their reported counselling needs were a reflection of those of the population.

One way round this is to use a variation of incidental sampling called quota sampling.

Quota sampling

Suppose you have found that there are two key variables that will have a significant impact on the counselling needs of quadriplegic patients; these are the cause of the quadriplegia (trauma or progressive illness) and the length of time spent in treatment (less than a year or more than a year). You then find out that 40% of all quadriplegic patients referred as a result of progressive conditions attend for clinical therapy for more than a year, while 60% discontinue before a year; 70% of quadriplegic patients referred as a result of trauma attend for clinical therapy beyond 1 year and 30% discontinue before 1 year (Table 3.1). Each of these subgroups might be expected to have quite different support and counselling needs, based on their previous progress and expectations of progress. For example, it might be predicted that those quadriplegics who have progressive diseases, for which the prognosis is especially poor, might have particularly pronounced needs for counselling support.

Table 3.1 Clinical therapy history and current diagnosis of quadriplegic patients taking part in a counselling needs survey

Diagnosis	Clinical therapy <1 year	Clinical therapy >1 year
Trauma	30%	70%
Progressive disease	60%	40%

Having this information you would then collect your sample by quota, ensuring that:

1. 40% of the quadriplegic patients in your sample with progressive conditions attend for clinical therapy beyond a year.
2. 60% of the progressive condition sample discontinue treatment within a year.
3. 30% of your sample who are quadriplegic as a result of trauma discontinue clinical therapy within a year.
4. 70% of your sample who are quadriplegic as a result of trauma receive clinical therapy for more than a year.

However, this approach means that you must know what particular characteristics are likely to be important in your study (in the above example, these were assumed to be length of time in clinical therapy and aetiology) and, secondly, you have to know what proportions of quadriplegic patients fall into these categories. These pieces of information may be difficult or even impossible to obtain, and this makes proper quota sampling problematic.

There are other non-probability sampling techniques which are:

- Accidental sampling (use of anyone who is available and willing)
- Purposive sampling (the researcher identifies specific people to take part)
- Volunteer sampling (individuals voluntarily respond to requests for participants)
- Snowball (participants invite people they know to take part who, in turn, invite others and so on).

RANDOM SAMPLING METHODS

Random sampling is also called probability sampling and the methods that fall within this category are perhaps the most commonly used and best ways of selecting a sample. They are also a fundamental requirement of the randomised controlled trial (see Chapter 6 for a description of this method). The basic concepts were referred to in the section 'Inferential statistics' in the previous chapter (pp. 20–21) and consequently only a review will be presented here. The fundamental principle underpinning random sampling is that every member of the target population should have an equal chance of being selected for study. There are a number of ways in which this can be achieved, some of which are highly sophisticated and beyond the requirements and reach of the lone researcher. For instance, in simple random sampling, you can put the names of all members of the population into a hat and then draw out the number you need for your sample, just like a raffle. Alternatively, you can use random number tables. This involves giving a number to every member of the population and then using a set of random number tables to select the sample size you need. [Random number tables can be found in a number of research texts, e.g. Robson (1999).] Essentially, the process works like this. Random number tables consist of the numbers 0–99 occurring with the same probability at any point in the table. If you wanted to select 25 hallux valgus patients from a population of 100 such patients then you would assign each one of the numbers from 0 to 99 to a patient, shut your eyes and stick a pin into the random number table. From that number you work in any direction you like and, keeping to that direction, make a note of the first 25 different numbers you encounter. You then tally these up with the corresponding numbers assigned to your patients and you have your random sample. Remember not to change direction once you have started; also, if you need to select another random sample then you should enter the table at a different point and move in another direction. There are also software packages that can generate random number tables (e.g. http://www.decisionanalyst.com) which can be downloaded free.

Two variations of random sampling are worth a brief mention: stratified random sampling and systematic sampling.

Stratified random sampling

This is akin to quota sampling in that it involves the researcher defining relevant subgroups of the population. A random sample, using either the 'raffle' or the random number technique, would then be drawn from each subgroup. This approach ensures that all the important subsets of a population are represented in the sample but, like random sampling, it requires the names

of all members of the population and is therefore costly, difficult and time-consuming.

Systematic sampling

This involves choosing every third, seventh, thirteenth or whatever, member of the population. While this is not a truly random technique, it usually provides a sample that is adequately representative of the population. The intervals should be decided in advance.

There is also cluster random sampling, which is used when the target population falls into natural clusters that might affect the results of your study if each cluster is not adequately represented. For instance, you might be concerned with conducting a survey of the attitudes of all the staff employed by a large hospital trust to moving to foundation hospital status. The target population might fall into the following groups: medical staff, nursing staff, professions allied to medicine, domestic staff, health care assistants, etc. These groups also fall into medical and surgical areas, in-patient and out-patient provision, clinical specialty and so on. To select a cluster sample, you would first need to identify the members of each possible group and then randomly pick your sample from these. So, you have to identify nurses who work in medical in-patient areas, nurses who work in surgical in-patient areas, nurses who work in medical out-patient areas, nurses who work in surgical out-patient areas, domestics who work in medical in-patient areas, domestics who work in surgical in-patient areas, etc. The researcher must identify the core groups of the target population and then, using the techniques of random sampling described above, select a sample from each cluster.

Random samples have an important advantage over other sampling techniques in that the sample, because it is more representative of the population, does not have to be a very large one. (Sample size will be dealt with later in this chapter and in Chapter 8.) However, there are major disadvantages. The researcher should theoretically be able to access all the population members before a random sample can be selected. If we think about the prospect of doing this with the topic of diabetes or cardiovascular disease, the task becomes impossible. Allied to this are the cost and resource implications; it is much cheaper and less labour intensive to use an incidental sample simply because they are, by definition, easily accessible.

SAMPLE SIZE

When you have chosen an appropriate method for selecting your sample you then have to decide how many people you want to survey.

Many would-be researchers are deterred from undertaking research because they believe they need hundreds of people to participate in it and, indeed, the meteoric rise of the randomised controlled trial as the gold standard of health care research has tended to confirm in many researchers' minds that large-scale, multi-site projects are the only valid means of conducting research. This is not necessarily so, and indeed in many situations it may be inadvisable to have crowds of people taking part, particularly if painful procedures or ethical issues are involved. There is no easy way of establishing the best size of sample since this decision depends very largely on the research that is being undertaken. However, as a general rule of thumb, a larger sample is more likely to be representative of the population than a smaller one; moreover, where techniques of inferential statistics are being used, small sample sizes are corrected by an increase in the stringency with which the analysis is conducted. In crude terms, then, if you have only a small sample, your results have to be 'better' before you can draw any conclusions from them.

The procedures for calculating appropriate sample sizes depend on whether an experiment or a survey is being conducted. The method that applies to surveys will be discussed here, while that which applies to experimental methods will be presented in Chapter 8. More detailed guidelines can be found on the following website which also provides a quick and easy way of calculating sample size for surveys (http://www.decisionanalyst.com).

The issue of sample size has become a salient one in recent years. Clearly, it is very important to use a sample that is big enough to reflect with reasonable accuracy the views of the population from which it is drawn. If the sample is too small it runs the risk of being unrepresentative, which might lead the researcher to draw inaccurate conclusions. A recent personal example illustrates the case perfectly. I had to chair a PhD viva, at which there were four people present: the candidate, the two external examiners and me. Afterwards, I went with the examiners for lunch. Of the four people at the viva, three were left-handed. All three people at lunch were vegetarian. If I had believed that these two samples were representative and of adequate size, I would have come to the conclusion that 75% of the population is left-handed and 100% of them vegetarian; both conclusions are clearly nonsensical.

On the other hand, it is also important from a resource perspective not to target more people than you need. If a sample of 300 would provide a representative view, to use 400 or 1000 would be an unnecessary waste of resources, since the additional numbers do not provide a commensurate increase in accuracy of the results. In other words, if the appropriate sample size is calculated to be 300, using 600 people might increase the representativeness, but it won't double it. Thus, the law of diminishing returns applies to sample size calculation: where time, money and resources are limited, it is important not to waste them on unnecessarily large samples. Yet it is also important that the sample is sufficiently big to reflect the views of the population from which it was drawn; calculating the correct sample size can therefore help to achieve both representativeness and cost effectiveness. It should also be noted that, besides wasting resources, an unnecessarily large sample may obscure valuable information. For example, if you had conducted a survey of 1000 stroke patients' satisfaction with occupational therapy (OT) services, the extreme views of a few (say 10) outliers would be hidden by 990 other perspectives. But had you used a sample of 100, these outlying views would stand out more clearly. If you then looked at these respondents more closely, you might find that the outliers were all very negative about the OT services, but, moreover, that the respondents all had something in common that set them apart from the rest of the sample. For example, these respondents might all be elderly Asian women whose OT was carried out by the same young white male. It could be that their extreme dissatisfaction with service provision was a product of this particular OT's cultural insensitivity, which would need to be addressed as a staff training issue. These illustrations should demonstrate the importance of obtaining a suitable sample size for your survey.

Determining how large your survey sample should be depends on a number of factors, such as potential sources of bias, sampling methods and the like. The method presented here will provide a conservative estimate (i.e. the largest number you would need) and is consequently suitable for the majority of surveys. In order to calculate the figure, you need two key pieces of information:

- What you predict the sample's response will be to your question
- The standard error of your sample.

This information is expressed as the following equation:

$$\frac{P_y \times P_n}{(\text{standard error})^2} = N$$

where P_y and P_n are the expected answers to your question and N is the number of participants you need. These terms will be explained in more detail.

P_y and P_n

These terms refer to the responses the researcher anticipates will be obtained from each of the questions in the study. So, for example, if we continue with the illustration of stroke patients' satisfaction with OT services, we might, on the basis of previous research, anticipate that 70% (or 0.7) of our respondents will be dissatisfied with the frequency of sessions with the OT (and therefore, 30% or 0.3 will be not be dissatisfied). If P_y stands for the not dissatisfied proportion (0.3) and P_n stands for the dissatisfied proportion (0.7), then we would multiply these values to get the numerator (number above the line) of 0.21. (It doesn't matter which proportion is represented by P_n or by P_y). However, within the same questionnaire, there might be a question relating to the respondents' satisfaction with the OT's communication skills. Let us suppose we have no expectation of how the patients might respond to this. On this basis, we would assume a 50/50

split. Therefore P_y and P_n will both equal 0.5, which would give us a numerator of $0.5 \times 0.5 = 0.25$. In essence, the more confident the researcher is about the potential responses to the questionnaire, the fewer the number of people required to take part. Where the researcher has no idea about the likely outcome, a larger sample will be required. The explanation behind this may be more evident from an actual example. In the 2000 US elections, George W. Bush was eventually confirmed as President following several recounts of the votes. The margin of difference between Bush and Gore was so small that the outcome of the election could not be predicted in advance. Any opinion polls prior to the election would have had to sample virtually the whole of the electorate in order to establish with any accuracy who the winner would be. In contrast, in the 2001 UK general election, Tony Blair got in by a massive margin, which all the opinion polls had consistently predicted. The outcome was potentially so clear-cut that only relatively small samples of the voting public needed to be polled in order to forecast the outcome with a high degree of accuracy. In other words, it is much harder to accurately predict the outcome of a close election than it is a landslide, so much larger samples are needed in close calls to achieve any semblance of precision.

While the calculation of the numerator may be mathematically easy, the underlying principles and implications are rather alarming, for two reasons. First, there will be many occasions when the researcher has no information that will enable him/her to anticipate the outcome to a question; and secondly, it is a laborious activity to calculate the required sample size for each question in the survey questionnaire, especially as the same number of respondents will be answering each question. Since many questionnaires will contain questions about which the researcher cannot make predictions, it obviously makes logical sense to calculate the sample size on the basis of those questions about which the researcher cannot make informed forecasts. This is a fail-safe or conservative position and is the basis of the guidelines provided here. Therefore, if we assume that our questionnaire will have at least one question about which we cannot anticipate the results, we must then conclude that P_y and P_n

both equal 0.5 (i.e. half the respondents will respond in one way and half in the other). This means that whenever you use a questionnaire in which the direction of responses to at least one of the questions is completely unknown, the numerator will always be 0.25. If, on the other hand, you can predict the outcomes of all the questions, then you can use informed and relevant proportions for P_y and P_n.

Standard error

I have already outlined the reasons why the researcher needs to ensure that the sample selected for the survey should be reasonably representative of the population from which they were drawn. Any findings from a representative sample are also likely to apply to the whole parent population. The degree to which a sample reflects the relevant characteristics of the parent population is central to both surveys and experiments because the closer the sample and the population are with regard to these characteristics, the more generalisable and accurate the results are likely to be. If this is illustrated with our example of stroke patients' satisfaction with OT services, we might find from our sample that 65% are dissatisfied with the quality of provision. This figure should approximate the views of the whole population of stroke patients. It has already been noted that the discrepancies between the responses of different samples and from the population are known as sampling errors. The usual acceptable sampling error is 5% or 0.05, which means that the researcher wants to be 95% confident that the results from his/her study are accurate to within 5% of the population's results. Sometimes a researcher needs greater accuracy and so will reduce the acceptable sampling error to 1% (99% confident). More information about confidence limits and intervals is provided in Chapter 18. When calculating the numbers needed for your survey, you need to decide in advance how accurate you want your results to be (i.e. the acceptable size of the sampling error). The following calculations are given for the two error levels indicated above: 5% and 1%.

To obtain the standard error value for the denominator in the above equation using a 5% error limit and 95% confidence, you need to

divide 5% (or 0.05) by 1.96, which is a constant value to be used with this accuracy level:

$$0.05 \div 1.96 = 0.0255102$$

This figure of 0.026 is the standard error and needs to be squared for use in our sample size formula above:

$$0.0255102^2 = 0.0006507$$

If we now substitute our values into the sample size formula we get:

$$\frac{0.25}{0.0006507} = 0.384$$

Therefore, 384 is the maximum sample size required when the researcher cannot predict the outcome of at least one question in the questionnaire and when an error limit of 5% is appropriate. However, please note that this is the number required for completed questionnaires. As there will always be non-returns, it is essential that this is built into the total number of questionnaires you send out in the first place, so that you can ensure the required number are returned. A reasonable return rate for a postal questionnaire is 40%, so you would need to send out around 1000 questionnaires, to ensure that you obtained the 384 required.

Should you ever wish to reduce the error limit to 1% (or 99% confidence), then the constant value which should be substituted is 2.576.

Once you have collected your results you then have to make sense of them. Some ways in which this can be done are described in the next chapter.

It may be worth pointing out that decisions concerning surveys or any other type of research approach can never be perfect; because of the practical difficulties and complexities of field and applied research, compromises in design always have to be made. However, it is important that the researcher knows the pros, cons and implications of any decision before implementing it, and this text is an attempt to provide some of this basic information.

If you are interested in finding out more about survey methods, the books listed in Further reading might be useful:

Key Concepts

- Surveys are a research approach which involves collecting data from a large number of people, either by questionnaires or interviews, so that an overview of that group can be obtained.
- Surveys can be prospective in design or retrospective. Retrospective surveys are more commonly used but, as they rely on people's recall of events, they may be flawed by selective or inadequate memory.
- Deciding on who takes part in your study is called sampling. The general idea behind sampling is that you can generalise the results from your sample to the rest of the population from which they were drawn.
- There are a number of different sampling methods, each of which has its own advantages and disadvantages.
- The appropriate size for the sample is not easy to determine, since it depends very much on the subject being studied, as well as on the researcher's knowledge of the relevant population's characteristics.
- Calculating an appropriate sample size for a survey requires the researcher to have some information about the probable responses to the questions in the survey instrument; where the researcher cannot make an informed prediction, the most usual required sample size will be 384 participants.

FURTHER READING

In addition to the general research texts cited at the end of Chapter 1, the following are particularly useful:

Surveys

Abramson JH, Abramson ZH 2008 Survey methods in community medicine, 6th edition. Churchill Livingstone, Edinburgh

De Vaus D 2002 Surveys in social research, 5th edition. Routledge, London

Kelly B, Long A 2005 The design and execution of social surveys. Online. Available http://nurseresearcher. rcnpublishing.co.uk/resources/archive/GetArticleById. asp?ArticleId=6151

May T 2003 Social research: issues, methods and process, 3rd edition. Open University Press, Buckingham

Watson R, McKenna H, Cowman S, Keady J 2008 Nursing research: designs and methods. Edinburgh, Churchill Livingstone

Interviews

Polgar S, Thomas S 2007 Introduction to research in the health sciences. Edinburgh, Churchill Livingstone

Robson C 2002 Real world research: a resource for social scientists and practitioner-researchers. Oxford, Blackwell Publishing

Questionnaire design

Boynton P 2004 Administering, analysing and reporting your questionnaire. BMJ 328:1372–1375

Boynton P, Greenhalgh T 2004 Selecting, designing and developing your questionnaire. BMJ 328: 1312–1315

Foddy W 1994 Constructing questions for interviews and questionnaires: theory and practice in social research. Cambridge University Press, Cambridge.

Gillham B 2000 Developing a questionnaire (real world research). Continuum, London

Kelly B, Long A 2005 The design and execution of social surveys. Online. Available http://nurseresearcher. rcnpublishing.co.uk/resources/archive/GetArticleById. asp?ArticleId=6151

Oppenheim A 2000 Questionnaire design and attitude measurement. Continuum, London

Watson R, McKenna H, Cowman S, Keady J 2008 Nursing research: designs and methods. Edinburgh, Churchill Livingstone

Analysing qualitative data

Attride-Stirling J 2001 Thematic networks: an analytic tool for qualitative research. Qualitative Research 1(3):385–405

Gibbs GR 2002 Qualitative data analysis: explorations with NVivo. Open University Press, Buckingham

Pope C, Ziebland S, Mays N 2000 Analysing qualitative data. BMJ 320:114–116

Stevenson C 2005 Theoretical and methodological approaches in discourse analysis. Online. Available http://nurseresearcher.rcnpublishing.co.uk/resources/ archive/GetArticleById.asp?ArticleId=5936

Watson R, McKenna H, Cowman S, Keady J 2008 Nursing research: designs and methods. Edinburgh, Churchill Livingstone

Randomisation

Altman DG, Bland JM 1999a Treatment allocation in controlled trials: why randomise? BMJ 318: 1209

Altman DG, Bland JM 1999b How to randomise. BMJ 319: 703–704

Jadad A 2007 Randomised controlled trials, 2nd edition. Blackwell, BMJ Books, Oxford

Sampling

Parahoo K 2006 Nursing research: principles, process and issues, 2nd edition. Macmillan, London

Robson C 1999 Experiment, design and statistics in Psychology, 3rd Edition. Harmondsworth, Penguin

Robson C 2002 Real world research: a resource for social scientists and practitioner-researchers, 2nd edition. Blackwell Publishing, Oxford

Saks M, Allsop J 2007 Researching health: qualitative, quantitative and mixed methods. Sage Publishing, London

Chapter 4

The nature of the data

LEVELS OF MEASUREMENT

Whatever sort of research you're interested in, whether it's a survey or an experiment, you will be involved in measuring something (e.g. exam performance, distance walked, vital capacity, range of movement and so on). These measurements form your data or results. If we look at the above examples a bit more carefully, we can see that each of them involves a different sort of measurement:

- Exam performance may be measured as marks out of say, 20 or 100.
- Distance walked may be measured in yards or metres.
- Vital capacity may be measured in litres.
- Range of movement may be measured in degrees.

You can doubtless think of other sorts of measures that might be involved in your own area of health research and it might be useful to make a list of these.

Key Concepts

When you carry out research you will be involved in measuring something. These measurements form your data or results and fall into one of four main categories of measurement. You need to be able to identify which category your own measurements come into, because this will affect the way in which you analyse your data, since some statistical tests can only be used with certain categories of measurement.

However, any measurement you use belongs to one of four main categories of measurement. It is important to be able to distinguish which category your data belong to because it will affect the way in which you analyse your results, since some analyses can only be used with particular categories of measurement.

The four categories are called 'levels of measurement' and each category gives us a different amount of information:

1. *Nominal level*: the most basic level which gives us least information.
2. *Ordinal level*: the next level which provides all the information of the nominal scale plus some additional information.
3. *Interval level*: a higher level of measurement which provides all the information of the nominal and ordinal scales but which offers additional information.
4. *Ratio level*: the highest level of all which provides all the information of the nominal, ordinal and interval scales but which offers further information still.

For the purposes of statistical analysis, the interval and ratio scales are combined to form a single category, and this is how we will be dealing with them in this book.

NOMINAL LEVEL

Let's take the nominal level first of all. As you may have guessed, this is simply a 'naming' category, in that it only gives names or labels to your data without implying any order, quality or dimension. So, for example, you might want to ascertain how many of the applicants for places at a school of osteopathy come from particular areas. You call one region Area A, another Area B, and another Area C and count up how many applicants fall into each category. This is a nominal level of measurement, because it has simply allowed you to allocate your data into one of three named categories.

Two important points are worth noting here. I have just said that this level of measurement has no implication for degree, order or quality of the data, which means that we could very easily alter the headings of the categories in any way, without affecting the results. So, for instance, Area A could just as easily have been called Area C or D, or X, Y or Z or Banana or Apple, since it will not affect the number of applicants who have come from that region.

Second, the categories are mutually exclusive, in that an applicant can only come from one area. Thus, once we have allocated a subject to one particular nominal category, they cannot be allocated to any other category.

Let's take an example. If you were looking at the final exam success of two different chiropractic schools, you might take School A and School B and count up the number of passes and fails at each.

What you are measuring here is exam success, but all you have done is to use two labels – 'pass' and 'fail' – and have counted up how many students in each school achieved more than 50% (pass category) and how many achieved less (fail category). You might end up with the data in Table 4.1.

A student who comes into the pass category cannot also come into the fail category and so this level of measurement involves mutually exclusive categories.

Measurement at this level gives us very little information about our data. You don't know how well the students have passed; all School A's pass students may have achieved 90%, while all School B's passes may have been 50–55%. You also don't know how bad the fails are (e.g. 0% or 43%). All you know is that a certain number of students can be labelled 'pass' and a certain number 'fail'. Therefore, this is a nominal level of measurement and, as you can see, it doesn't

Table 4.1 Students categorised according to 'pass' or 'fail'

	Pass	Fail
School A	29	11
School B	33	7

tell us a great deal. For example, if you had to recommend one of these schools on the basis of nominal data, you would probably suggest School B because it achieved 33 passes to School A's 29. But if School A had pass marks of 90% as opposed to School B's 50–55%, you might want to change your recommendation. However, you wouldn't know this from nominal data alone, since all this category allows you to do is to classify your data under the broad headings of 'pass' and 'fail'.

Political opinion polls which simply categorise people into Conservative, Labour, Liberal Democrats and Don't Knows are nominal scales. Voting on a particular issue in a meeting categorises people into 'For', 'Against' and 'Abstain', and so is a nominal scale. We don't know how Conservative a respondent in a poll is, or how 'against' a voter in a meeting is; we just know that they can be allocated to a particular category.

The following are also examples of the nominal level of measurement:

- The number of male and female applicants for speech therapy places at School A may be 39 males to 123 females. You don't know how old the applicants are, how good their 'A'-level results are, or how suitable they are; all you know is that you have 39 male applicants and 123 females.
- You send a questionnaire to all the podiatrists in a district asking them to indicate:

Do you smoke? Yes _____   No _____

You get a set of replies, which suggests that 42 people smoke and 101 do not. But you do not know how many cigarettes the smokers get through; it may be 5 per day or 65. All you know is that 42 podiatrists in a particular district smoke and 101 do not.

It may be worth noting that the nominal level of measurement is referred to as 'categorical' data in some text books.

ORDINAL LEVEL

The next category of measurement is the ordinal scale which tells us a bit more about our data. The ordinal scale allows us to rank order our data according to the dimension we are interested in, for example:

most preferred – least preferred
most improved – least improved
most competent – least competent.

Suppose you asked a clinical supervisor to

Activity 4.1 (Answers on p. 359)

Look at the following measures you might use in a piece of research, and indicate how these might be measured using a nominal category of measurement:

1 improvement in lumbar movement following physiotherapy
2 reduced incidence of chest infections following breathing exercises
3 increased range of movement in a leg, following manipulation
4 keeping appointments at a chiropractic clinic
5 perceptions of the quality of osteopathy treatment.

---

rank order a set of students on their competence during a placement. The supervisor might come up with the list in Table 4.2.

What we have is a rank ordering of these students in terms of the dimension we're interested in: their competence. We still don't have a great deal of information about them, however, because we don't know how much better Catherine A. is than Parveen B., or how much worse Susan D. is than the rest (or, in fact, whether any of them are competent at all). All we know is that Catherine A. is better than Parveen B. who in turn is better than Jack S.; but we don't know how much better. In other words, we have a relative and not an absolute measure of competence. It is also important to note that the differences

Table 4.2 Students arranged in order of competence

Competence position	Student
1 (Most competent)	Catherine A.
2	Parveen B.
3	Jack S.
4	Carol R.
5 (Least competent)	Susan D.

between each pair of ordinal positions is not necessarily the same; i.e. the difference in competence between Catherine A. and Parveen B. may not be the same as the difference between Parveen B. and Jack S.

POINT SCALES

Another example of an ordinal scale of measurement is the point scale. For example, in the previous study, with another set of students, you might alternatively have asked the clinical supervisor to indicate on the following scale how competent each student was:

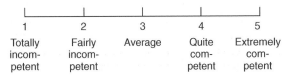

Here we have a dimension of most competent to least competent on a 5-point scale, (although we could use fewer or more than 5 points; using more than 7 points is not advisable) and on which each student may be rated. Therefore, had we asked the clinical supervisor to assess students using this scale, we might have found the results shown in Table 4.3.

Again, the difference between each pair of scores must not be assumed to be the same. The difference in competence between:

5 (extremely competent)
and
4 (quite competent)

may not be the same as between:

1 (totally incompetent)
and
2 (fairly incompetent)

Table 4.3 Students categorised using a point scale

Competence score	Students
5	Laura B.
4	Julie N., Paul S.
3	Chris D.
2	Jill F., Jaz H.
1	Sally C.

In our earlier example on the smoking questionnaire, we could modify our question from:

Do you smoke? Yes _____ No _____ to:

What sort of smoker would you classify yourself as:

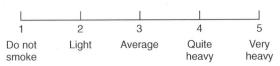

We would provide some bandwidth definitions of each of these points, such that

'light' means 1–10 cigarettes
'average' means 21–30
'quite heavy' means 31–40
'very heavy' means 40

Again, we don't know whether the podiatrist who selects 'very heavy' smokes 41 or 100 cigarettes a day, but we do know that s/he smokes more than the light smoker. Similarly, someone who scores 4 may not smoke twice the number of cigarettes as someone who scores 2. All we know is that someone with a score of 4 does smoke more than someone with a score of 2. This sort of bandwidth category is often used to collect age data, presumably so as not to embarrass the respondents, for example:

18–25 years   [ ]
26–35 years   [ ]
36–45 years   [ ]
46–55 years   [ ]
56–65 years   [ ]
65 + years   [ ]

The respondent who puts a tick in the 56–65 years box could be aged anywhere in that range, and therefore could be 21 years older than someone who ticked the 26–35 box or 39 years older, but the researcher wouldn't know; all they would know is that one respondent is older than another.

We can see particularly clearly from this example how the ordinal scale gives us more information than the nominal scale. If we use this rank ordering technique, we can count up the number of non-smokers (anyone who scores 1) and the number of smokers (those who score 2, 3, 4 and 5) and this gives us the information provided by the nominal scale. However, the ordinal scale adds a dimension to the label of 'smoker', in that it allows us to measure people according to whether they are very heavy, heavy, average or light smokers. In other words, it gives us a bit more information than the nominal level.

It should be noted, though, that the ordinal scale is a rather imprecise measurement. It is commonly used to assess subjective things like pain, levels of agreement on an attitude scale (when it's often called a Likert scale) etc; consequently, it relies on very personal interpretations and so cannot be assumed to have any absolute meaning.

Activity 4.2 (Answers on pp. 359–360)

Look back at the examples given in Activity 4.1 on p. 39, and convert each of these to an ordinal level of measurement.

INTERVAL/RATIO LEVEL

The interval level or scale of measurement is like the ordinal scale, except that it does assume equal intervals in its measurement. Interval scales are measures such as percentage in an exam, temperature, etc.

Interval and ratio measurements have two things in common. First, they assume equal intervals, such that it is possible to say that the difference between scores of 30% and 60% (i.e. 30%) is half the difference of that between scores of 30% and 90% (i.e. 60%). Similarly, the difference between marks of 40% and 50% on an exam is exactly the same as the difference between 80% and 90% (i.e. 10%). If we look back to the ordinal scale of measurement, we cannot make these statements because we simply don't know whether the difference between scores of 1 and 3 on a 5-point scale is the same as the difference between 3 and 5. In order words, on an ordinal scale the gap between 'no smoker' and 'average smoker' is not necessarily identical to the gap between 'average smoker' and 'very heavy' smoker (see above).

The second point to note is that the interval scale does not have an absolute zero point although sometimes one is arbitrarily imposed.

Table 4.4 Test marks of students

Mark	Student
44	Laura B.
39	Julie N.
36	Paul S.
30	Chris D.
22	Jaz H.
20	Jill F.
11	Sally C.

This means that a zero score on an interval scale does not necessarily mean an absence of the quality being measured. A good example of this is temperature on the Celsius scale, where zero temperature does not mean an absence of temperature, but rather that the temperature is at freezing point.

The ratio level of measurement is like the interval level except that it does have an absolute zero. It includes measures such as distance, height, weight, time, etc. Do not worry about this point, because for the purposes of statistical tests, interval and ratio scales are treated as the same. From now on, these two levels of measurement will be collapsed to form one category, which will be referred to as the interval/ratio level. (Interval/ratio data are sometimes referred to as continuous or scale data.)

If, then, we look back at the example of students' competence on clinical placement, our clinical supervisor could have given the students a test (marks out of 50, say), rather than rank ordering them. The results might have looked like Table 4.4.

From the data, we can see that the difference between Laura B. and Jaz H. is twice the difference between Jaz H. and Sally C. In addition, from the data we could rank order the scores to find each student's position in the group (ordinal level of measurement), and also we could classify the students into pass/fail (nominal level of measurement). Therefore, the interval/ratio level of measurement gives us more information than the ordinal scale, which in turn tells us more than the nominal scale.

Again, if we look at our smoking example, we could modify our questionnaire again and simply ask 'How many cigarettes do you smoke per day?' We might get a range of answers from 0 to 60, and, from this, we can say that someone who smokes 60 daily, smokes twice the amount of the person who smokes 30, three times the amount of the person who smokes 20, four times the amount of the person who smokes 15, and so on. We could also:

- Rank order the replies from heaviest smoker to lightest (ordinal scale).
- Classify the replies into smokers and non-smokers (nominal scale).

As a result, it can be seen that the interval/ratio level of measurement gives us all the information of the nominal and ordinal levels, plus a bit more. Other examples of interval/ratio data include temperature, blood pressure, time measures, length, weight, volume, degree of movement and heart rate.

POINT SCALES: ORDINAL OR INTERVAL?

It should be mentioned here that sometimes researchers treat point scales as though they were interval scales rather than ordinal scales, because when constructing the point scale they have assumed equal intervals between the points. Sometimes this is entirely legitimate (e.g. when analysing questionnaire data). As a broad rule-of-thumb, if you construct a point scale with at least seven points on it, and are assuming that the distances between the points are comparable, then you may wish to classify this as an interval scale for the purposes of analysis.

This point is highlighted by the visual analogue method of measuring pain. This commonly used technique involves presenting patients with an unmarked line of length exactly 10 cm, with 0 cm representing no pain and 10 cm representing excruciating pain:

```
0 ——————————————————————— 10
No                          Excruciating
pain                        pain
```

(Note: this line must be *exactly* 10 cm.)

The patient is then asked to mark on this line how much pain s/he is experiencing. The line up to the mark is then measured. In this way, one

---

Activity 4.3 (Answers on pp. 360–361)

1–5 Look back at the five examples given in Activity 4.1 on p. 39 and convert the measures to interval/ratio scores.

6 Suppose that you wanted to look at the incidence of low back pain among welders at the local car factory, you could measure:
  (i) How many had experienced low back pain and how many had not experienced low back pain over the last 2 years (nominal).
  (ii) Frequency of back pain, using a 5-point scale, by asking the question:
  How often have you experienced back pain over the last 2 years? (ordinal):

```
|_____|_____|_____|_____|
Never   Rarely  Sometimes  Quite    Very
                            often    often
```

  (iii) Frequency of back pain using absolute number of incidents (interval/ratio) by asking:
  How many times have you experienced back pain over the last 2 years?

Using the same format, construct nominal, ordinal and interval/ratio levels of measurement for the following:
  (i) accuracy of shooting an arrow at a target
  (ii) improvement in mobility after a hip replacement operation
  (iii) relief of neck and arm pain following use of remedial massage.

7 Look at the following measurements and say whether they are nominal, ordinal or interval/ratio:
  (i) Number of attenders vs. non-attenders at an out-patients' clinic.
  (ii) Patients' ratings of the degree of confidence they have in their clinical therapist, on a 7-point scale.
  (iii) Number of work hours lost through back injury in clinical therapists working with long-stay, high-dependency patients.
  (iv) Percentage of knee movement regained following therapy for leg fractures.
  (v) Recovery time in days following physiotherapy for thoracic surgery patients.

---

patient may report 54 mm of pain, and another 19 mm and so on. The problem then emerges as to how to classify the data. Pain is subjective, so should this be called an ordinal scale? However, length measurement in centimetres or millimetres is an interval/ratio scale, so how can the issue be resolved? There is no right answer here and it must be left to the researcher. However, as a general rule of data collection, it is usually advisable to use the most sophisticated level of measurement you can, since more detailed analyses can be performed. Therefore, it may be preferable to treat visual analogue data as interval/ratio.

It should be pointed out that the visual analogue method is a very versatile and valuable approach to data collection. It can be modified to suit most questions simply by altering the descriptions of the pole positions. In this way, it can be used to replace an ordinal scale in a questionnaire. You should always ensure that the left hand (0) pole represents the total absence of the quality you're measuring, while the right hand (10) end should represent the total presence of the quality. So, if you were measuring patient satisfaction, the 0 end would mean totally dissatisfied, and the 10 end totally satisfied. The data can be treated as interval/ratio, which means that you have far greater scope for analysis.

Remember that you need to be able to distinguish between nominal, ordinal and interval/ratio levels of measurement, because the level of measurement will affect how you analyse your data. More information about this will be given throughout the text.

Finally, it is generally advisable to use the highest levels of measurement you can (i.e. interval/ratio rather than ordinal, ordinal rather than nominal) because not only do the higher levels provide you with more information than the lower levels, but also the type of analysis that can be carried out with the higher levels is more detailed and sophisticated. Clearly, there will be occasions when you have no choice but to use nominal or ordinal levels of measurement. For instance, if you're collecting information about the number of left hip replacements versus right hip replacements, you would have to use the simple nominal categories of 'left hip' and 'right hip', since nothing else would be appropriate. However, as a general rule-of-thumb, use the higher levels of measurement whenever you can.

Key Concepts

There are four levels of measurement, each of which gives us a different amount of information about our data.

- Nominal scales give us least information and simply allow our data to be labelled or categorised, e.g. pass/fail, male/female, over-60/under-60, improvement/no improvement. The response categories are mutually exclusive.
- Ordinal scales give us a bit more information in that they allow us to put our data into a rank order, according to the dimension we are interested in, e.g. most competent to least, heaviest smoker to lightest, greatest movement to least, etc. The intervals between the scale points are not assumed to be equal.
- Interval/ratio scales give us more information, in that they deal with actual numerical scores, e.g. weight, height, time, percentage, pressure, capacity, etc., which allow direct mathematical comparisons to be made. The intervals are assumed to be equal.
- The interval and ratio levels are combined to form a single category for the purposes of data analysis.

FURTHER READING

Belcher J 2005 Nonparametric methods. Online. Available http://nurseresearcher.rcnpublishing.co.uk/resources/archive/GetArticleById.asp?ArticleId=6172

Brink PJ, Wood MJ 2001 Basic steps in planning nursing research, 5th edition. Jones and Bartlett Publishers, Sudbury, Massachusetts

Coolican H 2004 Research methods and statistics in psychology, 4th edition. Hodder Arnold, London

Coolican H 2006 Introduction to research methods in psychology. Hodder Arnold, London

Crichton N 2005 Principles of statistical analysis in nursing and healthcare research. Online. Available http://nurseresearcher.rcnpublishing.co.uk/resources/archive/GetArticleById.asp?ArticleId=6171

Eaton N 2005 Parametric data analysis. Online available: http://nurseresearcher.rcnpublishing.co.uk/resources/archive/GetArticleById.asp?ArticleId=6063

Field A, Hole G 2004 How to design and report experiments. Sage, London

Greene J, D'Oliveira M 2005 Learning to use statistical test in psychology, 3rd edition. Buckingham, Open University Press

http://www.socialresearchmethods.net/kb/measlevl.php December 11 2008

http://cnx.org/content/m10809/latest/ Connexionsat Rice University, Texas, USA

Lunsford BR 1993 Methodology: variables and levels of measurement. American Academy of Orthotists and Prosthetists. 5(4): 121–124. Online. Available http://chss.montclair.edu/sociology/statbooklevels.htm Montclair State University, New Jersey, USA

Parahoo K 2006 Nursing research: principles, process and issues, 2nd edition. Macmillan, Basingstoke

Polgar S, Thomas S 2007 Introduction to research in the health sciences. Edinburgh, Churchill Livingstone

Watson R, McKenna H, Cowman S, Keady J 2008 Nursing research: designs and methods. Edinburgh, Churchill Livingstone

Chapter 5

Techniques of descriptive statistics

The information or data collected from your project have to be interpreted, in order to make sense of it. It was noted in Chapter 2 that there are two main techniques you can use to interpret your data: inferential statistics, which are used to check whether your results support your hypothesis; and descriptive statistics, which are methods of describing your results in terms of their most interesting features. Descriptive measures about a sample of people are referred to as descriptive statistics, while the same measures of the parent population from which the sample was drawn are called population parameters. Techniques of descriptive statistics are commonly used to make sense of survey data, where large quantities of information are collected. Once these data have been organised and presented in a more accessible way, it is then possible for the researcher to formulate hypotheses from the data base. These hypotheses can then be tested using the appropriate inferential statistics. In this way, descriptive statistics are sometimes thought of as the first stage in analysing data sets, and inferential statistics the second stage. This chapter is concerned with some frequently used techniques of descriptive statistics.

ORGANISING DATA INTO A TABLE

It is very difficult to make any sense out of a large amount of information simply by looking at the raw data. However, if the data are organ-

Table 5.1 Frequency of causes of leg fractures seen at a sports injuries clinic over a period of 1 year

Cause of injury	Frequency
Football	52
Rugby	21
Skiing	11
Motorcycle racing	14
Athletics	19
Other	9
Total	126

Table 5.2 Frequency of pain levels among leg fracture patients at a sports injuries clinic over a period of 1 year

Pain level (score)	Frequency
No pain (1)	0
Mild pain (2)	5
Moderate pain (3)	29
Severe pain (4)	76
Excruciating pain (5)	16
Total	126

ised into a table, then they are much easier to understand.

Let's imagine you have been conducting a survey of your sports injuries patients and you have a mass of information concerning the nature of the injuries, the pain levels, types of treatment and progress rates. This information can be tabulated to make the key points clearer. To focus, for example, on leg fractures, the first set of information you have concerns the causes of injury, which are mainly football, rugby, skiing, motorcycle racing and athletics, i.e. nominal data. This information can be represented as in Table 5.1.

From Table 5.1 you can see at a glance the most common, as well as the least common, source of injury. In order to construct this sort of table, then, you must group the data into the relevant nominal categories, which here are the sources of the injury. The numbers of patients falling into each category are counted up and this information is then represented in a table.

You then decide to look at the reported pain levels of the leg fracture patients. In order to collect these data you have asked every patient on admission, to rate how much pain they experienced, using a 5-point ordinal scale:

1	2	3	4	5
No pain	Mild pain	Moderate pain	Severe pain	Excruciating pain

You tabulate this information as in Table 5.2.

Therefore, you needed to count up all the patients in each ordinal pain category before presenting the figures in table form.

The next set of data you need to interpret is the distance each patient could walk unaided

Table 5.3 Frequency of distance walked by leg fracture patients at a sports injuries clinic immediately upon removal of plaster cast

Distance (metres)	Frequency
Less than 1	1
2	3
3	5
4	8
5	13
6	16
7	16
8	12
9	15
10	11
11	15
12	5
13	3
14	1
15	2
Total	126

immediately the plaster cast had been removed. The raw data range from less than a metre to 15 m. You may recall from the previous chapter that length measurements are of an interval/ratio type. The data are organised as in Table 5.3.

Again, to arrive at this table, you would need to count up the total number of patients falling into each distance interval; these intervals should be arranged in order from lowest to highest and then set out accordingly.

However, if there are a lot of intervals, as there are in Table 5.3, then the table can be large and unwieldy and rather difficult to interpret. Conse-

Table 5.4 Frequency of distances walked by leg fracture patients at a sports injuries clinic, immediately upon removal of the plaster cast

Distance (metres)	Frequency
0–3	9
4–7	53
8–11	53
12–15	11
Total	126

Table 5.5 Geographical distribution of babies born with talipes

Geographical district	No. of babies with talipes
Bridgetown	15
Henley-by-the-sea	32
North Downs	26
Wallsend	10
Brick Lane	6

quently, it may be better in such cases to group the intervals (Table 5.4). These are known as class intervals.

While Table 5.4 may be a neater table, it should be noted that a lot of detailed information is lost by collapsing the data in this way. If you decide to combine your data intervals like this, you should ensure that the grouped intervals are of an equal size.

It can be seen by looking at Tables 5.1–5.4, that they provide at-a-glance information about your patients, and consequently they are a valuable technique for describing your results. Remember, though, that all tables should be clearly labelled and self-explanatory.

GRAPHS

Sometimes it is easier to make sense of a set of data if they are presented as a graph rather than as a table of results. While a graph tells you no more than a table of figures, it often shows trends and other features of the data more clearly. There are many software packages available that will give you a choice of graph designs, such as SPSS and Excel, and this together with the fact that we have all drawn graphs in school and elsewhere, the principles pertaining to graph-drawing will be outlined only briefly here.

For the purpose of clinical therapy research the frequency distribution graph is probably the most important. A frequency distribution refers to how often a particular event occurs; for instance, how many cardiac care patients in a particular age group have heart rates of the order of:

60–65 beats per minute,
66–70 beats per minute, or
71–75 beats per minute, etc.

The most common forms of frequency distribution graph are the histogram and related bar graphs, pie charts and the frequency polygon. The features of each will be outlined shortly, and some general rules for drawing graphs will be presented at the end of this section.

HISTOGRAMS AND BAR GRAPHS

These two graphical techniques are very similar, though many people feel the bar graph is clearer. Bar graphs are typically used to present nominal and ordinal data, and histograms for interval/ratio data. Each technique presents the data in a series of vertical rectangles, with each rectangle representing the number of scores in a particular category. However, with the histogram, the vertical bars are directly adjacent to one another, whereas with the bar graph there are spaces between them.

These techniques can best be demonstrated by illustrations. Suppose you want to find out what the distribution of babies born with talipes is within districts in your particular health region; you might come up with the figures in Table 5.5.

The frequencies for the nominal categories in Table 5.5 can be represented in a bar graph as in Figure 5.1. Note that the categories of event go along the horizontal or X-axis and the frequency with which they occur goes along the vertical or Y-axis.

If the categories along the horizontal axis have no natural order, then they may be arranged in order of size, with the greatest frequency on the left and the smallest on the right. Figure 5.2,

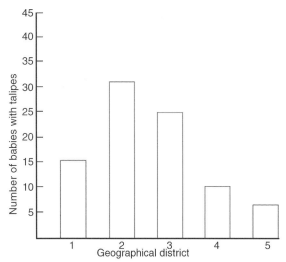

Key 1 = Bridgetown 2 = Henley-by-the-sea 3 = North Downs 4 = Wallsend 5 = Brick Lane

Figure 5.1 Bar graph showing distribution by district of babies born with talipes within a health region.

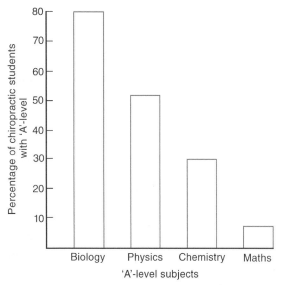

Figure 5.2 Bar graph showing comparative frequency of 'A'-level subjects among chiropractic students.

showing the 'A'-level subjects of chiropractic students, is an example of this.

Histograms

The histogram, which is usually used to represent interval/ratio data, can be illustrated by the following example. You are interested in carpal tunnel syndrome, and in particular its relation-

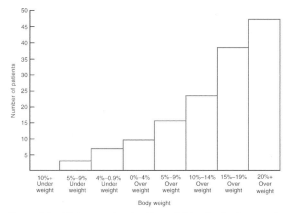

Figure 5.3 Histogram showing the weights of patients presenting with carpal tunnel syndrome.

Table 5.6 Body weight of patients with carpal tunnel syndrome

No. of patients	Body weight
0	10% or more underweight
3	5–9% underweight
7	0.9–4% underweight
9	0–4% overweight
15	5–9% overweight
23	10–14% overweight
38	15–19% overweight
47	20% or more overweight

ship to the body weight of the patient. You make a note of the weight of every person presenting with carpal tunnel syndrome (interval/ratio data) and find the data shown in Table 5.6.

Table 5.6 can be presented as a histogram, as in Figure 5.3.

It should be noted that the individual weights of patients have been allocated to categories, or class intervals, for the purpose of simplifying the data and drawing the histogram. Clearly the category size should be appropriate for the range of data available; a small number of categories will lose much of the detailed information of the data, while too many will complicate the table or graph. No more than nine categories are used as a rule.

PIE CHARTS

Nominal data can also be represented graphically using pie charts. A pie chart is a circle that

Table 5.7 Percentage of total of babies born with talipes in each district

District	No. of babies with talipes	Percentage
Bridgetown	15	16.85
Henley-by-the-sea	32	35.96
North Downs	26	29.21
Wallsend	10	11.24
Brick Lane	6	6.74
Total	89	100.00

Table 5.8 Age of disease onset for pneumonia patients within the health authority

Age of onset (years)	No. of pneumonia patients
15–24	21
25–34	30
35–44	17
45–54	10
55+	11
Total	89

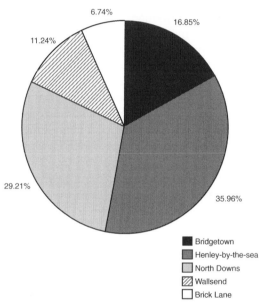

Figure 5.4 Pie chart of the distribution by district of babies born with talipes.

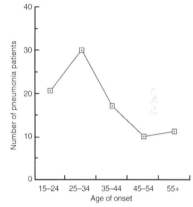

Figure 5.5 Frequency polygon showing age of onset of pneumonia within a particular region.

The value of a pie chart lies in its immediate visual appeal and the ease with which proportions can be compared. However, if there are a lot of categories, pie charts can be confusing and difficult to construct and interpret accurately.

FREQUENCY POLYGONS

Data of an interval/ratio type can also be plotted as a frequency polygon, in which the frequency of occurrence of each unit or event on the horizontal axis is plotted at the midpoint of the unit, and these points are then joined by a continuous straight line.

Imagine that you have conducted a survey of pneumonia patients which has included the age of onset of the illness (interval/ratio data), as in Table 5.8.

This can be represented by a frequency polygon as in Figure 5.5.

In this example the graph does not touch the horizontal axis. Some people are of the opinion

is divided into sections, each section representing proportionately the number in each category or event. In order to do this, the figures in each category must be converted to percentages of the total number first.

Let's imagine you wish to represent the data in Table 5.5 as a pie chart rather than as a bar graph. You would need to convert the figures for each district into a percentage of the total number of babies born with talipes in the region (Table 5.7).

The pie chart would look like Figure 5.4. To construct the pie chart, the percentages for each district must be converted to degrees. Each 1% equals 3.6 since 100% is the equivalent of 360.

Table 5.9 Average final exam marks in clinical therapy departments

Average final exam mark	No. of departments attaining mark
31–40	0
41–50	1
51–60	3
61–70	4
71–80	1
81–90	1
91–100	0

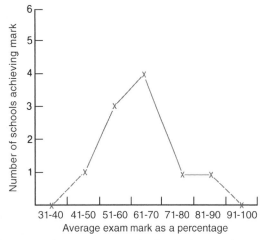

Figure 5.6 Frequency polygon showing distribution of average final examination marks, in 2002, across a number of departments of clinical therapy.

that this gives a rather odd appearance to the graph, and so, in cases where it is appropriate, you can add a class to either end of the units with scores on the horizontal axis.

To give an example, you might wish to plot the frequency of average final examination marks across a number of clinical therapy departments for 2002. The results you obtain are shown in Table 5.9. Your graph might look like Figure 5.6.

There are no departments that achieve an average mark of 31–40% or of 91–100%. Therefore, to give this graph a more complete appearance, the line can be extended to the values for the categories 31–40% and 91–100% (dashed lines in Figure 5.6).

Obviously, more than one set of data can be plotted on a frequency polygon, so that direct comparisons can be made. In the above example, you might want to plot the average marks for the year 2001 as well, so that you can compare performances.

WHICH TYPE OF GRAPH SHOULD YOU USE?

Whether you decide to use a histogram, bar graph, pie chart or a frequency polygon depends on the nature of the data you wish to present. Nominal data, for instance, should not be plotted as a frequency polygon, but rather as a bar or pie chart.

Generally, the frequency polygon is more suitable if two or more sets of frequencies are to be compared, since a number of lines can be represented in different colours or styles on the same graph. A similar comparison using bar graphs or histograms can be very confusing, since it will involve overlapping rectangles. However, that being said, lay people often find histograms and bar graphs easier to interpret, when they are not familiar with the subject area.

In short, which technique you use will depend on what your objectives are, and the nature of your data.

PRODUCING A SMOOTHER GRAPH

There is one further point of interest when plotting frequency distributions. Generally, the larger the amount of data to be plotted, the smoother the resulting frequency distribution curve and, conversely, the fewer the scores plotted, the more irregular and uneven the resulting graph. If you are concerned to identify trends, patterns and regularities in your data, you will obviously be keen to produce a smooth frequency distribution. If you cannot achieve this because you have only a limited number of scores to plot, you can obtain greater regularity by reducing the number of categories along the horizontal axis.

Let's suppose, for example, you were interested in the bed turnover rates of patients admitted to hospital following right hemisphere strokes. Having looked at some patient records over a 6-month period, you find that:

4 patients were discharged after 4 days
6 patients were discharged after 5 days

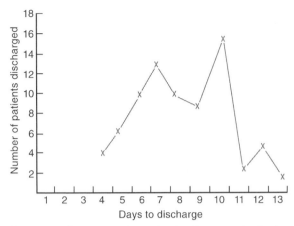

Figure 5.7 Frequency polygon showing frequency distribution of bed turnover rates for hospitalised stroke patients.

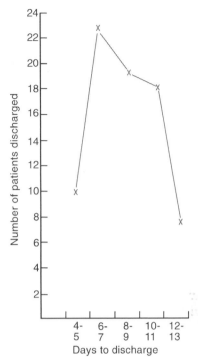

Figure 5.8 Frequency polygon showing frequency distribution of bed turnover rates for hospitalised stroke patients. The categories in Figure 5.7 have been collapsed.

10 patients were discharged after 6 days
13 patients were discharged after 7 days
10 patients were discharged after 8 days
 9 patients were discharged after 9 days
15 patients were discharged after 10 days
 3 patients were discharged after 11 days
 5 patients were discharged after 12 days
 2 patients were discharged after 13 days

If these data are plotted as presented, we get the graph shown in Figure 5.7.

However, if we collapse the data into appropriate class intervals along the horizontal axis, as shown in Figure 5.8, we achieve a rather smoother graph.

You can see from the above illustration that reducing the categories along the horizontal axis makes the graph appear more regular, and in so doing allows you to get a clearer idea of the trends in the data. (A word of caution, though! Reducing the categories in this way may also distort your data, and obscure important features.)

TEN RULES FOR DRAWING GRAPHS OF FREQUENCY DISTRIBUTIONS

1. The horizontal axis, also known as the X-axis, must be used to represent the categories or events.
2. The vertical axis, also known as the Y-axis, must be used to represent the frequencies with which the events occur.
3. The intervals along the axes must be of a suitable size, so that the graph may be drawn and interpreted accurately.
4. The intersection point of the axes conventionally should be zero. If this does not suit your purposes, ensure you make a note of this so that it is clear to the reader.
5. All graphs should be clearly labelled and self-explanatory. Both axes should also be labelled.
6. Nominal and ordinal data are usually described in bar graphs or pie charts.
7. Interval ratio data are usually described in histograms and frequency polygons.
8. Interval ratio data can be combined so that the graph can be inspected for trends.
9. If the categories are to be combined to form larger subgroups (class intervals) you should not use too many groups, otherwise the graph may be difficult to interpret. Similarly, you should not use too few subgroups, otherwise a lot of information will be lost.

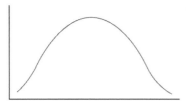

Figure 5.9   Normal distribution.

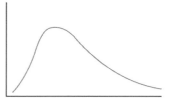

Figure 5.10   Skewed distribution (1). This is also known as a positive skew.

10. If you subgroup your data, the subgroups should be of equal size, otherwise you will distort the information.

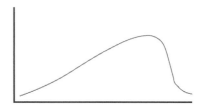

Figure 5.11   Skewed distribution (2). This is also known as a negative skew.

Key Concepts

- Data can be represented by drawing graphs.
- Histograms and bar graphs can describe frequency distributions by columns or vertical bars to represent the numbers obtained in each category or event.
- Pie charts can represent data pictorially by using a circle, which is divided into segments, the size of which represents the numbers in each category or event.
- Frequency polygons are graphs which use a single line to connect the numbers in each event.
- Nominal and ordinal data are best described using bar graphs and pie charts.
- Interval/ratio data are best described using histograms and frequency polygons.

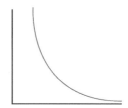

Figure 5.12   J-shaped distribution.

SHAPES OF FREQUENCY DISTRIBUTION CURVES

If you plot a large number of graphs over a period of time, you will notice that some shapes of frequency distribution tend to occur time and again. It may be useful to outline some of these briefly.

Normal distribution (Figure 5.9)

This is probably the most important frequency distribution shape of all and has numerous implications for statistics. So important is it that the next section will be devoted entirely to a more detailed description of it. For the time being, suffice it to say that it is typically a symmetrical bell-shaped curve, and were we to plot heights or heart rates of a population as a frequency dis-

tribution, we would find that both are normally distributed.

Skewed distribution (1) (Figure 5.10)

This is also known as a positive skew. It is skewed to the left and is the sort of graph that might result from an overly difficult exam, i.e. too many students achieving marks near the bottom end of the score range.

Skewed distribution (2) (Figure 5.11)

This is also known as a negative skew. The graph is skewed to the right and might have been derived from a set of results from an exam that was too easy.

J-shaped distribution (Figure 5.12)

This is the sort of frequency distribution which might result from monitoring the number of gastric contractions of a group of patients over a period following a meal. The vast majority of

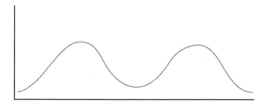

Figure 5.13   Bimodal distribution.

Table 5.10   Number of physiotherapists recording a given degree of movement

Degree of movement	No. of physiotherapists who recorded this score
11–20	0
21–30	1
31–40	3
41–50	5
51–60	4
61–70	1
71–80	1
81–90	0

patients would show very few contractions since they would presumably be satisfied; they are represented by the highest part of the graph on the left. However, a few people would show rather more activity and they are represented by the flattened tail of the graph to the right.

Bimodal distribution (Figure 5.13)

This distribution is characterised by two distinct peaks and might have been obtained by the attitudes of a group of health care professionals on a controversial issue, such as privatising a significant part of the NHS. Such a survey would be unlikely to produce many neutral attitudes, with most people either being very much in favour of privatisation or very much opposed to it. The respondents opposed to privatisation would be represented by the left-hand peak and the respondents in favour of it, by the right-hand peak.

MEASURES OF CENTRAL TENDENCY

Activity 5.1 (Answers on p. 361)

In order to look at the consistency of measurements taken on a goniometer, you ask 15 physiotherapists to measure the knee joint mobility of a post-fracture patient. You obtain the results in Table 5.10.

1 Draw (a) a histogram, and (b) a frequency polygon to show these results.
2 In order to identify trends in the results, reduce the units along the horizontal axis and re-draw the frequency polygon.

As has already been stated, any results from a piece of research must be presented in a way that can be clearly understood by the reader. Besides making tables of the results and drawing graphs,

the data can be presented in terms of measures of central tendency.

Measures of central tendency involve describing a set of data in terms of the most typical scores within it. This approach may be valuable to the clinical therapist in three ways:

1. A comparison of some capacity of a group of patients with an established norm or standard for that capacity. For instance you may wish to compare the mobility of a group of laminectomy patients, with the normal or average mobility of people of a comparable age group who have not undergone this operation.

2. Establishing a standard or norm not previously known. For example, if a new piece of equipment was introduced to stimulate muscle contraction, which you thought might be useful for patients with muscular dystrophy, you would need to establish the level of stimulation provoked in normal muscles by the apparatus, as well as in patients' muscles, in order to establish what could normally be expected from this piece of equipment.

3. Comparing different treatment techniques or different groups of patients, e.g. the comparison of two different types of prosthetic training for lower limb amputees.

In order to answer the questions, three measures of central tendency can be used: the arithmetic mean, the median and the mode.

ARITHMETIC MEAN

This is the average of a set of scores and is derived from adding all the scores together and dividing the total by the number of scores. It is usually denoted by the symbol $\bar{x}$. It is an extremely valuable concept in statistics, and enables the researcher to appraise a set of results at a glance.

For example, in the illustrations given above, the mean mobility for the laminectomy group can be compared with the mean mobility for the non-patient group to examine the differences. Similarly, the mean mobility of each of the two prosthetic training groups for lower limb amputees can be compared, to give an estimate of which programme is more effective.

While the arithmetic mean is undoubtedly one of the most useful concepts in statistics, it can be misleading. If we take the third example above, relating to prosthetic training, we can demonstrate this. Supposing you had the choice of giving a lower limb amputee one of two training programmes. In order to help you make your choice, you turn to some statistics and find that programme A produces an average walking distance of 40 m within 4 weeks, while programme B produces an average of 51 m in the same period. From this information alone you would almost certainly favour training programme B. But let us suppose you were to look at the original data as shown in Table 5.11.

Although programme A certainly produces, on average, less ambulatory movement, the results are much more consistent than those from programme B. Furthermore, with the exception of the three 100-m distances, the remaining

results from training programme B are lower than all the distances obtained by patients in programme A. In other words, the presence of three extreme scores in programme B has distorted the mean and could have been misleading had you not looked at the original data. Having examined the raw data, you would probably now choose training programme A.

However, if you were conducting a large-scale survey, you might have thousands of data points and consequently it would be impossible to inspect the raw data thoroughly. Therefore, the arithmetic mean, while an essential component of statistics, is insufficient in itself to provide the necessary information about a set of results, and other forms of descriptive statistics are required as well.

MEDIAN

The median is simply the mid-score in a set of results, such that there are as many scores above it as below it; i.e. 50% of the scores in the data base lie below the median and 50% lie above it. To compute the median, arrange the scores in order of magnitude; then, if there is an odd number of scores, the middle score becomes the median. So, for example, if you had five scores:

$$14 \quad 9 \quad 28 \quad 5 \quad 11$$

you would arrange them in order of magnitude:

$$28 \quad 14 \quad 11 \quad 9 \quad 5$$

and the median is the third score from the end, i.e. 11. On the other hand, if there is an even number of scores, the median is the average of the two middle scores. So, if you had:

$$14 \quad 9 \quad 28 \quad 5 \quad 11 \quad 18$$

you would arrange these in order of magnitude:

$$28 \quad 18 \quad 14 \quad 11 \quad 9 \quad 5$$

and the median is the average of the two middle scores, i.e.

$$\frac{14+11}{2} = 12.5$$

Table 5.11   The results of two different prosthetic training programmes for lower limb amputees

Programme A		Programme B	
Patient no.	Metres walked	Patient no.	Metres walked
1	38	1	30
2	42	2	28
3	45	3	100
4	36	4	100
5	40	5	31
6	39	6	33
7	44	7	30
8	46	8	28
9	34	9	30
10	36	10	100
$\bar{x}$	40	$\bar{x}$	51

These examples oversimplify the calculation of the median, because they only involve a small number of scores and the median for each set of data is easily determined. Moreover, the above methods are very labour intensive, especially when the researcher has a large data set to sort out. In these instances, another formula is required. Let's return to the data presented in Table 5.11, but instead of having just two groups of 10 patients whose mobility is being measured, let's extend this to a total sample of 70. To find the median of these 70 scores, you first need to group your data into class intervals (see p 43). These class intervals should be of an appropriate size and of equal intervals. So, for our extended data base of 70 scores, we might use the following class intervals for number of m walked:

28–33, 34–39, 40–45, 46–51, 52–57, 58–63, 64–69, 70–75, 76–81, 82–87, 88–93, 94–99, 100–105

You could have used smaller class intervals (e.g. 28–30, 31–33, 34–36, etc.), or larger intervals (e.g. 28–35, 36–43, 44–51, etc.), but do ensure that the interval you use is manageable and suitable for the size and range of your data set. You now need to look at your data base and count up how many scores come within each class interval. From our hypothetical results, we might get the data shown in Table 5.12.

However, let us suppose that when we collected our data, rather than measuring the number of m walked to the nearest whole metre (28 m, 33 m, etc.), we had been much more precise and had measured the distances exactly as m and centimetres. We might have found that one patient walked 57 m and 66 cm, while another might have walked 39 m and 80 cm. How should we classify these results using the class intervals outlined above? At first glance, it would seem that the first patient should come into the class interval 52–57 m, because he didn't walk far enough to get into the 58–63 bracket. Likewise, the second patient looks as though he should come into the 34–39 class, because he hadn't quite walked far enough to qualify for the 40–45 class interval. And yet, if we look at the exact distances these two patients walked, we can see that they are closer to the lower limit of the next category than they are to their own (39 m 80 cm

Table 5.12 Table of cumulative frequencies of the mobility scores of a sample of patients following two types of mobility training.

Class intervals for metres walked	Number of scores in each class interval
28–33	2
34–39	4
40–45	4
46–51	5
52–57	7
58–63	8
64–69	11
70–75	12
76–81	6
82–87	5
88–93	3
94–99	2
100–105	1
	Total = 70

is closer to 40 m than it is to 39 m). Therefore, for greater precision, we should re-draw the class intervals to create exact class intervals, as shown in Table 5.13. These class intervals afford much greater precision (but note that, for simplicity, I haven't altered the numbers in each class interval, although, in reality, it would be quite likely that there would be some changes). We can now calculate the median value for our data set, by taking the following steps:

1. Because the median is the point at which 50% of scores lie below it and 50% above, we need to find the half-way score in our data set. Therefore, we have to divide the total number of scores (70) by 2, which equals 35. Therefore, the 35th score is the median score.

2. Working from the smallest class interval upwards (i.e. 27.5–33.5), count up the number of scores in each class interval until you reach the interval that contains the 35th (median) score. The 35th score is contained in the class interval 63.5–69.5. Therefore, the total number of scores up to, but not including, this interval is:

$$2 + 4 + 4 + 5 + 7 + 8 = 30$$

This value of 30 is called S.

Table 5.13

Exact class intervals for metres walked	Number of scores in each class interval
27.5–33.5	2
33.5–39.5	4
39.5–45.5	4
45.5–51.5	5
51.5–57.5	7
57.5–63.5	8
63.5–69.5	11
69.5–75.5	12
75.5–81.5	6
81.5–87.5	5
87.5–93.5	3
93.5–99.5	2
99.5–105.5	1
	Total = 70

3. Substitute the value for S in the following formula:

$$\text{Median} = L + \frac{\left[\dfrac{N}{2} - S\right]}{f} \times I$$

where

L is the lower limit value of the class interval that contains the 35th (median) score, i.e. the 35th score is contained in the class interval 63.5–69.5; therefore $L = 63.5$;

N is the total number of scores; therefore $N = 70$;

S (from step 2 above) $= 30$;

f is the number of scores in the class interval that contains the 35th (median) score; therefore $f = 11$;

I is the size of the class interval used; here we have used class intervals of 6 m (27.5–33.5, 33.5–39.5, etc.); therefore $I = 6$.

Using these values in the formula above:

$$\text{Median} = 63.5 + \frac{\left[\dfrac{70}{2} - 30\right]}{11} \times 6$$

$$= 63.5 + \frac{5}{11} \times 6$$

$$= 63.5 + 0.455 \times 6$$

$$= 63.5 + 2.73$$

$$= 66.23$$

Therefore the median score in this set of data is 66.23.

This formula therefore provides the researcher with an accurate method of calculating the exact median score from a large data set.

Disadvantages of the median

While the median obviously tells you the middle score out of a set of results, it tells you nothing about the range of the scores. For example, in the following sets of scores, the median in both cases is 10:

13 12 11 10 9 8 7

99 98 97 10 3 2 1

but the nature of the sets of scores is quite different, and the pattern of a set of scores may have important implications for their interpretation. For instance, if the first set of figures above referred to the ages of patients presenting with a particular disease, you may well think that the disease is one of childhood and early adolescence. You would not be inclined to think this if presented with the second set of figures. Thus, the nature of the scores is important in research if they are to be accurately interpreted.

So, the median alone gives insufficient information about the nature of a set of data. If it is used in conjunction with the mean, then more information can be derived about the total set of scores. For example, the more similar the mean and median, the smaller the range of scores. This can be illustrated with the above sets of figures. The first set has a mean and a median of 10 and the scores are all within a small range (13–7); however, the second set of figures also has a median of 10 but a mean of 44.3 and a range of scores from 99 to 1.

While the median may not be as valuable as the mean, if both techniques are used together they can be more useful in describing a set of data, especially where there are extreme scores.

MODE

The mode is the most commonly occurring score in a set of data. So, in the following two sets of scores, 15 is the mode:

15 15 14 10 15 18 15
15 15   3   2   1   4   5

However, within any set of scores, you may have more than one mode. Its value lies primarily in its ability to answer the question: Which one event occurs most often? So, for example, you might want to ask: What is the commonest age of onset of motor neurone disease or of childhood type 1 diabetes? To answer this question you would simply look at the ages at which the patients first presented with the symptoms of the condition and identify which was the most frequently occurring age.

A COMPARISON OF THE MEAN, MODE AND MEDIAN

Comparing the value of the arithmetic mean, the median and the mode, the mean is the most commonly used statistic and provides more information about a set of scores than the median and the mode. This is because the computation of the mean depends on the exact value of every score in a set of data and alteration of even one score will alter the mean. This is not necessarily the case for the median and the mode as illustrated by the following set of data:

3 14 10 19 8 5 15 20 3

The mean of these data is 10.8, the median is 10, and the mode is 3. If we alter the 20 to 40, the mean becomes 13, but the median and the mode stay the same.

In addition, the median and the mode may be totally unaffected by altering a large number of scores in a set of data. If the above set of figures is changed to:

3 34 10 39 2 1 45 17 3

although six out of nine numbers have been radically altered, the median remains 10 and the mode 3.

Conversely, the median and the mode may be drastically altered just by changing one number. To take the above set of numbers, if the first 3 is changed to 34, the median becomes 17 and the mode 34.

In other words, the median and the mode are less reliable than the mean when providing information about a set of scores, because they may not be altered by radical changes to a lot of scores, or they may be changed by altering just one score. The mean, on the other hand, will alter if any score is changed, however minimally.

However, as already pointed out, the mean may be less useful than the median or mode if there are extreme scores in a set of data, because it is easily distorted by the presence of very large or small scores. However, although all three concepts can be used in descriptive statistics to provide information about a set of data, it is advisable always to calculate the mean, and then to decide whether the median and the mode will provide you with relevant information about your particular set of data.

Key Concepts

Measures of central tendency are a form of descriptive statistics and allow the researcher to highlight features of a set of results in terms of the 'most typical values'. The three most commonly used measures of central tendency are:

- the arithmetic mean: the average of a set of scores
- the median: the mid-score in a set of results, such that there are as many scores above it as below
- the mode: the most commonly occurring score in a set of data.

Activity 5.2 (Answers on pp. 361–362)

1 Calculate the mean, median and the mode for the following sets of figures:
  (i) 91 87 90 76 51 48 72 76 80 44 89
  (ii) 25 39 17 41 24 17 37 31 27
  (iii) 44 43 51 54 60 71 39 41 55 43
2 Just by comparing the means and the medians, find out which of these sets of data have (a) the largest range and (b) the smallest range of scores.

MEASURES OF DISPERSION

If you look back at the measures of central tendency, you will see that it is possible to obtain the same or very similar means for sets of scores which are quite different. For instance, the mean for each of the following two sets of numbers is 10:

$$9 \quad 11 \quad 12 \quad 8 \quad 10 \quad 11 \quad 12 \quad 12 \quad 8 \quad 7$$
$$1 \quad 2 \quad 3 \quad 3 \quad 2 \quad 1 \quad 40 \quad 3 \quad 15 \quad 30$$

The scores in the first set are all quite similar to each other in that they only range from 7 to 12; the scores in the second set, however, range from 1 to 40. Just knowing the mean of a set of scores, then, can be quite misleading; we need to know how variable the scores are as well; in other words, what the spread of the data is. The statistics which describe the variability of scores are called measures of dispersion and are valuable to the clinical therapist for the same reasons as the measures of central tendency.

If you look back to p. 53, you will see that the first reason given is that the researcher can compare a group of patients with an established standard to discover how far their linguistic capacity, weight, mobility, functional skills or whatever resemble the norm. This can be carried out just using means, medians and modes, but we have already seen that similar means can be obtained from two totally different sets of scores. So, if we use the example on p. 53, you might find that four out of five of your laminectomy patients had extremely limited mobility, while one had much greater mobility than the non-patient group. If you simply combine the mobility scores of these five patients and take the mean, you may well find that, because of the one very mobile patient, the mean is very similar to that of the non-patient group and yet four of the patients were barely mobile. In other words you need to know what the spread of scores is.

Similarly, if you wish to establish norms for a new piece of apparatus, it is insufficient just to use measures of central tendency, because they can be misleading unless you know how consistent the scores are. Obviously a piece of equipment which produces uniform results will be much more use than one which produces erratic results from poor to excellent, even though the mean performances may be similar.

In addition, measures of dispersion can identify patients who respond particularly well or particularly poorly. This information may be useful when selecting treatments. And similarly, when comparing two or more treatment types,

the treatment which produces homogeneous results, i.e. where the range of scores is small, will be regarded quite differently from the treatment which produces erratic results which cover an enormous range. So, in descriptive statistics, not only do you need to use measures of central tendency, you also need to describe the results in terms of how variable they are; to do this you use techniques called measures of dispersion.

There are three measures of dispersion which are valuable to the clinical therapist: the range, deviation and variance and the standard deviation.

RANGE

The range is quite simply the difference between the lowest and highest scores in a set of data. To compute it, simply find the smallest score in the set of data and subtract it from the highest score. Thus in the following set of data:

$$14 \quad 22 \quad 5 \quad 11 \quad 12 \quad 19 \quad 31 \quad 27$$

the range is:

$$31 - 5 = 26$$

Obviously, when used in conjunction with measures of central tendency, it can provide useful additional information, in the way already outlined. However, the information produced by the range gives a limited picture since a range of 45–3 may describe a set of scores such as:

$$45 \quad 44 \quad 43 \quad 42 \quad 7 \quad 6 \quad 5 \quad 4 \quad 3$$

or

$$45 \quad 40 \quad 35 \quad 30 \quad 15 \quad 10 \quad 5 \quad 3$$

In other words, the range provides no insight into how the scores are distributed. One way of getting round this problem is to use deviation and variance measures.

DEVIATION AND VARIANCE

A description of the spread of scores, as we've seen, is important in understanding the implications of a set of data. A picture of the distribution of the scores can be presented by expressing the scores in terms of how far each one deviates from the mean.

In order to calculate the deviation of a set of scores, the mean is subtracted from each score. Thus, for the following set of scores:

$$10 \quad 15 \quad 21 \quad 8 \quad 11 \quad 12 \quad 14 \quad 5$$

the mean is 12, and the deviation of each score is:

$$10 - 12 = -2$$
$$15 - 12 = +3$$
$$21 - 12 = +9$$
$$8 - 12 = -4$$
$$11 - 12 = -1$$
$$12 - 12 = 0$$
$$14 - 12 = +2$$
$$5 - 12 = -7$$

In subtracting the mean from each score, you can find the position of each score relative to the mean. So, for example, the score of 15 is +3 deviation points above the mean.

However, as you can probably see, expressing each score as a deviation from the mean is just as long-winded as setting out all your scores and the mean. What is needed is some shorthand method of expressing how varied and dispersed the scores are.

While many students assume that the obvious way would be to add together all the deviation scores, the answer is always 0, because the positive and negative numbers cancel themselves out (try it for yourself and see), so this clearly tells us nothing. One way of getting round this problem is to square each deviation score (this obviously gets rid of all the minus signs) and then to add these squared deviation scores up. The result is then divided by the number of scores you added, to give the mean. The result is called the variance.

If we compute the variance for the set of scores above, we get:

$$\frac{\left(-2^2\right)+\left(3^2\right)+\left(9^2\right)+\left(-4^2\right)+\left(-1^2\right)+\left(0^2\right)+\left(2^2\right)+\left(-7^2\right)}{8}$$

$$= \frac{4+9+81+16+1+0+4+49}{8}$$

$$= \frac{164}{8}$$

$$= 20.5$$

The variance of a set of scores tells us by definition how dispersed or varied the scores are.

Obviously, the smaller the variance, the more similar the scores, while the greater the variance, the more disparate the scores. If you look back to the example on p. 54 about the prosthetic training programmes, you can see that knowledge of the spread of scores would be a very useful piece of information here, since the smaller the variance the more reliable and consistent the treatment procedure.

STANDARD DEVIATION

Although the variance score gives you the average of the squared deviation scores, it has been obtained, obviously, by using such varied squared deviations as 81 and 0 (see the previous set of numbers). Sometimes you may want to find out what the average or standard degree of deviation is for a set of scores, rather than the average of the squared deviations. To do this you need a very useful statistic called, not unreasonably, the standard deviation (or SD).

To calculate it, you simply take the variance figure (i.e. the mean of the squared deviation scores; in the above case, 20.5), and then take the square root of this, to give you the standard deviation of the scores from the mean. The formula then is:

$$SD = \sqrt{\frac{\sum (x-\bar{x})^2}{N}}$$

where
$\sqrt{}$ = square root of all the calculations under this symbol
x = the individual score
$\bar{x}$ = the mean score
Σ = total, or sum, of every calculation to the right
N = the total number of scores.

So, for the figures above, the standard deviation is:

$$= \sqrt{\frac{164}{8}}$$

$$= \sqrt{20.5}$$

$$= 4.528$$

Sometimes you will find the SD formula given as:

$$SD = \sqrt{\frac{\sum(x-\bar{x})^2}{N-1}}$$

The $N - 1$ is used if you want to infer the standard deviation of the population from which your sample is drawn, whereas using just N gives the standard deviation of the sample only.

This means that the standard degree of deviation of this set of scores from the mean is 4.528. Such information gives you a picture, in a single figure, of how dispersed or variable a set of scores is. As we've already pointed out, this is particularly useful in determining the consistency of a set of numbers.

All of this may seem rather confusing to you when deciding how to describe a set of data. As a rule of thumb, I would recommend that you always calculate the mean, range and standard deviation of a set of scores and then decide which of the other measures provides you with information that is relevant to the aims of that particular piece of research.

Key Concepts

Measures of dispersion are a branch of descriptive statistics which allow the researcher to describe a set of data in terms of how variable the scores are.

The measures of dispersion which are of particular importance to the clinical therapist are:

- the range is the difference between the lowest and highest scores in a set of data.
- the deviation provides information about the extent to which each score deviates from the mean, and is calculated by subtracting the mean from each score.
- the variance is the mean of the squared deviations. It is calculated by squaring each deviation score, adding the results up and dividing the total by the number of scores you added together.
- the standard deviation (SD) is the average amount of deviation and is computed by taking the square root of the variance score.

Activity 5.3 (Answers on p. 362)

1 Find the range, deviation, variance and standard deviation of the following sets of scores:
   (i) 14   9   21   23   18   17   33   28   12
   (ii) 71   50   48   64   80   81   79
2 You are concerned about one of the weighing scales in use in your department, since you are not sure how reliable it is. How might you assess its reliability using descriptive statistics?

MEASURES OF RELATIVE ACHIEVEMENT

Throughout this chapter, I have pointed out that descriptive statistics are very useful for providing information about relative achievement, performance or capacity; in other words, how well a given individual is performing relative to the group. So you might be interested in assessing how well a student is doing relative to the rest of the year, or how long it takes an elderly patient with osteoarthritis to move from sitting to standing, compared with other similar patients. There are also national averages against which the health professional might wish to compare an individual, such as the relative progress of a baby with cerebral palsy relative to national normal developmental milestones, or the fitness level of a coronary heart disease patient compared with national norms. So the health professional might want to ask the question: Is this neonate abnormally long or abnormally short? To answer the question, the baby's length at birth would be compared with national norms to establish where it lay relative to other babies. To make these comparisons, the researcher can use percentiles and deciles.

Percentiles

A percentile point (p) represents the scores that lie below a given percentage point. Therefore, a percentile point of 15 cuts off the bottom 15% of scores in a data set, and a percentile point of 72 cuts off the bottom 72% of scores in the data set. So if you had a sample of 200 patients who had been assessed for their mobility following total joint replacement, the range of scores in m might look like this (smallest scores to the left, highest to the right):

2.3 2.5 3.1 3.1 3.7 .... 23.6 23.7 24.8 25.6

The first percentile in this data set cuts off the bottom 1% of the scores, which, as our sample contains 200 patients, is the bottom two scores (i.e. 2.3 and 2.5). The 10th percentile cuts off the bottom 10% of scores, which here would be the lowest 20 scores. The 35th percentile cuts of the bottom 35% of scores, which here would be the lowest 70 scores and so on. We can see from this that the median is the same as the 50th percentile, because it cuts off the bottom 50% of the scores. Identifying percentile points is easy in this hypothetical example, because we conveniently have 200 scores. Where the number of scores is neither 100 nor a multiple of 100, things obviously become more difficult: where would the cut-off be if we had 167 patients in our sample? This obviously needs a different approach, but, before we go on to calculate these percentiles, another commonly used term of relative achievement will be mentioned briefly: the **decile**. The decile is equivalent to 10 percentile points, so that the first decile is the same as the 10th percentile, and the 4th decile is the same as the 40th percentile and so on. Obviously, then, the median is the same as the 5th decile. Sometimes the term '**quartile**' is referred to in research reports. The quartile is the same as 25 percentile points. So the 1st quartile cuts off the bottom 25% of scores (the equivalent of the 25th percentile), the second quartile cuts off the bottom 50% of scores (and is the same as the median, the 50th percentile and the 5th decile) and the 3rd quartile cuts off the bottom 75% of scores (the equivalent of the 75th percentile). The most commonly used measure, however, is the percentile.

I have already noted that percentiles are easy enough to calculate if the data set is straightforward, but how would we calculate percentiles if we had 763 patients, many of whom obtained the same score? The method used is a variation on the formula used to calculate the median (see pp. 54–56) and we will continue with the example provided there, which related to the mobility of amputees with prostheses. First, you need to construct a frequency table like Table 5.14, using exact class intervals to group your data. Now you have to calculate cumulative frequencies for the data and add this in another column. So,

Table 5.14

Exact class intervals for metres walked	Number of scores in each class interval	Cumulative frequency
27.5–33.5	2	2
33.5–39.5	4	6 (i.e. 2+4)
39.5–45.5	4	10 (i.e. 2+4+4)
45.5–51.5	5	15 (i.e. 2+4+4+5)
51.5–57.5	7	22 (and so on)
57.5–63.5	8	30
63.5–69.5	11	41
69.5–75.5	12	53
75.5–81.5	6	59
81.5–87.5	5	64
87.5–93.5	3	67
93.5–99.5	2	69
99.5–105.5	1	70
Total = 70		

starting with the lowest class interval, add the frequencies together.

Usually, when assessing relative achievement, every 10th percentile point is used (this is the same as the decile, but the term is less commonly used). So a health professional would typically use the 10th, 20th, 30th, 40th, 50th, 60th, 70th, 80th and 90th percentile points to compare an individual's performance. In our example, this would enable a given patient's mobility to be compared with the rest of the group, to establish how well or how badly the patient was doing. So for example, a patient's mobility might be below the 10th percentile, which would mean that, compared with the others, he isn't making much progress. Another patient might be above the 90th percentile, which would indicate very good mobility relative to the others. To make comparisons of an individual's performance with that of the rest of the group, we need to calculate every 10th percentile point for our data set.

For the 10th percentile (p10)

1. Multiply the desired percentile point (i.e. 10) by the total number of scores (i.e. 70) and divide by 100

$$\frac{10 \times 70}{100} = 7$$

This is expressed as the formula:

$$\frac{p \times N}{100}$$

where

p = the desired percentile point
N = the total number of scores in the data set.

The value of 7 represents the 10th percentile point; this is the 7th score.

2. Look at Table 5.14 and, moving up the cumulative frequencies, identify the class interval in which the 7th score lies, i.e. 39.5–45.5. Note the lower limit of this class interval, which is 39.5; this is called L.

3. Note the number of scores that are contained in the class interval in which the 7th score lies, i.e. 4. This value is called f and therefore f = 4.

4. Count up the number of scores *below* the class interval that contains the 7th score, i.e. 4 + 2 = 6. This value is called S and therefore S = 6.

5. Make a note of the size of the class intervals we have used, i.e. 6 (27.5–33.5, 33.5–39.5, etc). This value is called I and therefore I = 6.

6. Substitute these values in the formula:
p10 (required percentile point) =

$$= L + \left[\frac{\left(\frac{p \times N}{100} \right) - S}{f} \times I \right]$$

Therefore

$$p10 = 39.5 + \left[\frac{7-6}{4} \times 6 \right]$$
$$= 39.5 + 1.5$$
$$= 41$$

Therefore the 10th percentile (p10) = 41 m.

For the 20th percentile (p20)

$$\frac{p \times N}{100} = \frac{20 \times 70}{100}$$
$$= 14$$

$$L = 45.5$$
$$f = 5$$
$$S = 10$$
$$I = 6$$

Therefore

$$p20 = 45.5 + \left[\frac{14-10}{5} \times 6 \right]$$
$$= 45.5 + 4.8$$
$$= 50.3 \, \text{m}$$

For the 30th percentile (p30)

$$\frac{p \times N}{100} = \frac{30 \times 70}{100}$$
$$= 21$$

$$L = 51.5$$
$$f = 7$$
$$S = 15$$
$$I = 6$$

Therefore

$$p30 = 51.5 + \left[\frac{21-15}{7} \times 6 \right]$$
$$= 51.5 + 5.142$$
$$= 56.642 \, \text{m}$$

For the 40th percentile (p40)

$$\frac{p \times N}{100} = \frac{40 \times 70}{100}$$
$$= 28$$

$$L = 57.5$$
$$f = 8$$
$$S = 22$$
$$I = 6$$

Therefore

$$p40 = 57.5 + \left[\frac{28-22}{8} \times 6 \right]$$
$$= 57.5 + 4.5$$
$$= 62 \, \text{m}$$

For the 50th percentile (p50, i.e. the median)

$$\frac{p \times N}{100} = \frac{50 \times 70}{100}$$
$$= 35$$

$L = 63.5$
$f = 11$
$S = 30$
$I = 6$

Therefore

$$p50 = 63.5 + \left[\frac{35 - 30}{11} \times 6 \right]$$
$$= 63.5 + 2.73$$
$$= 66.23 \, \text{m}$$

For the 60th percentile (p60)

$$\frac{p \times N}{100} = \frac{60 \times 70}{100}$$
$$= 42$$

$L = 69.5$
$f = 12$
$S = 41$
$I = 6$

Therefore

$$p60 = 69.5 + \left[\frac{42 - 41}{12} \times 6 \right]$$
$$= 69.5 + 0.498$$
$$= 69.998 \, \text{m}$$

For the 70th percentile (p70)

$$\frac{p \times N}{100} = \frac{70 \times 70}{100}$$
$$= 49$$

$L = 69.5$
$f = 12$
$S = 41$
$I = 6$

Therefore

$$p70 = 69.5 + \left[\frac{49 - 41}{12} \times 6 \right]$$
$$= 69.5 + 4.002$$
$$= 73.5 \, \text{m}$$

For the 80th percentile (p80)

$$\frac{p \times N}{100} = \frac{80 \times 70}{100}$$
$$= 56$$

$L = 75.5$
$f = 6$
$S = 53$
$I = 6$

Therefore

$$p80 = 75.5 + \left[\frac{56 - 53}{6} \times 6 \right]$$
$$= 75.5 + 3$$
$$= 78.5 \, \text{m}$$

For the 90th percentile (p90)

$$\frac{p \times N}{100} = \frac{90 \times 70}{100}$$
$$= 63$$

$L = 81.5$
$f = 5$
$S = 59$
$I = 6$

Therefore

$$p90 = 81.5 + \left[\frac{63 - 59}{5} \times 6 \right]$$
$$= 81.5 + 4.8$$
$$= 86.3 \, \text{m}$$

Therefore we can now say that:

10% of the scores lie below 41 m
20% of the scores lie below 50.3 m
30% of the scores lie below 56.642 m
40% of the scores lie below 62 m
50% of the scores lie below 66.23 m
60% of the scores lie below 69.998 m
70% of the scores lie below 73.5 m
80% of the scores lie below 78.5 m
90% of the scores lie below 86.3 m.

So an amputee with prostheses who walks 48.7 m after training comes within the bottom 20% of the group, while one who walks 81.3 m is doing better than 80% of the group.

However, an individual who comes between the 10th and the 20th percentile points may be absolutely at the mid-point between these two percentiles, or he may be close to either limit, but a simple comparison with a group using percentile points will not provide you with this more detailed information. If you want to be more specific about exactly where an individual lies in percentile terms, you need the following formula:

$$P = \frac{\left[\frac{f}{I}\right] \times \left[P_p - L\right] + S}{N} \times 100$$

The symbols here mean exactly as they did in the previous percentile calculations. So, for the examples just used (two patients walking 48.7 and 81.3 m), we can calculate exactly the percentile point at which these scores lie as follows:

For the score of 48.7, locate the class interval in which 48.7 lies and substitute the relevant values. The score of 48.7 lies in the class interval 45.5–51.5.

Therefore,

L = the lower limit of this class interval = 45.5

f = the number of scores in that class interval = 5

I = the size of the class intervals used = 6

P_p = the score we're using = 48.7

S = the number of scores below the class interval that contains P_p = 10.

Therefore

$$P = \frac{\left[\frac{5}{6}\right] \times \left[48.7 - 45.5\right] + 10}{70} \times 100$$

$$= \frac{[0.833 \times 3.2] + 10}{70} \times 100$$

$$= \frac{2.666 + 10}{70} \times 100$$

$$= 0.181 \times 100$$

$$= 18.1$$

Therefore 48.7 m is at the 18th percentile (rounded to the nearest whole number).

For the score of 81.3 m, locate the class interval in which 81.3 is located and repeat the procedure.

Therefore

$$P = \frac{\left[\frac{6}{6}\right] \times \left[81.3 - 75.5\right] + 53}{70} \times 100$$

$$= \frac{[1 \times 58] + 53}{70} \times 100$$

$$= \frac{5.8 + 53}{70} \times 100$$

$$= 84$$

Therefore, a score of 81.3 m is at the 84th percentile.

The use of percentile points to gauge relative performance, development or achievement is widespread, because it can give the health professional a clear idea of where an individual lies relative to the group or to national norms. But while this is very useful as an indicative measure, it can also be rather misleading. If you look back to p. 63, where the percentile points are related to the m walked by the amputees, we can see that the differences in metres associated with the percentile points are quite varied. For example, the gap between the 10th and the 20th percentile is 9.3 m, whereas the gap between the 60th and the 70th percentiles is only 3.502 m. This means that a patient who walks 41 m needs to walk another 9.3 to move up 10 percentile points, while another patient who walks 69.998 m only needs to walk another 3.502 to move up the same number of percentile points. Therefore, the difference in metres walked by two patients located at the 25th and the 28th percentiles is not necessarily the same difference in metres as two patients located at the 67th and 70th percentiles, even though both pairs differ by three percentile points. This means that percentiles are simply ordinal scales which provide a measure of relativity or rank; they cannot provide any information about the actual difference between the scores. If the researcher needs greater accuracy in establishing exactly where a particular score lies relative to the rest of the group, we need to use standard, or z, scores. This procedure will be described after the next section because the properties of the normal distribution relate directly to z scores.

Key Concepts

- When the researcher is interested in assessing the relative achievement of a participant compared with group or national norms, percentile or decile points are used.
- A percentile point represents those scores in a data set that lie below it; for example, a percentile point of 15 cuts off the bottom 15% of the scores and a percentile point of 71 cuts off the bottom 71% of scores.

- By identifying the percentile point at which a given score lies, the researcher can assess the relative position of that score within the total data set.
- Deciles are equivalent to 10 percentile points, so for example, the 3rd decile is the same as the 30th percentile.
- The median is the 50th percentile point and the 5th decile.

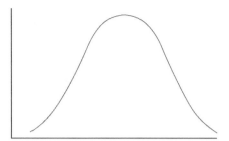

Figure 5.14   Normal distribution curve.

Activity 5.4 (Answers on p. 362)

The following hypothetical data set refers to the number of words in the vocabularies of 140 5-year-old children with cerebral palsy. Calculate the 10th, 20th, 30th, 40th, 50th, 60th, 70th, 80th and 90th percentile points.

Exact class intervals for vocabulary size	Number of children in each class interval
51.5–58.5	3
58.5–65.5	10
65.5–72.5	8
72.5–79.5	9
79.5–86.5	12
86.5–93.5	15
93.5–100.5	13
100.5–107.5	20
107.5–114.5	16
114.5–121.5	11
121.5–128.5	10
128.5–135.5	8
135.5–142.5	3
142.5–149.5	2
	Total = 140

Activity 5.5 (Answers on p. 362)

Three children (A, B and C) from this sample have vocabulary sizes of 63, 77 and 138 words, respectively. Calculate the exact percentile point for each child's performance.

NORMAL DISTRIBUTION

It was pointed out earlier that there are a number of frequency distribution shapes which occur commonly in statistics. The most common of all these is the so-called normal distribution curve (sometimes known as the Gaussian distribution, after Gauss, the astronomer and mathematician who investigated it). The normal distribution curve is a symmetrical bell-shaped distribution (Figure 5.14).

It possesses a number of important mathematical properties:

1. It is symmetrical.
2. The mean, median and mode all have the same value.
3. The curve descends rapidly at first from its central point, but the descent slows down as the tails of the curve are reached.
4. No matter how far you continue the tails of the curve, they never reach the horizontal axis.
5. The normal distribution curve occurs in data drawn from a wide range of subjects: mathematics, physics, engineering, psychology, etc. For example, height, IQ and the life of electric light bulbs all have normal distributions. In other words, if we collected, for example, height data from a large number of people randomly drawn from the population and drew a frequency distribution of it, we would end up with something that resembled a normal curve.
6. If the mean and standard deviation of a normally distributed set of data are known, then we can draw the normal distribution curve. The reason we can do this is a result of the relationship between the standard deviation and the normal distribution curve.

THE STANDARD DEVIATION AND THE NORMAL DISTRIBUTION CURVE

When a set of data is normally distributed, a fixed percentage of the scores always falls in a

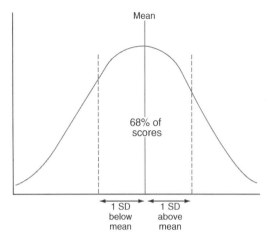

Figure 5.15 The standard deviation and the normal distribution curve.

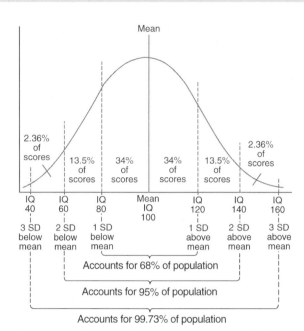

Figure 5.16 Hypothetical normal distribution curve for IQ.

given area under the curve. If we take the central point of the curve shown in Figure 5.15 and then move 1 standard deviation above and below the mean, then 68% of the scores will always fall within this range. This is a constant fact of the normal distribution, i.e. that 34% of scores fall within 1 standard deviation above the mean, and 34% of scores fall within 1 standard deviation below.

If we move on, we find that a further 13.5% of the scores fall between standard deviations 1 and 2 above the mean, and 13.5% fall between standard deviations 1 and 2 below the mean. Thus, the two standard deviations on either side of the mean account for a total of 95% of the scores (13.5 + 34 + 34 + 13.5).

Going on to standard deviations 2–3 above and below the mean, we find that 2.36% of scores fall within each category, thereby allowing a total of 99.73% of the scores to be accounted for by 3 standard deviations above and below the mean (2.36 + 13.5 + 34 + 34 + 13.5 + 2.36 = 99.72, represented normally as 99.73 as a result of calculating further decimal places).

So, to take an example, suppose we know that the mean IQ of the population is 100 and the standard deviation is 20; then 68% of the population have IQs between 80 and 120, 95% have IQs between 60 and 140, and 99.73% have IQs between 40 and 160. We can see this more clearly in the normal curve in Figure 5.16.

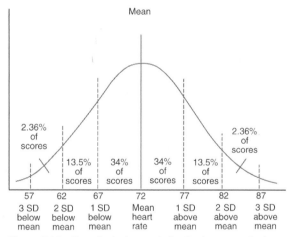

Figure 5.17 Hypothetical normal distribution curve for heart rate.

THE VALUE OF THE NORMAL DISTRIBUTION

The value of the normal distribution is twofold. First, it allows the researcher to describe a set of data and to predict (from knowledge of the properties of the normal curve) what proportions of people possess certain characteristics.

For example, if we know that the average heart rate is 72, with a standard deviation of 5, and that heart rate is normally distributed, we can draw the curve shown in Figure 5.17.

Now, because we know that 68% of people are accounted for by scores within 1 standard deviation either side of the mean, we know that 68% of the population must have heart rates between 67 and 77 beats per minute. Furthermore, we know that another 13.5% of people fall within standard deviations 1 and 2 above the mean and another 13.5% fall within standard deviations 1 and 2 below the mean. This means 13.5% of the population have heart rates of 77–82 beats per minute and 13.5% have heart rates of 62–67 beats per minute. Finally, we know that 2.36% of the population fall within standard deviations 2–3 above the mean and a further 2.36% within standard deviations 2–3 below the mean. This means 2.36% of people have heart rates of 82–87 beats per minute and 2.36% have heart rates of 57–62 beats per minute.

This information also allows us to 'work backwards'; if a patient presents with a heart rate of 86, then you can ascertain just how statistically unusual this is, since you know that only 2.36% of the population come within this range.

The second function of the normal distribution curve relates to its role in inferential statistics. Many of the tests used in inferential statistics require that the results being analysed are normally distributed (see section on 'parametric' statistics); if they are not, then these tests are inappropriate and other sorts of test (i.e. 'non-parametric') should be used. This will be explained in more detail in Chapter 9.

The normal distribution curve also underlies some of the theoretical assumptions of inferential statistics, although these need not concern us unduly here. However, the normal distribution will be referred to again in the chapter on estimation, as it is fundamental to understanding this concept.

STANDARD SCORES OR Z SCORES

Standard scores are also referred to as z scores and tell us how far above or below the group mean a given score is located. Because z scores can only be used with data that are approximately normally distributed, it is important that you read the previous section about normal distributions. This section noted that a fixed per-

centage of scores (68%) in a set of normally distributed data lies within 1 standard deviation either side of the mean; 13.5 % of scores lie between 1 and 2 standard deviations above the mean and 13.5% between 1 and 2 standard deviations below the mean. Thereafter the percentages are 2.36 and 0.14 (see Fig. 5.17). If we continue with the IQ example, we can say that a child with an IQ of 130 is 1.5 standard deviations above the mean (because this score comes exactly midway between standard deviations 1 and 2), while a child with an IQ of 50 is 2.5 standard deviations below the mean (because the score comes halfway between standard deviations 2 and 3). These two examples are straightforward because they conveniently fall at the mid-point between 2 standard deviations. But what if a child had scored 137 or 53? We cannot make any claim about exactly where this child comes relative to the mean without converting the IQ to a z score.

To calculate z scores, two further values are needed: the mean and the standard deviation for the data set. These terms have already been discussed on pp. 53–60. In the IQ example outlined above, the mean was 100 and the standard deviation 20 (see p. 66). Using these values we can convert the IQs of 137 and 53 to z scores, by using the following formula:

$$z = \frac{R - \bar{x}}{SD}$$

where
R = the raw score
$\bar{x}$ = the mean score
SD = the standard deviation

Therefore, for a raw IQ score of 137:

$$z = \frac{137 - 100}{20}$$
$$= 1.85$$

This means that an IQ of 137 is 1.85 standard deviations above the mean.

For an IQ score of 53

$$z = \frac{53 - 100}{20}$$
$$= -2.35$$

Therefore, an IQ of 53 is 2.35 standard deviations below the mean (below is indicated by the minus sign). The z scores, then, allow the researcher to plot exactly where an individual score lies in relation to the group or national data.

Key Concepts

The normal distribution curve is a commonly occurring frequency distribution which possesses certain mathematical properties:

- If the mean and the standard deviation of a set of scores are known, then the researcher is able to predict what proportion of the population has scores within a certain range. This is possible because a fixed proportion of the population will fall within a certain scores range, as long as those scores are normally distributed.
- The normal distribution curve is of fundamental importance in the theory behind inferential statistics.
- In a set of normally distributed data, the researcher can identify exactly where a given score lies relative to the mean using z scores.
- z scores will give a precise statement of how many standard deviations above or below the mean a particular score lies. This is valuable in assessing the relative performance of an individual.

Activity 5.6 (Answers on p. 362)

To compare the age at which the same three children acquired their first word with a normative data base (see Activity 5.5), you find that the national norms for language acquisition for non-disabled children are normally distributed, with a mean of 18.0 months and a standard deviation of 1.75 months. Child A first spoke at 24.25 months, child B at 22.5 months and child C at 19.25 months. Using z scores, find out how these three children compare with the national database.

Activity 5.7 (Answers on p. 362)

If we know that heart rate during weeks 10–20 of pregnancy is normally distributed, with a mean of 82 and a standard deviation of 8, then:

1 What percentage of patients will have heart rates between 66 and 98?
2 What percentage of patients will show heart rates of 99–106?
3 If a patient presents with a heart rate of 57, how common is this in terms of percentages?

FURTHER READING

Coolican H 2004 Research methods and statistics in psychology, 4th edition. Hodder and Stoughton, London

Coolican H 2006 Introduction to research methods in psychology, 3rd edition. London, Hodder Arnold

Crichton N 2005 Principles of statistical analysis in nursing and healthcare research. Online. Available http://nurseresearcher.rcnpublishing.co.uk/resources/archive/GetArticleById.asp?ArticleId=6171

Hallett C 2005 The use of descriptive statistics in nursing research. http://nurseresearcher.rcnpublishing.co.uk/resources/archive/GetArticleById.asp?ArticleId=6062

Watson H, McFadyen A 2005 Non-parametric data analysis. Online available: http://nurseresearcher.rcnpublishing.co.uk/resources/archive/GetArticleById.asp?ArticleId=6064

Parahoo K 2006 Nursing research: principles, process and issues, 2nd edition. Basingstoke, Macmillan

Pearson L 2005 Quantitative analysis: the principles of data presentation. Online. Available http://nurseresearcher.rcnpublishing.co.uk/resources/archive/GetArticleById.asp?ArticleId=6065

Polgar S, Thomas S 2007 Introduction to research in the health sciences. Churchill Livingstone, Edinburgh

Robson C 2002 Real world research: a resource for social scientists and practitioner-researchers, 2nd edition. Blackwell Publishing, Oxford

Watson R, McKenna H, Cowman S, Keady J 2008 Nursing research: designs and methods. Edinburgh, Churchill Livingstone

Chapter 6

Testing hypotheses

We have briefly covered the topic of descriptive statistics, which provide the researcher with one method of presenting data. However, this approach is typically used to make sense of data derived from some form of survey, and is not always appropriate for analysing results from an experiment where an hypothesis has been tested. What is needed here, is a second branch of statistics known as inferential statistics.

There will be many occasions when you do not want simply to collect a lot of data about a broad topic area, but wish, instead, to test out an idea; for instance, comparing the effectiveness of two treatment techniques, or monitoring the progress of a specific group of patients. In such cases, you would carry out an experiment and analyse the results from this using a statistical test. This sort of data analysis is called inferential statistics, because it allows you to infer that the results obtained from your experiment, which used a small sample of people, may also apply to the larger population from which the sample was drawn. Look back to pp. 20–21 to refresh your memory on this.

However, before you can reasonably start inferring anything from the results of an experiment, it is essential that the experiment is properly designed, otherwise false inferences may be made. This chapter and the next are concerned with outlining the principles of good experimental techniques.

When carrying out any research which involves testing an idea or hypothesis, the following steps have to be taken:

- An hypothesis must be devised and stated clearly.
- A research project must be designed which will test the hypothesis.
- Results from the research have to be analysed using an appropriate statistical test.
- A report must be prepared on the research for future reference.

We shall deal with each of these stages in turn. This chapter will be concerned with the principles involved in devising hypotheses and some basic concepts about research design.

THE EXPERIMENTAL HYPOTHESIS

The starting point of any research is an idea known as the experimental or research hypothesis, sometimes referred to as H_1. This is usually based on some theory or article that the researcher has read or it may result from some observations that the researcher has made. You may, for instance, have noticed in the course of your work that certain patients seem to respond better to particular types of treatment. An observation of this type would form the basis of an experimental hypothesis. Examples of experimental hypotheses include such ideas as:

1. Male clinical therapy students perform better on clinical placements than do female clinical therapy students.
2. Leg fracture patients make quicker recoveries with traction than with cast-bracing.
3. Job satisfaction is greater among private practice podiatrists than among NHS podiatrists.

You probably have a number of such ideas that you are interested in looking at, and it would be useful to write them down at this stage.

If we look at the above hypotheses, we can see that what the experimental hypothesis does is to predict a relationship between two things, which are known as variables. It is possible to construct hypotheses that predict a relationship between three or more variables, but the conduct and analysis of such studies is very complex and outside the range of this text. This book will only deal with hypotheses that predict a relationship

between two variables. Therefore, the first hypothesis predicts a relationship between gender of the clinical therapy student (male or female) and performance in clinical assessments. The two variables here, then, are gender of student and performance. The second hypothesis predicts a relationship between type of treatment (traction or cast-bracing) and speed of recovery. The two variables here are type of treatment and recovery rate. The third hypothesis predicts a relationship between degree of job satisfaction and private/public podiatry practice. The two variables, then, are job satisfaction and type of podiatry employment.

The relationship predicted in the experimental hypothesis is assumed to be a consistent and reliable one. So, if we take the second of the hypotheses above, the underlying assumption is that leg fracture patients on traction will typically make more progress than those leg fracture patients with cast-bracing. This is not to say that traction is always more effective than cast-bracing, but rather that, if a patient is being treated with traction, the likelihood is that they will make greater progress than those patients treated with cast-bracing. What we do not anticipate is a rather random or unreliable outcome, such that sometimes traction patients do better, but sometimes they don't.

Key Concepts

The experimental hypothesis is the starting point of any research and predicts a relationship between two or more variables.

Activity 6.1 (Answers on pp. 362–363)

Look at the following hypotheses and write down what the two variables are in each case.

1 Children with scoliosis are more compliant with their exercise regime than are adolescents with scoliosis.
2 Men and women with arthritis differ in their responsiveness to remedial massage.
3 Girls with torticollis make quicker progress on therapy programmes than do boys.

4 Outpatients' clinics achieve better recovery rates for leg fractures than specific sports injuries clinics.

5 There is a difference in professional competence between clinical therapists with degrees and those with diplomas.

Now think about the research project you would like to carry out. State the experimental hypothesis, making sure it predicts a relationship between the two variables. Write down what the variables are.

When formulating your experimental hypothesis, there are some points which would be useful to bear in mind. First, your hypothesis should be testable. As an extreme example, you might have predicted that comatose patients report less pain than non-comatose patients when undergoing the same therapeutic intervention. How would you assess the reported pain levels of the comatose group? It would be an almost impossible task and consequently the hypothesis would not be testable.

Second, your hypothesis should be realistic in its aims. This means you should not be over-ambitious; for example, trying to compare the entire population of insulin-dependent diabetics with non-insulin-dependent diabetics for signs of neuropathy would be a gargantuan task. A project of that size would be not only unnecessary but beyond the scope of any individual researcher or even of a robust cohort of researchers. Consequently, the aims of your experiment should be confined to something more do-able.

Third, you must define what your variables mean. In the above example, 'comatose' patients is a very loose concept. Why are they comatose? What is their medical condition? How old are they? Who are they? You must be able to clarify exactly what your terms mean.

Finally, few researchers push back the frontiers of science with their projects. Most people, for whatever reason, have to undertake small-scale studies, but this does not necessarily imply that their value is limited. Many such projects can have far-reaching implications for health care policy and practice and contribute a great deal to our knowledge base.

The next step is to find out whether the relationship predicted in your hypothesis does, in fact, exist, which means you must design and carry out a suitable project to test your hypothesis. Any results you get from the research are then analysed using the appropriate statistical test. But, before we move on to talk about how you proceed, one very important point must be made.

THE NULL HYPOTHESIS

It must be logically possible for the relationship predicted in your experimental hypothesis to be wrong, otherwise there is no point in wasting your time carrying out any research. For example, anyone who hypothesised that all chiropractors who were born in 1940 are older than those born in 1945 and then spent 3 days amongst the record books trying to support their hypothesis would be indulging in a pointless exercise, since there would be absolutely no possibility that their prediction would be wrong. Therefore, to make any research project worthwhile, the results must not be a foregone conclusion; there has to be a chance that the predicted relationship does not exist.

To show that there is a possibility that the relationship predicted in the experimental hypothesis does not exist, we have to state a second hypothesis called the null hypothesis. This is sometimes referred to as H_0. So, while the experimental hypothesis predicts that there **is** a relationship between two variables, the null hypothesis says there is *no* relationship and that any results you get from your research project are due to chance and not to any real and reliable relationship between the variables.

Let's take an example. Supposing in the course of your work you have noticed that patients are more likely to follow oral rather than written instructions for exercises following coronary bypass surgery. You decide to carry out some research to see if your hunch is right. The first step is to state the experimental hypothesis clearly: i.e. 'Patients are more likely to comply with oral exercise instructions than with written exercise instructions following coronary bypass surgery'. So, you are predicting a relationship between the type of instructions given and degree of compliance. But, because it is possible that your observations are wrong, you must also state the null hypothesis that there is no relationship between the type of instructions and degree of compliance. The null hypothesis also implies that, should any differences in degree of compliance be found, then these are simply due to chance fluctuations and not to any real and consistent relationship. The usual way of stating the null hypothesis is simply to predict no relationship between the two variables. Therefore, here, your null hypothesis would be: 'There is no relationship between type of instructions and degree of compliance'.

If you ever get stuck when formulating the null hypothesis, the easy way to get round the problem is by:

1. Identifying the relationship in the experimental hypothesis, by stating: 'There is a relationship between *a* and *b*' (*a* and *b* being the two variables).
2. Changing the first part to: 'There is no relationship between *a* and *b*'. This gives you your null hypothesis.

It is very important to note that the null hypothesis predicts no relationship; it does not predict the opposite of the experimental hypothesis. Many students get confused over this, and in the example just given would assume that the null hypothesis says the reverse of the experimental hypothesis, i.e. that written instructions are more likely to be followed than are oral ones. (Just refresh your memory and check that this is the opposite of our original hypothesis.) This assumption is incorrect, because, if we look at it, a relationship is still being predicted between type of instructions and compliance. So, the null hypothesis says that there is no relationship between the two variables; in this case, between type of instruction and degree of compliance.

Activity 6.2 (Answers on p. 363)

To see whether you are happy with this concept, look at the experimental hypotheses in Activity 6.1 on pp. 70–71 and write down what the null hypothesis is for each one. State the null hypothesis for the research project you would like to carry out.

Why do we need to state the null hypothesis at all? Could we not just assume that there is a chance that our experimental hypothesis may be wrong without having to spell it out? The answer to this lies in a convention, which has its roots in the philosophy of scientific method. (For further details on this the reader is referred to Chalmers 1999 and Brown et al 2003.)

Essentially, this convention states that when we carry out any research we do not set out to find direct support for our experimental hypothesis (or at least we shouldn't!) but, conversely, to falsify the null hypothesis. In other words we still hope to find the relationship we predicted in the experimental hypothesis, but we do this by stating the null hypothesis and setting out to reject it. It should be noted here that the words 'prove' and 'disprove' in relation to the hypotheses are not being used. This is because we cannot really ever prove or disprove anything in physiotherapy, chiropractic, education, psychology or whatever; all we can do is find evidence that supports or fails to support our prediction.

The intending researcher need not worry unduly about all this, since it is sufficient simply to state the experimental and null hypotheses at the outset of any experiment. The relevance of the null hypothesis will be discussed further in different parts of the book.

Key Concepts

The null hypothesis states that the relationship predicted in the experimental hypothesis does not exist, and implies that any results found from the research are simply due to chance factors and not to any real and consistent relationship between the two variables. In any research project, the experimenter sets out to reject the null hypothesis and therefore, by implication, to support experimental hypothesis.

BASIC TYPES OF DESIGN

Once you have sorted out the experimental and null hypotheses for your research project, you then have to decide on the best way to find out whether your predicted relationship actually exists.

In other words you have to design a suitable research project. It should be noted that there are often a number of designs that can be used to test an hypothesis, and it is up to the researcher to select the most appropriate one. As there is usually no single correct way of testing an hypothesis, the researcher must take into account a number of design considerations, and it is with these that this chapter and the following one are concerned. It is important to reiterate that, in applied research, there is rarely any such thing as the perfect research design; more usually compromise decisions have to be made, which must be both informed and justified. The point about justification is a hugely important one and the reasons for your choice of design and conduct of the research should always be clearly stated in your dissertation, research report or article.

There are two basic sorts of research designs: experimental designs and correlational designs. Both designs start off with an experimental hypothesis which predicts a relationship between two (or more) variables, but the aims and methods of each approach are different. These differences can be best illustrated by an example. Let's take the hypothesis that the professional rank of the physiotherapist affects the degree of job satisfaction that is experienced. The relationship that is being suggested is between professional rank of the physiotherapist and degree of job satisfaction. This hypothesis can be tested either by an experimental design or by a correlational design, but in essence the experimental design will look for differences in job satisfaction between different ranks of physiotherapists, while the correlational design is interested to see if there is any pattern between the rank of physiotherapist and the degree of job satisfaction experienced. Let's see, in a very brief overview, how experimental and correlational designs would each approach the problem of trying to find out whether this relationship does, in fact, exist (fuller descriptions and explanations of each type of design will be provided in the next section). It should be noted that the following outlines are only suggestions, since there are other possible ways of using both types of design to test our hypothesis.

EXPERIMENTAL DESIGN: AN EXAMPLE

The experimental design might take a group of senior physiotherapists and a group of junior physiotherapists, measure the reported job satis-

Table 6.1 A correlational design investigating job satisfaction and professional rank

Subject	Level of physiotherapist	Job satisfaction score (on a 10-point scale)
1	District	9
2	Superintendent I	8
3	Superintendent IV	5
4	Senior	4
5	Physiotherapist	4

faction expressed by each group and compare the two groups to see if there is any difference between them.

We would have the following design:

Group 1
Senior physiotherapists ⎫ compared on
Group 2   ⎬ expressed job
Junior physiotherapists ⎭ satisfaction for
                           differences between
                           the groups

CORRELATIONAL DESIGN: AN EXAMPLE

The correlational design, on the other hand, might select a number of physiotherapists who represented the whole range of professional ranks, from most junior through to most senior levels, and measure their reported job satisfaction to see if there is any patterning in the data. For instance, is higher status associated with higher corresponding job satisfaction?

The correlational design would be as shown in Table 6.1.

The data on both status and job satisfaction would be examined to see if there is any pattern or association between them.

Experimental and correlational designs will be discussed more fully in the next two sections. It should be stressed, however, that for the hypothesis we are looking at, either design would be appropriate. This illustrates the idea that was mentioned earlier: for any hypothesis there may be a number of suitable designs to test it, and it is up to the researcher to think carefully about the aims, objectives and the relevant design considerations of the research, and to devise the most appropriate method of testing the hypothesis. It is also important for the researcher to be able to justify this choice.

Key Concepts

- Experimental designs look for differences between sets of results.
- Correlational designs look for patterns or associations between sets of results.
- Therefore, each approach has a different objective and will consequently use a different method to test the hypothesis.

We will deal with the basic principles involved in each design separately, starting with experimental designs.

EXPERIMENTAL DESIGNS

We have already noted that the experimental hypothesis predicts a relationship between two variables. The simplest way to find out whether this relationship actually exists is to alter one of these variables to see what difference it makes to the other. This is the basis of experimental design. This alteration is known as manipulation of variables and is actually something we do in everyday life, often without being aware of it.

This can be illustrated by a mundane example. Suppose you were babysitting for a friend and had decided to watch their television. You turn it on and discover that the sound is too low. Because you aren't familiar with the controls on this set you aren't sure how to adjust the volume, but you think it might be the knob on the front right of the set. Unwittingly, you have formulated an hypothesis: that there is a relationship between the knob and the volume. In order to test this hypothesis, you have to manipulate one of the variables; in other words, you alter the knob to see what effect it has on the sound. You have just performed a very simple experiment, which involved hypothesising a relationship between two variables and manipulating one to see what difference it made to the other. This is the basis of experimental design.

These variables have names. The variable that is manipulated is called the **independent variable or IV**. The variable that is observed for any changes in it resulting from that manipulation is called the **dependent variable or DV**. People

sometimes get confused about which variable is which. The easiest way to identify the IV and the DV is to ask the question: 'Which variable depends on which?' In the above example with the television the question is: 'Does the knob depend on the volume or does the volume depend on the knob?' Clearly in this case the volume depends on the knob, and thus the volume is the dependent variable. The knob is therefore the independent variable.

Some important points emerge out of this. If, after turning the knob, the volume did increase, you might have concluded (though perhaps not consciously) that twiddling the knob *caused* the volume to increase, and therefore the increase in volume could be seen as the *effect* of twiddling the knob. In this way, the IV can be thought of as the cause and the DV as the effect. Any changes that you note in the dependent variable which result from manipulating the independent variable constitute your data in an experiment.

Just to clarify this idea, let's take the hypothesis that leg fractures improve more quickly with traction than with cast-bracing. The two variables are: (1) type of treatment, and (2) speed of recovery. Which variable is which? Does the type of treatment depend on speed of recovery? Or does speed of recovery depend on type of treatment? Clearly, the second suggestion is correct. Type of treatment is the independent variable and speed of recovery is the dependent variable because how quickly a patient recovers depends on the treatment received. What is meant here, then, when we talk about manipulating the independent variable is simply assigning some patients to traction and some to cast-bracing. Their progress is then compared.

However, the problem is not always quite as simple as this. Supposing we hypothesised that there is a difference between the attitudes of nursing and physiotherapy students to shared learning in the undergraduate programmes. Here the dependent variable is the difference in attitudes to shared learning, so the independent variable must be the type of student (nursing or physiotherapy). But how does the experimenter manipulate the type of student? Obviously, in the previous example, it was easy (at least theoretically) for the experimenter to decide which treatment a fracture patient should receive, but in the latter case we cannot possibly take a group of students and decide which course they should follow. In this case the experimenter would simply select a group of nursing students and a group of physiotherapy students, and compare their attitudes to shared learning. The independent variable is still being manipulated but in a slightly different way. Obviously, this sort of manipulation is essential when the independent variable is of a 'fixed' nature, such as race, age, type of patient, etc. This point will be referred to again later.

One final point before moving on to discuss some basic principles of design: there may be many changes in your dependent variable that you wish to measure. For example, if we look at the hypothesis above, we predicted that there was a relationship between type of treatment for leg fractures (IV) and the speed of improvement (DV). Speed of improvement can be measured in several ways: how long it takes before the patient achieves a specified range of movement, how long before the patient walks a particular distance, levels of pain, etc. It would be legitimate to use any or all of these measures as your dependent variable. In other words, there may be a number of different, but relevant outcome measures you wish to take; you don't have to confine yourself to just one and, indeed, the measurement of a number of relevant outcomes is often advantageous.

Key Concepts

Experimental designs involve manipulating the independent variable and measuring the effect of this on the dependent variable. The independent variable can be thought of as cause and the dependent variable as effect.

Activity 6.3 (Answers on p. 363)

Look at the following hypotheses and decide which is the independent variable and which is the dependent variable. When you have done that, decide how you would manipulate the independent variable. If you find that you are having difficulty deciding which variable is which, just ask yourself which variable depends on which.

---

1. Men and women differ in their tendency to complain about pain during osteopathic treatment.
2. Walking frames are more effective than walking sticks in aiding the mobility of arthritis patients.
3. Absenteeism is greater amongst occupational therapists working in psychiatric hospitals than amongst occupational therapists working in general hospitals.
4. Chiropractors are able to establish greater rapport with male patients than with female patients.
5. Podiatry schools that require 'A'-level physics have higher pass rates on the final exam than schools that do not require 'A'-level physics.

MORE THAN ONE INDEPENDENT VARIABLE

So far we have assumed that all experimental hypotheses have just one independent variable. However, as mentioned earlier, this is not always the case and some more complex hypotheses may predict a relationship between more than one independent variable and the dependent variable.

An example of this sort of hypothesis would be a predicted relationship between the age of a patient and his/her compliance with one of two sorts of medical regime, e.g. that there is a difference between children and adolescents with scoliosis in terms of their compliance with oral or written instructions regarding their recommended exercises. Here the dependent variable is compliance with exercises, and the independent variables are the age of the patient and the type of instructions they receive. This hypothesis requires a rather more complicated design, which is outside the scope of this book, but the reader is referred to Polgar & Thomas (2007), or Greene & D'Oliveira (2006) for more details on experimental designs with more than one independent variable.

As has already been noted, in this book we shall deal only with experiments that test hypotheses with just one independent variable.

SOME BASIC PRINCIPLES OF EXPERIMENTAL DESIGN WITH ONE INDEPENDENT VARIABLE

To recap, experimental designs require the experimenter to manipulate or alter the independent variable and to measure the effect of this on the dependent variable. In other words, you alter one variable and measure the difference it makes to the other. Hence experimental designs are said to look for differences in the dependent variable that result from the manipulation of the independent variable. It is important to note that this applies only to experimental designs and not to correlational designs which we shall look at in the next section.

So, having formulated your experimental hypothesis and null hypothesis, the next task is to design a suitable experiment to find out whether the relationship predicted in your hypothesis exists. The basic concepts involved in this are best explained by an example.

Suppose you wanted to test the hypothesis that chiropractors who completed a counselling course run by the local college developed improved communication skills with their patients. The independent variable is attendance on a course and the dependent variable is communications skills. To test this hypothesis you decide to assess the communication skills of those chiropractors who have completed a counselling course. Therefore you would have the following design:

Independent variable   *Dependent variable*
Attendance on course   Measurement of
                           communication skills

What could you conclude from the skills scores? Could you assume that the chiropractors' communication skills had changed or not? You have probably quite correctly decided that we cannot conclude anything from this study, since we don't know what the chiropractors' skills levels were in the first place. So an essential feature of an experiment is a pre-test measure, where possible, of the dependent variable. Let's revise our design to include this:

Pre-test   Attendance on Post-test
measure of   course (IV)   measure of
communication   communication
(DV)   (DV)

What could you conclude from this experiment now? You could certainly decide on the basis of some statistical comparison of the pre-test and post-test scores whether there had been a significant change in communication skills but you couldn't ascribe it necessarily to course attendance, since it is quite possible that there are other explanations for any observed change.

Activity 6.4 (Answers on p. 363)

Can you think of any possible alternative reasons for these results?

In other words, we cannot conclude that attendance causes a change in communication (remember that experimental designs provide evidence of cause–effect relationships). It should be pointed out at this stage that it is not always possible to take a pre-test measure of the DV. To take an example: supposing you wanted to look at the effect of TENS used as pain relief during labour, on the baby's APGAR scores (a measure of the neonate's health and condition at birth, as a score out of 10). Your hypothesis predicts a relationship between the use of TENS (IV) and the babies' APGAR scores (DV). You decide to select a group of women who have opted for TENS during labour and to look at the APGAR scores of their babies immediately after birth (this is not a good design for all the reasons outlined earlier in the paragraph, but it is for illustration only). How could you take a pre-test measure of APGAR scores? It would not be possible, since the baby can only be assessed on this scale after birth and therefore, you could not pre-test the DV before the mothers received TENS. Therefore, there will be some occasions when a pre-test measure of the DV is impossible.

Certainly, from the previous study, attendance on the course would be just one possible explanation of any change in communication skills, but there could be other reasons for this. It is conceivable that the chiropractors in the study might have become more skilled anyway, simply because they were just a bit older and a bit more experienced. They might also have changed jobs, got promotion, attended other courses or had any one of a number of experiences which might account for their changes in communication. How, then, can we ever be sure that the results in our experiment are caused by the independent variable? The only way to do this is to select another group of chiropractors who do not experience the independent variable, i.e. do not attend the course. We then have to make sure that the only difference between the groups is whether or not they experience the independent variable. So, going back to our example, we would select two groups of chiropractors, of which just one group had attended a counselling course, and we would compare their post-test communication skills. Our revised design looks like this:

Group 1	Chiropractors who attend a counselling course	
Pre-test measure of communication skills (DV)	Attendance on course (IV)	Post-test measure of communication skills (DV)
Group 2	Chiropractors who have not attended a counselling course	
Pre-test measure of communication skills (DV)	No attendance on course (no IV)	Post-test measure of communication skills (DV)

These two groups are given names: the group that receives the independent variable (a treatment, intervention or in this case, attends a counselling course) is called the experimental (or treatment) group or condition. The group that does not receive the independent variable (no treatment, no intervention or in this case, does not attend a counselling course) is called the control group or condition. The control group is therefore a 'no-treatment' group. Any changes in each group's communication skills at the post-test stage are then compared using a statistical test to find out if there are any significant differences between them. The concept is a logical one: if the only difference between the two groups is the fact that one group experienced the IV and the other did not, then any differences between the groups in terms of communication skills at the end of the study must have been caused by the IV. However, while the idea is logical, in practice it is very difficult to achieve, because it implies a level of control over the participants' lives that is not feasible, desirable or ethical. The best that can realistically be achieved

is that the two groups are as similar as possible. However, the more we can eliminate the influence of other factors and variables on the outcomes of our study, the more *internal validity* we can say the study has.

Placebos

Sometimes a control group is used slightly differently. While the proper definition of a control group is a 'no-treatment' group, there may be occasions when it is more appropriate to give this group some 'pretend' treatment.

Let's take an example. Imagine a situation where community podiatry services for the elderly are being audited. A question arises as to whether there is any evidence to suggest that podiatry has any benefit for patients who have ingrowing toenails. One way of testing this (as long as the ethics were acceptable) would be to have an experimental group receiving podiatry and a control group having no treatment. However, it occurs to you that one of the factors that may contribute to any benefits that might derive from the podiatry is the patient's expectation that the pain levels resulting from the ingrowing nails will improve if they are given some treatment. In other words, any improvement the patient demonstrates may be the result not of the podiatry itself, but rather of the power of expectation and auto-suggestion.

In order to establish whether or not this is the case, you decide to give the control group some dummy treatment which involves the same amount of one-to-one attention coupled with some non-invasive treatment that has no value (e.g. foot massage). If, at the end of the study, you found that the experimental group has made more progress than the controls, then you could conclude that podiatry was beneficial to these patients and the audit commission's question would have been answered.

The dummy treatment is called a **placebo**. This technique is used a lot in drug trials, where some patients are given the real drug and other patients are given a useless salt or sugar tablet. However, so great is the power of the mind and the patient's expectations that the group on the placebo usually shows a marked improvement, which is known as the **placebo effect**. The whole topic of placebos is a fascinating one; a Discovery

Channel programme (*Placebos: cracking the code*, 26 October 2002) reported that big placebo pills are more effective than small ones, that two placebo pills are more effective than one and that red placebo pills are more effective than white ones. While the use of placebos is probably outside the range of most non-medical research, the issue is an important one, not only because of their widespread use in randomised controlled trials (or RCTs), which have become the gold standard of health care research (see Chapter 7), but also because they involve deception, which is a major ethical problem. This point will be expanded in the next section.

There are still many flaws in our design, but we will talk about ways of eliminating them and refining the experiment in the next chapter. Nonetheless, the key concepts that have been outlined should give you an idea about some of the fundamental issues involved in experimental designs.

Key Concepts

- The subjects in the experimental condition are subjected to the independent variable. The experimental condition can therefore be thought of as the 'treatment condition'.
- The control condition subjects are not subjected to the independent variable. The control condition can therefore be thought of as the 'no-treatment' group.
- Sometimes the control group is given a dummy treatment called a placebo.

SOME ETHICAL ISSUES

By now you might be wanting to raise some ethical issues. The type of design described above, which uses a control or no-treatment group, is fine when we want to look at something like the effects of a counselling course on communication skills. In this instance, there is no real moral dilemma about not giving chiropractors a counselling course. But supposing your hypothesis was that cystic fibrosis patients would improve significantly on a new exercise regime. The IV here is the treatment and the DV is the improvement. You select your two groups of patients, and you give the experimental group your new treatment, but, according to the above principles of experimental design, the other group of cystic fibrosis patients should receive no treatment. Is this ethical? Surely we cannot possibly leave a group of patients with no treatment while we are busily testing out our ideas?

In cases such as this, you would compare two experimental groups rather than one experimental group and one control group. So, instead of comparing your new treatment with no treatment, you would compare it with the conventional treatment or another form of treatment.

Our design would look like this:

Experimental condition 1
Pre-test   New exercise   Post-test
measure of DV   regime (IV)   measure of DV

Experimental condition 2
Pre-test   Conventional   Post-test
measure of DV   treatment (IV) measure of DV

In this case, both groups are subjected to a version of the independent or treatment variable and their progress compared, to find out whether there are any differences between the groups. This is a perfectly legitimate design, but because it doesn't employ a control group it is sometimes referred to as a quasi-experimental design. (It is also worth noting that health care research that focuses on the comparison of new treatment regimens with existing protocols often refers to the 'standard' or usual treatment as the control. This is not strictly correct, but is common practice.) While this design modification gets round the problems of the control, there are many other ethical issues to consider. Because of their importance in research, a separate section is dedicated to the topic at the end of this chapter.

One final point: it is possible to obtain a control group without violating ethical principles, although the quality of the research design would be compromised to a degree. For example, there are often naturally occurring control groups such as people who do not want any treatment for their condition, or alternatively people who are on the waiting list for treatment. However, while using participants from these types of group may be more ethically acceptable, they may also differ from the experimental group in a number of key respects. For example, waiting list patients may not have the severity of condition that the experimental group has and therefore they are not directly comparable. Nonetheless, if a true control group is essential to the study, then this may be a design compromise worth making.

Activity 6.5 (Answers on p. 363)

Look at the following hypotheses and set out the experimental design you would use in each case, using the sort of format and headings shown above:

1. Patients who are given information about the value of clinical therapy exercises are more likely to do those exercises than are patients who receive no information.
2. Osteopaths who have been hospital patients are more sympathetic than those who have not.
3. Chiropractors who have qualified in the last 5 years are more motivated to do research than those who have been qualified for more than 10 years.

MORE COMPLEX DESIGNS

The sort of design we have been looking at is the most simple experimental design of all: a pre-test measure of the dependent variable, manipulation of the independent variable and a post-test measure of the dependent variable. Two groups are used, of which one may be a control condition or, alternatively, both groups may be experimental conditions.

However, you may become a bit more ambitious and decide that you would like to look at something a little more complex than this. If we look back to the hypothesis that cystic fibrosis patients make significant improvements on a new exercise regime, we used a design which involved the comparison of two experimental groups. But you could, if you wished, add further conditions to this design. If you managed to resolve any ethical problem in your mind, you might decide to add a control condition as well, and so your design would look like this:

Experimental condition 1

Pre-test measure of DV	New exercise regime (IV)	Post-test measure of DV

Experimental condition 2

Pre-test measure of DV	Conventional treatment (IV)	Post-test measure of DV

Control condition

Pre-test measure of DV	No treatment (no IV)	Post-test measure of DV

So you still have two experimental conditions, or levels of the independent variable, but you now have a control condition as well.

Alternatively, you might feel that it would be useful to compare three types of therapy instead of two, perhaps adding heat treatment to the exercise regime and conventional therapy.

Therefore, your hypothesis would be something like 'exercise, heat treatment and conventional therapy are differentially effective in helping cystic fibrosis patients'. The dependent variable is degree of improvement and the independent variable is still type of treatment, but this time we have got three types of treatment. Therefore, the independent variable has three experimental conditions or levels: exercise, heat treatment and conventional therapy. Our design would look something like this:

Experimental condition 1

Pre-test measure of physical condition	New exercise regime (IV)	Post-test measure of physical condition (DV)

Experimental condition 2

Pre-test measure of physical condition	Heat treatment (IV)	Post-test measure of physical condition (DV)

Experimental condition 3

Pre-test measure of physical condition	Conventional therapy (IV)	Post-test measure of physical condition (DV)

You could extend this further and add a control condition thus:

Experimental condition 1 ⎫ compared on the
Experimental condition 2 ⎪ dependent variable to
Experimental condition 3 ⎬ assess whether there
Control condition ⎪ are any differences
⎭ between the groups

Or you could go on adding experimental conditions involving different forms of treatment.

In all these cases we still have only one independent variable, i.e. type of treatment, but we have varying numbers of experimental conditions or levels of it.

So, it should be clear by now that hypotheses which predict a relationship between one independent variable and a dependent variable may be tested by comparing:

1. One experimental condition and one control condition
2. Two experimental conditions
3. Two experimental conditions and one control condition
4. Three experimental conditions
5. Three experimental conditions and one control condition
6. More than three experimental conditions, etc.

Each of these designs requires a different statistical test to analyse the results, since, unfortunately, there is no multi-purpose test for all experiments. Matching the design with the appropriate statistical test is something that we shall look at in Chapter 9.

CORRELATIONAL DESIGNS

Not all research has to take the form of manipulating an independent variable to see what effect it has on the dependent variable. Sometimes a researcher is not interested in looking for differences between groups or conditions in this way, but instead is concerned to find out whether two variables are associated or related. (Look back to pp. 73–74 to refresh your memory on the distinctions between experimental and correlational designs.)

Let's suppose we are interested in finding out whether there is a relationship between students' grades on clinical assessments and their performance in theory exams, since we have noticed that students who get high grades on one tend to get high grades on the other. Our hypothesis might be that: 'There is a relationship between performance on clinical assessments and performance in theory exams, high marks on one being associated with high marks on the other'. The two variables are clinical assessment and theory exam performance.

A major difference in the research design needed to test this hypothesis is that the experimenter does not manipulate one of the variables, but simply takes a whole range of measures on one of the variables and assesses whether they show a pattern or relationship of some sort with the measurements on the other variable.

The correlational designs and analyses which will be covered in this book are only concerned with ordinal and interval/ratio data, since these levels of measurements provide a range or dimension for our data. It is possible to do a correlation with just nominal data, but such analyses are not always very informative. That having been said, Chapter 24 covers a correlational approach used when the study is concerned with the agreement between two raters, using nominal data.

In our example, then, we might take a group of clinical therapy students and collect their clinical assessment marks and their theory exam marks to see if the two sets of scores are linked; for example, high marks on one variable being associated with high marks on the other. Because the experimenter does not manipulate one variable, the concepts of independent and dependent variable are not appropriate in correlational designs.

Furthermore, because there is no manipulation of one variable and hence no measurement of the effect this has on the other variable, we cannot say, in a correlational design, which variable is cause and which effect. So returning to our example, we don't know whether clinical performance affects theory exam performance or vice versa. For instance, it may be that students who are good at clinical practice use their experience to answer their theory paper. Or it is possible that students who do well in theory use their knowledge in the clinical context. Alternatively, clinical performance and theory exam performance may both be related to a third variable. For example, good marks on both may be due to an 'easy' marker. Therefore, from any results we got from this study we do not actually know whether:

practice affects theory
or
theory affects practice
or
another variable affects both theory and practice.

You can see from this that, because we cannot ascertain which variable is having an effect on the other, there cannot be an independent or dependent variable or an identifiable cause and effect. Even in correlational studies where we feel we could make an educated guess as to which variable is cause and which effect, we still cannot draw causal conclusions. For instance, a parent might observe that their child's eczema got worse when the child's behaviour deteriorated. However, while there might indeed be a pattern in the data such that the severity of the child's eczema and naughtiness seemed to go together, it could not be ascertained from this study whether:

the eczema caused the bad behaviour
or
the bad behaviour caused the eczema
or
both were caused by a third, unknown factor, such as problems at school.

Therefore, a key feature of correlational designs is that they tell the researcher nothing about cause and effect and to make any such claim would be quite incorrect. Because of this inability to state categorically which variable is cause and which is effect in a correlational design, many researchers prefer the certainty of experimental designs. However, because the experimenter is not involved in manipulating anything (such as types of treatment), the correlational design is often thought to be more acceptable ethically.

As causal conclusions are often wrongly drawn from correlational studies, this point will be explored again at the end of the next section.

Key Concepts

- Experimental designs covered in this book have two variables in the hypothesis, one independent and one dependent. The independent variable is manipulated by the experimenter, and the difference or effect this has on the dependent variable is measured. Thus in experimental designs we can ascertain cause and effect.
- Correlational designs also have two variables in the hypothesis but neither is manipulated. Therefore, there is no independent and no dependent variable. As a result it cannot be ascertained which variable is having an effect on the other. All that can be established is whether or not the scores on the two variables are linked in some way.

CORRELATIONS BETWEEN MORE THAN TWO SETS OF DATA: RELIABILITY MEASURES

Note that correlational designs are not confined to seeing how far just two sets of data are related; they can also be used to look at the degree of similarity between three or more sets of data.

Let's imagine you want to observe a child with cerebral palsy on a number of features, such as speech clarity, spinal curvature, mobility, functional status, control, etc. If you observe the child just once, how will you know whether what you see is typical of what the child can do? Would it not be better to observe the child on a number of occasions in order to see whether there is a significant similarity in observed ability? This would mean that you need to assess the child on all the aspects of behaviour in which you're interested on several occasions. If you then analysed your data according to the principles of a correlational design, you would find out whether the observations were similar or not and from this you could get some reliable assessments of the child's capacities. This sort of 'self-checking' is useful in the clinical therapies and is called **intra-observer reliability measures**.

Let us take this idea a step further. Suppose you have been working with this child for several months and have grown very fond of her. This affection could bias your observations of her capabilities. Would it not be useful, therefore, to have a number of independent clinical therapists (say five) observing the child, according to your checklist of activities, to see if they were in agreement? If you then analysed their scores using a test for correlational designs, and found that the ratings given by the independent clinical therapists were significantly similar, you would have a better and more reliable basis for making your statements about the child's capabilities. This form of 'other-checking' is called **inter-observer reliability**, and again is a valuable tool for clinical therapists. Because of the relevance of inter-rater reliability for clinical therapy, more details on this technique will be given in Chapter 24.

THE CORRELATION COEFFICIENT

It should be noted here that the degree to which each variable is associated in a correlational design is determined using an appropriate statistical test. We will deal with these tests in more detail in Chapter 9 but it is important to look at the underlying concepts here. To do this, let's return to our earlier hypothesis about the relationship between students' theory and clinical assessments. Imagine that we have collected the students' clinical and theory exam marks; the next step is to find out whether there is a significant relationship between them, so we use the correct statistical test (see Chapter 9). When we have finished the calculations involved in this test, we will end up with a number somewhere on a range from −1.0 through 0 to +1.0.

This figure is known as a correlation co-efficient. The size of the correlation coefficient indicates the closeness of the relationship between the two variables. The closer the figure is to −1 or +1, the stronger the relationship, while the closer it is to 0 the weaker the relationship. This concept is illustrated by the continuum in Figure 6.1.

THE SCATTERGRAM

Let's explore this idea a bit further, using the hypothesis about the link between clinical assessments and theory exam marks. Supposing you had collected the clinical assessments and theory exam marks from 30 students (so you would have two scores for each student) you could plot their scores on a graph, known as a scattergram (Figure. 6.2) to see if there is any association between the marks.

In order to do this, you need to take a student's pair of scores (say, for the dot ringed in Figure 6.2, 58% on the theory exam and 66% on the clinical assessment) and to move along each relevant axis until you had located their score. You make a mark at the intersection point. This is repeated for each pair of scores.

Activity 6.6 (Answers on p. 364)

As practice, plot the scores in Table 6.2. as a scattergram.* The hypothesis is that there is a relationship between the number of cigarettes smoked daily and the rate of recovery following thoracic surgery.

Table 6.2   Number of cigarettes smoked daily and number of postoperative days to discharge

Subject	No. of cigarettes	No. of postoperative days to discharge
1	20	15
2	15	12
3	17	12
4	0	7
5	5	7
6	0	8
7	10	9
8	7	8
9	40	17
10	0	7

*In plotting a correlational graph, it does not matter which variable is plotted against the vertical axis and which against the horizontal one. However, should you ever wish to plot the data from an experimental design it is a convention that the independent variable scores are plotted along the horizontal axis and those from the dependent variable along the vertical axis.

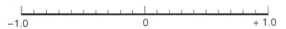

−1.0   0   + 1.0

Figure 6.1   The value of the correlation coefficient lies somewhere on a range from −1 to +1.

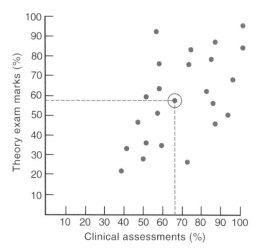

Figure 6.2   A scattergram showing the relationship between theory exam marks and clinical assessments.

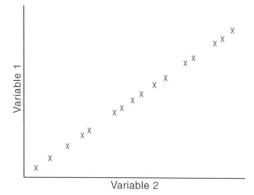

Figure 6.3   The upward slope in this scattergram indicates a positive correlation between variable 1 and variable 2.

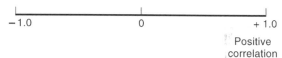

Figure 6.4   The correlation coefficient has a value towards the +1 end for a positive correlation.

POSITIVE CORRELATION

When you have plotted a scattergram you can see from the nature of the pattern of dots, whether there appears to be a relationship between the two variables. If the dots show a general upward or downward slope, it is likely that there is a relationship between the two variables. So in the example about theory and practice marks, it seems that there is a relationship, because the pattern of dots in Figure 6.2 shows a general upward slope. This is known as positive correlation.

A positive correlation means that high scores on one variable are associated with high scores on the other, and hence low scores on one variable are linked with low scores on the other. For example, we might hypothesise that there is a positive correlation between body weight and hypertension, such that the higher the weight the higher the hypertension. So a scattergram pattern which shows a general upward slope like the one in Figure 6.3 indicates a positive correlation.

It should be noted that the perfectly smooth upward slope in the graph in Figure 6.3 shows a *perfect* positive correlation (i.e. there is a one-to-one relationship between high scores on one variable and high scores on the other). However, perfect correlations are extremely rare, if they exist at all. But, the smoother and straighter the upward slope, the stronger the positive correla-

tion between the two variables. A positive correlation would be represented on our continuum somewhere around the +1.0 end, as in Figure 6.4.

NEGATIVE CORRELATION

The correlation coefficient just mentioned would have been derived from a statistical analysis and the nearer to +1, the stronger the relationship. This, however, is not the only sort of correlation that can occur. Sometimes it is possible that high scores on one variable are associated with low scores on the other. For example, we might hypothesise a relationship between body weight of an arthritic patient and distance that can be walked, such that the greater the body weight the shorter the distance. Our data may look like Table 6.3.

Plotting these results on a scattergram, we end up with the pattern in Figure 6.5. There is a general downward slope in the pattern of dots.

When this sort of pattern emerges, it suggests that high scores on one variable are associated with low scores on the other. This is known as a negative correlation and would be represented on our correlation coefficient continuum near the −1 end; the closer to −1, the stronger the negative

Table 6.3 Body weight and distance walked in arthritic patients

Patient	Weight (kg)	Distance (metres)
1	74	12
2	59	20
3	64	15
4	67	15
5	72	10
6	80	5

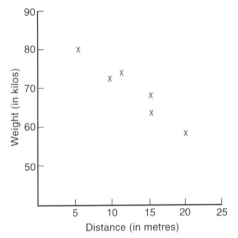

Figure 6.5 This scattergram has a downward slope, as the higher the body weight in arthritic patients, the shorter the distance that can be walked.

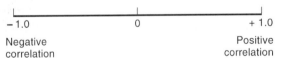

Figure 6.6 A correlation coefficient value near to −1 indicates a strong negative correlation.

correlation (Figure 6.6). On a scattergram, a negative correlation is indicated by the pattern shown in Figure 6.7. (Again this shows a perfect negative correlation, which is very unlikely ever to occur.)

It is very important to note that a negative correlation does not mean no correlation. This is a point that confuses some students. A negative correlation indicates a relationship between high scores on one variable and low scores on the other, while no correlation means that there is no relationship at all between the two variables. The following example demonstrates this:

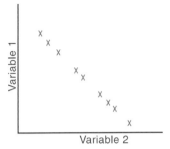

Figure 6.7 A scattergram pattern indicating a negative correlation.

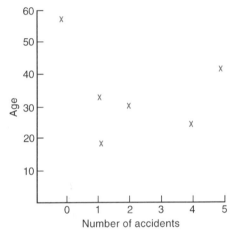

Figure 6.8 This scattergram pattern suggests there is no link between the two variables.

Table 6.4 Age of driver and number of road traffic accidents

Subject	Age	No. of road traffic accidents
1	19	1
2	30	2
3	57	0
4	41	5
5	25	4
6	32	1

Hypothesis There is a relationship between the age of driver and the number of road traffic accidents.

The data obtained are shown in Table 6.4.

Plotting these on a scattergram we get the picture shown in Figure 6.8. This shows a fairly random scattering of dots, suggesting there is no

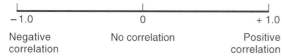

Figure 6.9 A correlation coefficient value around 0 indicates little or no relationship between the two variables.

link between the variables of age and the number of road traffic accidents.

In this case the correlation coefficient score from our statistical analysis would be around 0 (Figure 6.9).

A WORD OF WARNING

It should be reiterated that, even if you do find a strong positive or negative correlation, you still cannot conclude that the variables are causally related. However, many people do make this error. For example, when the AIDS problem started to reach public awareness a few years ago, one politician asked whether the condition was caused by Greek yoghurt, since he had noted that the amount of yoghurt appearing in supermarkets had risen alongside the number of reported AIDS cases. Almost certainly, had the data been analysed using the appropriate test, a positive correlation would have been found, but clearly Greek yoghurt was not responsible for causing the epidemic.

Key Concepts

- Positive correlations indicate that high scores on one variable are associated with high scores on the other.
  - They are represented by an upward slope on a scattergram.
  - They have a correlation coefficient near +1; the closer the coefficient to +1, the stronger the positive correlation.
- Negative correlations indicate that high scores on one variable are associated with low scores on the other.
  - They are represented by a downward slope on a scattergram.
  - They have a correlation coefficient of around −1; the nearer the coefficient to −1, the stronger the negative correlation.

- No correlation indicates that there is no relationship between the scores on the two variables.
  - They are represented by random clusterings on a scattergram with no obvious direction to the pattern.
  - They have a correlation coefficient of around 0, with the closer the coefficient to 0, the weaker the relationship between the two variables.

Activity 6.7 (Answers on p. 364)

1 Look at the following hypotheses and state whether they suggest positive or negative correlations between the variables. Also state how they would be represented on a scattergram, and where on a scale of −1 to +1 the correlation coefficient would be.
  (i) The older the patient, the longer the rehabilitation period following lower leg amputation.
  (ii) The further from an osteopathy clinic a patient lives, the less the likelihood of keeping an appointment.
  (iii) The lower the 'A'-level results of chiropractic students, the lower the exam mark in the final year.
  (iv) The higher the clinical therapist's occupational stress, the lower their job satisfaction.
2 Look at the following correlation coefficients and rank them from the strongest relationship to the weakest:

$$-0.73 - 0.42 + 0.61 + 0.21 - 0.17 + 0.09$$

Similarly, for several months, a Sunday newspaper made a deliberate mockery of assuming causality from statistical correlations. For example, it reported that over the previous few years the number of divorces had risen. Furthermore, it was noted that there had been an increase in the number of lofts that were being insulated. The paper concluded, tongue-in-cheek, that insulating lofts causes divorce. I'm sure you can see from this that, just because data are correlated, does not mean that they are also causally related.

MAKING PREDICTIONS

However, if you do find that two variables are correlated together, you can make predictions about one variable from information about the other. Therefore, if you found that two variables were negatively correlated, you could predict high scores on one variable from knowledge of low scores on the other and vice versa. Equally, if you found that two variables were positively correlated, you could predict high scores on one variable from a knowledge of high scores on the other or low scores could be predicted for one variable from a knowledge of low scores on the other.

For example, you might have established that there is a positive correlation between the degree of occupational stress a patient has and the level of spinal tension. If a patient then presents with a specified incidence of occupational stress, you would be able to predict from this knowledge how much spinal tension the patient was experiencing. This technique is known as linear regression and will be dealt with in more detail in Chapter 17.

There are other, more complex, ways of making predictions from correlated data, which are outside the scope of this book, because of the statistical complexities, but which have great value for health care professionals. For example, you might be interested in trying to establish risk factors for falls among the elderly, so that some sort of preventive action can be taken. Using techniques called **multiple** or **logistical regression** you could establish which of a range of correlated data were the best predictors of a fall (whether you use multiple of logistical regression depends on how you are measuring the variable you're predicting). You might find that age, living alone and early dementia were the best predictors of risk and therefore any elderly person who scored high on these risk factors might be targeted for some safety equipment (eg grip rails) at home. As a computer would be the best means of making these predictions, the reader is referred to Pallant (2007).

HOW CLOSE MUST THE CORRELATION BE?

We have already said that the nature of the scattergram and the correlation coefficient indicate the strength of the relationship between the two variables and that there is unlikely to be a perfect correlation. Therefore, how smooth must the scattergram slope be and how close must the correlation coefficient be to +1 or −1 before we decide that there is a relationship? Will +0.63 do? or −0.54? Because we cannot make an arbitrary decision like this, after we have calculated the correlation coefficient using a statistical test, we use a set of statistical tables to see whether the correlation coefficient is sufficiently big to indicate that the relationship between the two variables is significant. This will also depend on how many subjects you have used in your project.

We will deal with these concepts in more detail in Chapter 17.

ETHICS

We have already looked at some preliminary ethical issues as they relate to control or no-treatment groups. Ethical considerations go beyond the design of the study, however. Any piece of research that involves human subjects must endeavour to protect the rights, dignity, physical and psychological welfare of the participants; indeed, a project that compromises any aspect of a participant must be considered to be ethically questionable. Following some highly publicised scandals in the UK regarding the retention of human organs without consent, the issues of ethics and research probity have received a very high profile. In addition, the rise of the evidence-based care culture has created a concomitant rise in research studies within the health services. The pressure to conduct and publish research has resulted in a notable tightening of the research approval process, and most health organisations now require that every research proposal, whether the participants be patients, carers or staff, first go through an ethics committee. Ethical guidelines and procedures are available from the National Patient Safety Agency: http://www.nres.npsa.nhs.uk. There is also a comprehensive manual by Eckstein (2003), which readers might find useful.

Much has been written on ethics in research, but it may be worth outlining the six key principles (ICN 1996).

First is the principle of **beneficence**, which requires that the project should be able to demonstrate that there will be some benefit not only to those people participating in the study, but also to the wider population. This benefit might take the form of improved treatment procedures for a given condition, more screening or surveillance, etc.

The second principle is that of **non-maleficence**, which is a 'do no harm' rule. This aims to protect participants from physical or mental danger, which may be short or long term, permanent or temporary.

The third principle is **fidelity**, which is founded on the premise that, because the researcher must safeguard the participant, there must be trust between them. Central to this must be the participants' knowledge that the researcher will never put the research above their welfare.

The fourth principle is **justice**, which requires that all participants be treated equally and fairly. Enshrined within this is the notion that it would be inequitable to provide treatment to some patients whilst withholding it from others. This immediately challenges the methodological requirement for a control group, which demands that some participants will receive no intervention or treatment.

The fifth principle is **veracity**, which means that the participants should not be deceived at any stage of the study, especially its aims, processes, possible outcomes, side-effects, etc. Omission is just as culpable here as commission and therefore failing to tell the participants about any key aspect of the research may be just as unacceptable as proactively deceiving them. Since the use of double-blind procedures (see Chapter 8) and placebos is founded on a form of deception, their use may in some cases, be unethical.

The last principle is **confidentiality**, in that all the data collected during the research must be protected and all participants must be unidentifiable by anyone outside the research project. This has implications for dissemination of the research and its findings. This principle has further legal backing from the 1998 Data Protection Act. For further information, the reader is referred to: http://www.opsi.gov.uk/acts/acts1998/ukpga_19980029_en_1 or http://www.data-protection-act.co.uk/ for a more user-friendly interpretation.

As a good starting point to ensure that your study does not jeopardise the subject sample in any way, ask yourself the following questions.

What is the research topic?

Your research must start off with the assumption that its outcomes will be of benefit to someone other than the researcher. Research for its own sake, or which involves sensitive, embarrassing issues is unlikely to be permitted by ethical committees.

Who will undertake the research?

Any research involving human subjects must be conducted by someone who has sufficient skills and competence to undertake the necessary procedures without inadvertently harming the subjects, either physically or psychologically; moreover, the researcher should have fundamental respect for the participants. Remember, too, that the researcher is in a position of power and influence over the subjects; this authority must never be abused in order to coerce patients into taking part in a study against their will.

How will the participants be treated?

The protection of the participants must be the primary concern of every researcher; similarly, the major purpose of any ethical committee to which a research proposal is submitted is to ensure that no harm, of any sort, comes to the subjects. The particular ethical dilemma which faces health care researchers is the issue of informed consent, which demands that the participants knowingly, willingly, rationally and freely agree to take part. A great deal of health care research inevitably deals with vulnerable people (those in pain, the anxious, distressed, psychiatrically disturbed, elderly, young, confused, etc.) and, consequently, the problem of informed consent is magnified. Remember that the following guidelines must be adhered to:

- Never deceive or coerce the participants in any way.
- Always obtain their full and informed consent.

- Never embarrass or compromise the subjects; always preserve their dignity and wellbeing.
- Always ensure the participants' confidentiality and privacy.
- Always offer participants the right to withdraw from the research at any time, without jeopardising their current or future treatment.
- Always consult with and inform any relevant authority about the proposed research before embarking on it.
- Always discuss the methodology with experienced researchers to ensure that it is appropriate and that it can be carried out without damage to the patients.
- Be considerate, respectful and as objective as possible when conducting the research; always act with integrity.

How will the research be carried out?

Both qualitative and quantitative methodologies have ethical problems attached to them. The issue of control groups in experimental designs has already been discussed; in research designs where it would be unethical to withhold treatment for a group of subjects, or where a placebo condition is inappropriate, a second treatment group should be used instead. In qualitative studies, although there is no manipulation of treatment conditions, intrusive interviewing techniques that raise difficult, private and sensitive issues for the respondent create serious ethical concerns. Also, the interpretation that the researcher makes of qualitative data, such as free-response answers on a questionnaire, inevitably reflects the investigator's own values. This is not to suggest that the researcher deliberately distorts the subjects' responses, but rather that there will be an unavoidable degree of bias when making sense of any subjective database. This may mean that a subject's true intentions are misrepresented by the researcher's own perspectives and personal agendas. And, finally, observational studies that require the researcher to be present during any embarrassing intervention or examination process are clearly ethically problematic.

APPLYING FOR ETHICAL APPROVAL

The procedure for applying for ethical approval for a research project changes on a frequent basis, so it is difficult to provide definitive advice. The website http://www.nres.npsa.nhs.uk will evolve to provide updates on ethical procedures in the UK, but each country will have its own systems. However, the following information may be useful to anyone intending to undertake research in the UK and will provide general guidelines for anyone outside:

Ethical approval must be sought from an NHS Research and Ethics Committee, if the research involves:

- patients and users of health services; the personal and medical information of any patient past or present; their bodily material, including fetal material; anyone who has recently died on NHS property;
- their relatives or carers
- the use of NHS property
- NHS staff
- Using staff and inmates of any prison or young offenders' institution, if the project is health-based
- Patients, relatives and facilities of any private hospital or care home, if the participants have been referred by the NHS or the provider unit has a contract with the NHS.

(see http://www.nres.npsa.nhs.uk/applicants /apply/research-in-the-nhs)

If you have any doubts as to whether you need to apply for ethical approval for your study, then you can check the following website http://www.nres.npsa.nhs.uk/applicants/ apply/research-in-the-nhs/ or alternatively, you can send your proposal by post (see queries@nationaires.org.uk)

If you think you do need to obtain ethical approval, then the following guidance may be helpful; it is taken from http://nres.npsa.nhs. uk/applicants/apply/applying-for-ethical-review and also provides links to follow at each step:

1. Check that your project requires ethical clearance from an NHS Research and Ethics Committee (REC) – see http://www.nres.npsa. nhs.uk/applicants/apply/research-in-the-nhs

2. If it does, then you will need to complete the NRES online application form, ensuring that the Chief Investigator has signed it. Further

advice is provided on http://www.nres.npsa.nhs.uk/applicants/my-online-applications/

3. All applications must include the research protocol and the other relevant information noted; failure to supply all the material will mean that your proposal will not be reviewed.

4. The proposal then needs to be booked in with an NHS REC. Booking is normally done through a Central Allocation System (0845 270 4400).

5. The type of research may require you to make an additional application to further bodies eg if the study is a clinical trial of a medicine or product, then you would need to apply to the Medicines and Healthcare products Regulatory Agency (MHRA www.mhra.gov.uk). The details are available on the applying-for-ethical-review website cited above.

6. Your proposal will then be evaluated by an NHS REC, who all operate according to standardised procedures. There are different types of ethics committees, each of which deals with a different type of research. The applying-for-ethical-review website above provides a flowchart to show which sort of project should be submitted where.

7. The Central Allocation System will advise you of the first available slot for an appropriate REC to assess your proposal; you can take this first available space or you can opt to wait for a preferred REC.

8. REC meeting dates can be found on a link on the applying-for-ethical-review website. You must be prepared to attend the meeting or be available by phone.

9. You will be informed of the REC's judgement within 60 days of submitting a new proposal, or 35 days of submission of an amended proposal.

It would be unrealistic to suggest that applying for ethical approval is quick and easy; it isn't. However, at the time of writing (February 2008) a pilot scheme called the Integrated Research Application System (IRAS) is being trialled, in an attempt to streamline and simplify submissions. Its intention is to enable researchers to submit their proposal once and IRAS will collate all the information required to apply for ethical approval for a wide variety of research projects. Further information can be found on https://www.myresearchproject.org.uk. While this scheme is being piloted, the existing ethical processes described above will operate alongside.

Dissemination of the research

If a soundly conducted research study generates results that may have a beneficial impact on future patient care, then the researcher has a moral duty to publish the findings in a forum where optimal use can be made of them. In the process of publishing, though, the researcher must ensure that a full and fair account of the results is presented. It is unacceptable to reproduce only those aspects of the data set that support the original hypothesis. In addition, the results should be interpreted as objectively as possible, without making unrealistic or unsubstantiated claims that go beyond the actual data.

All health care research carries an obligation to respect and protect the welfare of its participants. Like other applied research areas, clinical therapy must ensure that its research studies maintain a suitable balance between ethical considerations and the validity of the research design.

FURTHER READING

Anthony D 2005 Regression analysis. Online. Available http://nurseresearcher.rcnpublishing.co.uk/resources/archive/GetArticleById.asp?ArticleId=6066

Brown B, Crawford P, Hicks C 2003 Evidence based research: dilemmas and debates in health care. Open University Press, Maidenhead

Chalmers AF 1999 What is this thing called science? 3rd edition. Hackett, London

Cohen L, Holliday M 1996 Practical statistics for students. Paul Chapman, London

Coolican H 2004 Research methods and statistics in psychology, 4th edition. Hodder Arnold, London

Coolican H 2006 Introduction to research methods in psychology, 3rd edition. Hodder Arnold, London

Eckstein S 2003 Manual for Research Ethics Committees, 6th Edition. Cambridge University Press, Cambridge

Field A, Hole G 2004 How to design and report experiments. Sage, London

Greene J, D'Oliveira M 2006 Learning to use statistical tests in psychology, 3rd edition. Open University Press, Buckingham

Greenhalgh T 1997 How to read a paper: statistics for the non-statistician II. BMJ 315:422–425

ICN 1996 Ethical guidelines for nursing research. International Council of Nurses, Geneva

Merrill Education 2006 A guide to ethical conduct for the helping professions, 2nd edition. Prentice Hall, London

National Patient Safety Agency. Online. Available http://www.nres.npsa.nhs.uk

Oliver P 2003 The students' guide to research ethics. Open University Press, Buckingham

Pallant J 2007 SPSS survival manual, 3rd edition. Open University Press, Buckingham

Polgar S, Thomas S 2007 Introduction to research in the health sciences. Churchill Livingstone, Edinburgh

Robson C 2002 Real world research: a resource for social scientists and practitioner-researchers, 2nd edition. Blackwell Publishing, Oxford

Walker W 2005 The strengths and weaknesses of research designs involving quantitative measures. Journal of Research in Nursing 10(50):571–582

Walley T 2007 Health technology assessment in England: assessment and appraisal. The Medical Journal of Australia 187(5):283–285

Watson R, Mckenna H, Cowman S, Keady J 2008 Nursing research: designs and methods. Edinburgh, Churchill Livingstone

Chapter 7

Designing your study

SOME BASIC CONCEPTS

DEFINITION OF SUBJECTS

When you carry out any research you will almost certainly recruit people (e.g. patients, clients or colleagues) to take part in it. The people who take part in research are called subjects; subjects are sometimes referred to as Ss, but are now more properly called participants. However, as most texts and many journals still use the term 'subjects', I will continue to use this words throughout the text. You will always have to decide what sort of subjects you need in your research, (e.g. trainee clinical therapists, elderly amputees, osteoporosis patients, etc.) and these subjects must be defined carefully and clearly. It is insufficient, for example, just to state 'hemiplegic patients' since the term covers a range of causes of problem and types of person. So you must be clear as to the precise nature of your subjects. The definition you use for who you are going to include is sometimes referred to as the 'inclusion criteria'. More will be said about this under the section on randomised controlled trials and in the next chapter.

GENERALISABILITY

Whoever you decide to use, there is a very important point to note: you don't want your results to apply only to the small group or sample of people you used in your experiment, as you need to be able to generalise your results. This is a crucial feature of research and central to the topic of inferential statistics. For example, supposing you had compared two different compensatory techniques (A and B) to aid the performance of basic self-help behaviours in elderly stroke patients, and had found much better results with the group using technique B. It is important that these results do not just apply to the small sample of subjects you used in your experiment, but that technique B will improve the skills performance in the majority of elderly stroke patients.

The point here is that, if your results can be generalised in this way, then predictions can be made, and this is another essential feature of research. So, when you have to treat a new elderly stroke patient, you can predict that self-help behaviours are more likely to be improved by technique B than by technique A, on the basis of the generalisability of the results from your research; this knowledge would support your choice of treatment.

But, short of carrying out your experiment on huge numbers of elderly stroke patients, how can you ascertain that your results are generalisable? We have already touched on this issue when the topic of inferential statistics was introduced. If you recall, inferential statistics allow the researcher to use a small sample of people in an experiment, and from the results of these experiments to infer that the same findings would apply to the larger population from which the sample comes. Now in order to be able to make this assumption, you must ensure that the sample you selected for study is sufficiently large and representative.

Sample size

The issue of sample size in relation to surveys has already been introduced in Chapter 3, but the whole problem of calculating an appropriate sample size for use in experimental work involves some different principles. These principles include many of the concepts that are introduced in the next chapter and so the topic of sample size will be dealt with there. It may, though, be worth reiterating the basic ideas here. A sample must be sufficiently large to ensure that it reflects the population from which it was derived.

Let's consider the situation whereby the manager responsible for hospital-based clinical therapy is thinking about altering the number of hours in the day shift. If she asks one clinical therapist out of the 30 under her, then it is less likely that she will receive a view which reflects the opinion of the whole group (or population) than if she asks 15 of the 30. In other words, the number of subjects you select for study must be sufficiently big for you to be able to generalise the results from your experiment.

What does this mean in practice? There is probably no simple answer to this, because an appropriate sample size depends upon a number of factors, in particular, the size of the effect of the IV and the power of the statistical test to detect the effect of the IV. These are quite complex points and are based upon some concepts that are covered in the next chapter. As a result, the details about sample size calculations will be dealt with there.

It should be noted that if you're dealing with a very rare condition, say, von Recklinghausen's syndrome, it will be unlikely that you will get many participants anyway, and therefore the whole point about calculating an adequate sample size is less relevant. In such instances, you may want to consider a single-case study instead. There are also situations where more subjects are required. Where this is the case, it will be pointed out in the relevant chapter. Similarly, in some of the worked statistical illustrations quoted in later chapters, only small sample sizes are used. This has been done simply for ease of calculation.

A representative sample

The sample must be representative of the population from which they come and so fairly typical. The easiest way to ensure reasonable typicality is to select your subjects randomly, for example. putting the names of all the elderly stroke patients you might have access to in a hat and randomly selecting 25 or 30. This point was covered in more detail in Chapter 3 and will be referred to again later in this chapter.

Before moving on though, it is important to recognise that you cannot always select your subjects randomly because there are practical problems or insufficient numbers of particular patients types. If you cannot obtain a proper probability sample then you must be aware of the limitations of generalising the results from your study.

TREATMENT OF YOUR SUBJECTS

Although ethical issues were discussed in more detail in the previous chapter, they are of sufficient importance to merit brief mention again, especially with regard to how you treat your subjects. You should never do anything to your subjects which would harm or upset them in any way. It is important that you treat your subjects well, that you do not deceive them or use your position to pressurise them to take part.

It is important that your subjects know what they are letting themselves in for before they agree to participate; in other words, they give their informed consent. In all events, your research project should be referred to the relevant ethical committee for consideration before you begin.

Failure to observe these guidelines would undoubtedly tarnish a researcher's reputation, has the potential to throw clinical therapy research into disrepute and could damage the participants physically or psychologically.

TYPES OF EXPERIMENTAL DESIGN

Whatever sort of participants are involved in your study, you will need to decide how to use them in the research design and this decision is a crucial one. Sometimes, to manipulate the IV the researcher has to select two or more groups of participants and compare them on the DV; at other times, it may be more appropriate to manipulate the IV by taking just one group of participants and measuring their responses on the DV on two or more occasions.

When two or more different groups of subjects are used and compared in a project, it is called an unrelated-, between- or different-subject design. When just one group of subjects is used in all conditions it is called a related-, within- or same-subject design. We will look at each of these more closely.

DIFFERENT- (UNRELATED- OR BETWEEN-) SUBJECT DESIGNS

It was said earlier that hypotheses could often be tested in different ways, using different types of experimental designs, and that it was the job of the experimenter to decide on the most suitable design for a particular hypothesis. However, for some hypotheses there is really only one obvious way to test them. Let's adapt the hypothesis given on p. 76 and predict that there will be an improvement in chiropractors' communication skills following either a counselling course or a social skills training course. We would need to use two different groups of chiropractors, one in each condition (i.e. type of course). The design looks like Figure 7.1.

At the end of the experiment the communication skills of the two groups would be compared to see if, in fact, the group who had attended the counselling course were significantly better.

This is a typical example of the sort of hypothesis which requires a different-subject design since it would have been totally inappropriate to use just one group for both conditions. If we think about this idea a bit more closely, it becomes clear that, if we had selected just one group of chiropractors to undertake both the counselling condition and the social skills training condition, all sorts of problems would have emerged.

Let's explore this a bit further. There are two possible ways of carrying out this experiment, using just one group of subjects. You could send your group of chiropractors either:

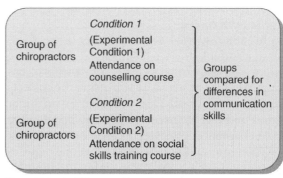

Figure 7.1   A different-subject design.

a. On a counselling course for 3 months
   followed by
   a social skills training course for 3 months

or

b. On a social skills training course for 3
   months followed by
   a counselling course for 3 months.

You can see from this that, although both conditions, or courses, have been assessed in each design, the results from the second condition would always be contaminated by the results from the first because the group had done both courses or conditions.

For example, in the first design, if we did find that there was a significant change in communication skills after going on a counselling course for 3 months and that there was no further change after the social skills training course, what could we really conclude about the second course? It may be that the social skills training course had no effect because the group's communication skills had changed as far as they could by the end of the counselling course, or because the second course provided a time for consolidating the skills already acquired. Alternatively, if we found that there was a change following the social skills training course, this may be due to the continued effect of the counselling course, or the effects of the social skills training course or the cumulative effect of both, but we wouldn't know which.

In the second design, the same argument applies: any change in communication skills found after doing the second course might simply be due to the combined effects of both courses, but we couldn't demonstrate that the difference in skills between the end of course 1 and the end of course 2 was exclusively the result of doing the second course.

In other words, whatever the order these designs adopt, any results obtained would have more than one explanation because we have contaminated the outcome by subjecting the subjects to both conditions. This is known as an order effect and will be discussed in more detail in the next chapter.

Therefore, an hypothesis like this one requires a different-subject design in order to eliminate the confounding effects of participating in both conditions. It is important to note here that, in this context, 'different' simply means 'separate'. In other words, in the previous example, while all the subjects were chiropractors and were therefore similar to each other, they were split into two separate or different groups.

There are many other hypotheses in clinical therapy research which necessitate using two or more different groups of subjects. For example, any comparisons of different races, ages, sexes, type of patient, health professionals, etc. all mean that different subjects have to be used. For example, if you wanted to compare the job satisfaction of the speech therapists and the occupational therapists working in a particular district, you would have to use one group of speech therapists and another group of occupational therapists. One subject group is quite obviously inappropriate here, since it is unlikely that someone would be simultaneously both a speech therapist and an occupational therapist.

In other words, if the manipulation of the independent variable simply involves the comparison of two or more inherently different groups of subjects (old vs. young, male vs. female, cardiac vs. carcinoma patients, etc.), you must use a different-subject design.

Remember that you don't need to confine yourself to the comparison of just two different or separate groups. It is perfectly acceptable to compare three or more groups. For instance, in the above example, a further group of physiotherapists and one of dieticians could also be compared with the speech and occupational therapists on job satisfaction, although the method of analysis will be different.

While it is sometimes essential to use different groups of subjects in your experiment, there is a major disadvantage in the design: that of individual differences among the subjects. If we look at the example regarding differences in job satisfaction between speech and occupational therapists, it is quite possible that some subjects will interpret the questions in an idiosyncratic way; a few might misunderstand the instructions for completing the questionnaires, while others may just have had a really difficult patient and consequently were feeling disenchanted at that moment; one or two may have just been promoted, while others may have been disappointed by the outcome of the same round of promotions. All these factors may influence how the subjects respond to the job satisfaction questionnaire and so will affect the results. For example, the speech therapist who has just seen a particularly difficult patient may be feeling frustrated and irritated at the time of completing the job satisfaction questionnaire. Therefore, his/her score may be low, but yet unrepresentative of how s/he normally feels about the work. While these individual differences may be evenly distributed among all the groups, thereby cancelling the effects out, it is also possible that more of the individual differences that affect the results may occur in only one of the groups and thus will artificially distort the results.

The problem of individual differences can be partly overcome by ensuring that the subjects are randomly selected and allocated to conditions if appropriate. Randomisation can mean one of two things in different subject designs. First, it can mean randomly selecting a group of subjects (e.g. knee replacement patients) and, second, it can mean randomly allocating half of participants to one treatment and half to the other, in order to compare the effects. Obviously, the second sort of randomisation cannot be done in our example about the job satisfaction of different clinical therapy professions, since it would not be possible to select a group of health carers and randomly allocate them to being speech therapists or occupational therapists. Here randomness means something different: that the subjects in each group should be a random, and therefore typical, selection of the group they represent. In other words, the subjects drawn from the speech therapy group should be reasonably typical of the speech therapists in the district, and not all particularly demotivated, overly conscientious, awkward or anything else. The same should be true of the subjects in the occupational therapy group. The ways in which random selection can be achieved are outlined in Chapter 3.

SAME- (RELATED- OR WITHIN-) SUBJECT DESIGNS

Some hypotheses, however, are not suited to using designs with different subjects in each con-

dition. Some hypotheses are more suited to being tested by designs which use only one group of subjects, but this group is measured under all the conditions and its performance in each condition is compared.

> ### Key Concepts
>
> When two or more different groups of subjects are used in an experiment it is called
>
> an **unrelated-subject** design
>
> or
>
> a **between-subject** design
>
> or
>
> a **different-subject** design.
>
> The advantages of this design are that it can overcome any problems associated with the order of conditions and it is also essential when 'fixed' differences such as race, sex, ages, types of patient are being compared.
>
> However, its major disadvantage is that individual differences among the subjects may distort the results. This can be partially overcome by randomly selecting the subjects and then randomly allocating them to conditions, where possible.

For example, you might be interested in looking at the level of confidence a group of elderly patients had in uniformed vs. non-uniformed community podiatrists. Here, you would randomly select a group of patients and ask them to indicate how confident they felt (a) when being treated by a uniformed podiatrist and (b) when being treated by a non-uniformed podiatrist. The design would look like Figure 7.2.

Thus, one group of subjects is tested under both conditions and the two sets of ratings are

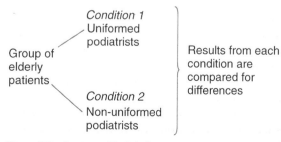

Figure 7.2 A same-subject design.

compared to see if there is any difference between them.

It would be inappropriate here to use two groups of patients, one to rate the uniformed podiatrists and the other to rate the non-uniformed, because the groups may differ inherently in a number of ways which would affect the outcome of the results. For example, one group may be generally more confident anyway, may love all uniforms, or may try harder to please the experimenter by inflating their ratings, etc., and we wouldn't know this because we have nothing against which to measure their ratings. Hence, there may be basic individual differences between the two groups which might affect the results and which would prevent us from establishing any baseline for comparison.

However, if we use just one group of patients, then whatever their idiosyncrasies and personal characteristics, they will at least be constant over both ratings. The subject group, then, serves as its own control. Therefore, one important advantage of a same-subject design is the fact that it overcomes the problem of individual differences inherent in different-subject designs. Because of this, it is especially useful in 'before and after' type experiments, where the researcher wants to look at the effects of a treatment procedure on a group of subjects. Common examples of this are the television advertisements for washing powder, showing viewers the dirty washing before being washed in the product and the same linen after being washed. The same clothes are used when the before and after assessments are made, and thus constitutes a same-subject design.

However, this design too has its snags. If we look at the example concerning podiatrists' dress, supposing we gave all the subjects the uniformed rating-task first and the non-uniformed rating-task second. It is quite conceivable that on the first task they didn't quite understand what was required of them and so filled in the questionnaire using the wrong criteria, while by the second task they had realised what they had to do. This may well distort the results. Alternatively, it could be argued that, by the time the second task had to be completed, the subjects were bored or tired and so filled in lower confidence ratings. In other words, the results may have been affected by the order in which the tasks were carried out. Therefore, to overcome this, half the subjects should do task A first, followed by task B, while, for the remaining subjects, the order would be reversed. This is called counterbalancing and is discussed more fully in Chapter 8.

It should also be noted that one group of subjects can be tested on more than two occasions. For example, you might wish to look at the pain levels experienced by a group of women in the first stage of labour using TENS (transcutaneous electrical nerve stimulation). To do this, you decide to select one group of, say, 20 women and you assess their pain levels before using TENS, 1 hour after using TENS, 2 hours after using TENS and 3 hours after using TENS. Your design would look like Figure 7.3.

You have here a same-subject design, with the subjects being measured under four conditions, to establish whether the use of TENS makes any difference to their pain levels.

Key Concepts

When one group of subjects is tested or measured on all the conditions and their performance compared, it is known as

a **related-subject** design

or

a **same-subject** design

or

a **within-subject** design.

The advantage of this design is that it eliminates the distorting effects of individual subject differences.

However, it has two disadvantages: firstly, it cannot be used when 'fixed' differences such as sex, race, type of ailment are being compared, and secondly, any effects deriving from the order of the conditions may have to be counterbalanced.

MATCHED-SUBJECT DESIGNS

One way of overcoming all the disadvantages of both different- and same-subject designs is to use two or more groups of subjects who are matched on a number of characteristics. Let's take an

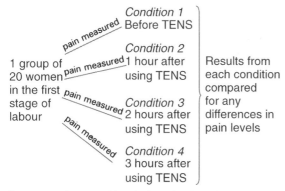

Figure 7.3 A same-subject design, with the subjects being measured under four conditions.

example. Suppose you wanted to compare the recovery times of leg fractures resulting from road traffic accidents (RTAs) and leg fractures resulting from sports injuries. Obviously you cannot use a same-subject design, since a patient's fracture cannot simultaneously be due to an RTA and sports injury, and, if you use a different-subject design, you might find a number of individual differences in the subjects which predisposed one group to recover more quickly than the other. For example, the sports injuries patients may be younger, male, fitter and stronger, whereas the RTA patients may be less fit, older, diabetic and include females. In addition, the amount and type of treatment may be different for each group. All these factors may influence recovery rates. In such cases, then, it is necessary to try to identify the characteristics which may bias the results of the experiment and to ensure that the groups are matched on these factors.

The way in which the matching is carried out involves, first, identifying all the possible characteristics which may influence the results, and then selecting a subject (for example, an RTA patient) and assessing how s/he rates on these characteristics. For example, in this case, you might note their age, sex, degree of fitness (perhaps by heart rate, pulse rate, blood pressure), previous fractures to the leg (and anything else you feel may bias the results). You must then find another patient in the sports injuries category who is the same age and sex, has the same fitness ratings, has had the same number of previous fractures to the leg and has other charac-

teristics similar to the RTA patient. You then need to find the next set of 'twins' and so on. These twinned patients do not need to be identical to the first pair selected, but they must be the same as each other. Therefore, in terms of the personal characteristics which are likely to influence the results from the experiment, each pair of subjects is like identical twins, with the only difference between them being the way in which the fracture occurred. Thus, for every subject in one group, there is an 'identical twin' in the other. However, the matching shouldn't stop there. You would also need to ensure that the quality, type and extent of treatment were also the same for each patient, together with any other factors which were likely to influence the study's outcomes.

When you are involved in comparing 'non-fixed' groups (e.g. the effects of two different treatments), you can match up a pair of subjects first and then randomly allocate one subject to one treatment and the 'twin' to the other treatment. Because of the similarity of the subjects, matched designs are treated like same-subject designs for the purposes of statistical analysis. Similarly, as with same-subject designs, the matched design overcomes the problem of individual differences, because of the 'twinning' of the subjects. Yet the matched-design has all the advantages of a different-subject design, since 'fixed' groups can be compared and there need be no order effects.

So why don't we always use matched designs if they're so good? I'm sure you will have realised already that it is often extremely difficult to match pairs of subjects in this way, usually because there are limited numbers of suitable subjects to choose from. Even if we allow ourselves a little leeway, say by matching an RTA patient aged 30 with a sports injury patient aged 28, there may still be many important differences between the subject pair that we either cannot identify or cannot match for (e.g. biochemical composition of bones and blood that affects healing rates). Thus, while these designs are theoretically very desirable, in practical terms they are extremely difficult to implement properly.

It must be stressed that it is not adequate simply to select 20 RTAs and 20 sports injury patients, all of whom are male and under 40, and say that you've matched them. For every subject in one group, there must be a 'twinned' subject in the other, matched on all the relevant variables which may influence the outcome of the experiment. Therefore, because of the difficulties involved in matching people, caused largely through our lack of knowledge of which factors are relevant, it is usually desirable to use a same-subject design in preference to a matched-subject design. As one eminent statistician notes:

> A matching design is only as good as the experimenter's ability to determine how to match the pairs, and this ability is frequently very limited. Sidney Siegel (1956, p 62)

While matched-subject designs can be used with more than two groups of subjects, because of the problems outlined above, it is very unlikely that you will ever be able to match subjects up in 'triplets' or 'quadruplets', and so this may be better avoided.

Key Concepts

Matched designs involve selecting pairs of subjects, matched on every variable which may influence the outcome of the experiment, and allocating one of the pair to one condition and one to the other.

This design has all the advantages of same- and different-subject designs.

It has the major disadvantage that it is very difficult to match subjects in this way, because, firstly, it is not always possible to find subjects who are sufficiently similar, and, secondly, you can never be sure that you have matched pairs of subjects on all the factors that may influence the results.

RANDOMISED CONTROLLED TRIALS

So far, in this chapter, we have covered the basic principles of experimental designs and, for most readers of this book, this may be sufficient. However, a text on research methods for health care professionals would no longer be complete without some discussion of the randomised controlled trial (RCT). Widely considered to be the gold standard of health research because of its capacity to eliminate bias, the results derived

from RCTs are used to inform clinical decision-making, treatment guidelines and protocols, nationally and internationally. RCTs, though, have been criticised as having only limited relevance in the evaluation of many health care interventions, but, because of their rigour and assumed objectivity, the value of the RCT is very highly rated and, consequently, the results from RCTs are considered to be invaluable in guiding health provision. It is unlikely that any reader will be interested in setting up an RCT single-handedly, simply because of the size, complexity and cost. But it is quite conceivable that some readers may be involved in a team which designs and conducts an RCT. Therefore, this section will outline some of the fundamental concepts that underpin these gold-standard research designs. Further details are available in Jadad (1998) and Duley & Farrell (2002).

The RCT embodies many of the principles of the experimental design, with its principal focus being the elimination of bias at all stages of the research study. Therefore, it demands that subjects are randomly allocated to conditions or treatment groups (see pp. 92–93), with each group receiving a different intervention. The results or outcomes of these interventions are compared for any differences between them. The outcomes are always measurable or quantifiable (as opposed to being qualitative). The RCT can be conducted with numerous treatment groups, or just with one treatment group and one control group (see pp. 76–77). In this sense, the RCT is an experimental design of the sort discussed earlier in this chapter.

However, the essential features that characterise an RCT are that:

- Participants are randomised to treatment groups.
- The characteristics of the participants in the groups are very similar, so that any differences in outcome can be more reliably attributed to the effects of the treatment.
- It uses a double-blind procedure, so that neither the participants nor the health professionals treating them know which treatment any given patient is receiving.
- It is controlled, in that one group receives either no treatment or a placebo treatment; in

this way, the effects of the intervention can be compared with the non-intervention.

- The outcomes are measurable in numerical terms.
- The procedures are standardised, such that the groups are all treated in an identical manner, with the obvious exception of the intervention itself.

We will take each feature in turn.

RANDOM ALLOCATION

The participants in an RCT must be randomly allocated to treatment groups. Random allocation is strictly defined to mean that all the participants have the same chance of being allotted to any of the groups in the study (i.e. the control and the treatment groups). Randomisation in RCTs demands certain procedures to be fulfilled, all of which are intended to minimise the effects of bias. First, the participants and the health carers involved must not be aware of the treatment group to which any patient has been assigned. This is called the double-blind procedure and will be discussed later and in Chapter 8. In essence it is a safeguard against any distortion in the outcome that may result from the knowledge of the type of treatment received. Second, the method of randomisation must be decided in advance. Third, this system must be adhered to throughout the study.

While the best way to achieve randomisation continues to be debated, the simplest method involves tossing a coin and allocating participants on the basis of the heads/tails results. Clearly, this can only be used when the RCT consists of a single intervention and control group. When more intervention groups are involved, rolling a dice or using random number tables are acceptable options (see pp. 30–31). Other forms of random sampling can be used, such as stratified random sampling (pp. 31–32), randomised block designs, which enable the investigator to allocate the same number of participants to each intervention, and weighted randomisation, which allows unequal numbers of participants to be allocated to each intervention. This procedure is useful when there are concerns about the safety of the intervention, because par-

ticipants can be kept to a minimum. For a more detailed description of these randomisation processes the reader is referred to Jadad (1998).

COMPARABILITY OF GROUPS

Random allocation also decreases the chances of individual differences distorting the outcomes. If participants are randomly allotted to groups, then there is a high chance that any quirks or individual differences that could influence or bias the results will be equally distributed across the groups (see pp. 93–95). Therefore, the groups are considered to be balanced at baseline. On this basis, any differences between the groups at the conclusion of the RCT can be more confidently attributed to the effects of the intervention. It should be noted that, while these randomisation processes reduce the risk of bias, they do not eliminate it.

Although the randomisation process is intended to ensure that the groups are balanced at baseline, the initial identification of suitable participants for a trial is also important. This requires the investigator to stipulate clear and explicit inclusion and exclusion criteria. For example, an RCT comparing the effects of electrical stimulation on the mobility of stroke patients might specify that only patients are eligible for inclusion if they are:

- Between the ages of 70 and 80 (excludes those younger than 70 and older than 80).
- Have right hemisphere lesions only (excludes those with left and left + right lesions).
- Have no co-morbidities (excludes those with cardiac problems, progressive illnesses, etc.).

These criteria must be made clear at the outset of the RCT and must be adhered to throughout the recruitment process. However, it should be noted that the results from the RCT will only be generalisable to other patients who are similar to the study group and not to the population of stroke patients as a whole. The problem of whether to be restrictive or permissive when deciding the inclusion/exclusion criteria is debatable and both options have their strengths and weaknesses.

DOUBLE-BLIND PROCEDURES

Two other points are important to randomisation. First, the nature of the intervention to which a participant has been allocated should be concealed from the health professionals delivering the treatment, as well as from the participants themselves (see pp. 105–106). This brings with it certain ethical problems, because duplicity and concealment of information compromises ethical principles and informed consent (see section on ethics, pp. 86–89). It is also worthy of note that blinding a participant to the nature of the treatment is at least practically possible when the intervention is pharmacological or physical, because the control group can be given a placebo pill or treated with a pointless exercise programme. It is not as easy when surgical interventions are being evaluated, because the patient will know quite clearly whether or not they have been operated on. Placebo operations, while they have been conducted, generate very serious ethical concerns.

Second, the individual responsible for the randomisation should not be a member of staff involved in conducting the RCT or in delivering care. Knowledge of the nature of the treatment can give rise to demand characteristics and bias (see pp. 105–106).

CONTROL GROUPS

The RCT, as its name suggests, partly depends for its success on the use of a control or non-treatment group. Non-treatment often takes the form of a placebo intervention, which, as has already been noted, brings with it serious ethical problems, in that denying a patient access to a treatment may well be morally indefensible. Consequently, the control group often takes the form of the standard treatment. So, for example in our study of stroke patients, the standard treatment might be a simple exercise regime and this would constitute the 'control' group in the study. In the strictest sense, this is not a true control group, because the patients are receiving some form of treatment; however, the use of the standard intervention as a control condition offsets many of the ethical problems.

NUMERICAL MEASUREMENT

The RCT is a quantitative methodology in that it collects numerical data for analysis. The analysis ascertains whether or not the intervention has had any effect on the outcomes. The larger the sample the more likely it is that an effect will be observed (see sample size calculations in Chapter 8); thus RCTs typically recruit large numbers of participants. However, statistical significance is not necessarily the same as clinical significance, and so the size of the required clinical effect should be stipulated in advance. This point is developed in Chapter 8.

STANDARDISATION OF PROCEDURES

This aspect of the RCT is also intended to minimise the potential for bias. In other words, all the groups must be treated in exactly the same way, with the obvious exception of the actual treatment itself. In the previous stroke patient example it would not be acceptable to give the electrical stimulation group additional occupational therapy help whilst withholding it from the standard treatment group.

The RCT, while being generally regarded as the most valuable source of health care research data, is not without its critics. While this is not the place to debate the arguments for and against the RCT, it may be worth pointing out that there are many topics within clinical practice that cannot easily be subjected to RCT scrutiny. For example, any holistic treatment that involves a variety of complex interpersonal interactions or inputs cannot be usefully reduced to an RCT. Take for example, the psychotherapeutic treatment of a patient with eating disorders. This intervention depends for its success on a multiplicity of dynamic, interactive contextual factors, such as the relationship between the client and the therapist, the relationship between the client and the family, the relationship between the client and the other patients, the relationship between the client and the peer group, the social context and history of the client, etc. It would be quite meaningless to select a single element of this picture and attempt to monitor and control it through an RCT.

Moreover, despite the protocols introduced to try to eliminate bias in RCTs, the human, political and economic framework which determines the health topics, patients and products to be evaluated by the RCT, as well as how the results are to be analysed and disseminated, all introduce an inevitable aspect of bias (see Rogers 2002, for a discussion of this). So, the RCT properly conducted can usefully inform the health care professional's choice of clinical interventions, but it is not as unbiased or as useful as its many advocates would suggest, and it is definitely inappropriate for some complex health care interventions which are holistic in nature. In other words, it has a valuable role in informing health care, but it is not the sole way of providing this information.

- The results are always quantifiable, as opposed to being qualitative.
- The procedures are standardised, such that the only difference between the groups is the nature of the intervention itself.
- While the RCT can provide valuable evidence that can inform health care, it cannot usefully investigate more holistic interventions.

Key Concepts

Randomised controlled trials (RCTs) are a rigorous form of experimental design; they are considered to be the gold standard of health research because of their ability to minimise bias.

They are characterised by:

- The random allocation of subjects to either the treatment(s) or control group using tightly defined randomisation procedures.
- The use of a control group, which can receive no treatment, a placebo or the standard treatment.
- The comparability of the groups at the outset of the RCT; this is known as being balanced at baseline.
- The use of double-blind procedures, whereby neither the participants nor the health professionals treating them know whether they are receiving the active or placebo/control intervention.

FURTHER READING

Brown B, Crawford P, Hicks C 2003 Evidence-based health; dilemmas and debates. Buckingham, Open University Press

Cohen L, Holliday M 1996 Practical statistics for students. Hodder Arnold, London

Coolican H 2004 Research methods and statistics in psychology, 4th edition. Hodder and Stoughton, London

Coolican H 2006 Introduction to research methods in psychology, 3rd edition. Hodder Arnold, London

Duley L, Farrell B (eds) 2002 Clinical trials. BMJ, London

Greene J, D'Oliveira M 2005 Learning to use statistical tests in psychology 3rd edition. Buckingham, Open University Press

Jadad AR 1998 Randomised controlled trials: a user's guide. BMJ, London

Peat J 2001 Health science research; a handbook of quantitative methods. Sage Publishing, London

Pett M 1997 Nonparametric statistics in health care research. Sage Publishing, London

Polgar S, Thomas S 2007 Introduction to research in the health sciences. Churchill Livingstone, Edinburgh

Rogers WA 2002 Evidence-based medicine in practice: limiting or facilitating patient choice? Health Expectations 5:95–103

Siegel S 1956 Nonparametric statistics for the behavioural sciences. McGraw Hill Kogakusha, Tokyo

Watson R, Mckenna H, Cowman S, Keady J 2008 Nursing research: designs and methods. Churchill Livingstone, Edinburgh

Chapter 8

Sources of error in research

There are a number of potential sources of bias or error which can creep into the design of an experiment. These may distort your results and therefore must be controlled for. We will look at each of these separately.

ORDER EFFECTS

When a piece of research is carried out that follows an experimental design, the experimenter manipulates the independent variable (IV) and measures the effect of this on the dependent variable (DV), in the hope that altering the IV will have a significant effect on the DV. Changes in the DV are called the experimental effect and constitute the data in your study.

Let's take an example. Suppose you had hypothesised that clinical therapy students perform worse on a neurological placement than on an orthopaedic placement during their second year of training; in other words you are predicting a relationship between type of placement (IV) and performance (DV). To test this, you set up the experiment shown in Figure 8.1.

This is a same-subject design, with one group of students being measured on two occasions and their performances in both placements compared (using the appropriate statistical test) to see if they differ.

Let us assume that you did in fact find that students seem to do better on orthopaedic placements; can we conclude that the results are the

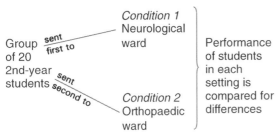

Figure 8.1   A same-subject design, with one group of subjects being measured on two occasions.

Table 8.1   A suggested order of three clinical placements

Subgroup	Placement		
	A	B	C
1	1	2	3
2	2	3	1
3	3	1	2

effect of some inherent difficulty associated with neurological clinical therapy? Or might there be some other explanation?

One obvious alternative explanation that we've already touched on, and you've probably thought of, relates to the sequence of the placements. If the students' first placement is on a neurological ward and their subsequent placement is on an orthopaedic ward, it is conceivable that their improved performance in the latter case may be due simply to the fact that it was second. In other words, the students may do better on any second placement (regardless of its nature) because they are more confident, more skilled, more familiar with hospital routines, etc.; they are more practised. Hence, this is known as a **practice effect**. It is, of course, equally likely that students do worse on their second placement because they are more jaundiced, more tired, less motivated, etc. This is known as a **fatigue effect**.

Regardless of which way performance is affected, the general issue is the same: that order effects, rather than the IV (in this case, the nature of the placement itself), could be influencing students' performance. Order effects are a common problem in experiments where one group of subjects is compared on two or more conditions, i.e. same-subject designs.

COUNTERBALANCING

To get round the problem of order effects, a technique called **counterbalancing** is used, where half the subjects do activity A first, followed by activity B, while the other half do activity B first, followed by activity A.

In our example, then, 10 students would do their neurological placement first, followed by the orthopaedic placement, while for the remain-

ing 10 the order would be reversed. At the end of the study, all the neurological ratings would be compared with all the orthopaedic ratings. In this way, any effects of order will be evened out. You can select which students do which placement first by randomising them, using any of the systems outlined on pp. 30–31. It is important to ensure that the students are randomly allocated. Don't put all your worst students into neurology first just to prove your point! The section on random selection (pp. 30–32) may clarify this point further.

So, by counterbalancing in this way, any bias in the results due to order effects is balanced out. One point is important here: we cannot eliminate order effects totally, because one activity must precede the other in designs like this. All we can do is to balance out the order effects as far as possible. Where you have more than two conditions, you will need to ensure that each subgroup of subjects is assessed in every position. So, if you had three placements (A, B and C), you would need to break your group down into three subgroups, using random allocation methods, and then allocate them as shown in Table 8.1.

This would still not eliminate completely the possible effects of order. There are much more complex methods of counterbalancing which would do more to control order effects. For example, in the above example, the sample could be randomly broken down into six subgroups, such that every possible combination of placement order can be covered: e.g. group 1 = ABC, group 2 = BCA, group 3 = CAB, group 4 = ACB, group 5 = BAC and group 6 = CBA. For a lot of research, the simpler techniques should suffice.

So, one explanation for the results from the experiment described above is the possible influence of order effects. However, even if you had counterbalanced these, there are still other variables which could account for your results.

Key Concepts

If one group of subjects has to be measured in all the conditions then the order in which they do these conditions may influence the results. For example, they may perform better on the last activity because of **practice effects**, or they may perform worse on the last activity because of **fatigue effects**.

In order to eliminate these sources of bias, the order in which the subjects carry out the activities should be counterbalanced, such that half the subjects do activity A first, followed by B, while for the remainder, the order is reversed.

EXPERIMENTER BIAS EFFECTS

Suppose, like all experimenters, you are very committed to your research and are very keen that your hypothesis will be supported – in this case, that students will do worse on neurological wards. It is conceivable that, in your anxiety and enthusiasm to obtain the predicted outcome, you will unwittingly influence the results.

I don't mean by this that you will cook the books, but that you may unintentionally use a slightly different set of criteria when assessing the students on each placement, perhaps ignoring some negative things on the orthopaedic placement, or putting more emphasis on other factors while carrying out the evaluation. In other words, you may have a set of expectations about the outcome of the experiment which will influence what you perceive, how you behave, etc.

Alternatively, you may unconsciously influence your subjects' responses by using a set of non-verbal cues. Imagine in the present example, you had decided, as an additional outcome measure, to elicit the students' subjective evaluations of their placements. You interview the first student on the neurological placement and s/he starts to say how awful it was, how incompetent and unskilled they felt, etc. This is exactly what you want to hear because it supports your hypothesis! And when we hear something we like we automatically respond with a set of non-verbal cues which the other person quickly picks up; for instance, we might smile, nod our head, lean forward into the conversation, all of which

encourages the other person to go on saying similar things. When we hear something we don't like, we might frown or lean back (symbolically rejecting the content of the discussion) and this has the effect of discouraging further comments of that type.

In addition, the subjects may take a dislike to the experimenter and so deliberately say things they know will not support the hypothesis; conversely, they may like the experimenter and distort their responses to help him/her.

In all cases, there is the potential for bias, particularly where the data involve subjective report. Such influences are very common and are known as **experimenter bias effects**. Other sources of experimenter bias include the personal characteristics of the experimenter, such as status, sex, class, race, age and so on, all of which may have some effect on the subjects and their performance.

It should be emphasised that normally such experimenter influences are quite unintentional and unconscious, but there is a great deal of documented evidence to show that they exist. How can we get round this problem?

'BLIND' PROCEDURES

The usual solution is to operate a **'blind' procedure**, whereby you ask someone who does not know what your hypothesis is to collect your data; in this case, to assess the students. Because the data collector is not aware of what you have predicted, s/he will also not know how the students are meant to behave in each placement and so the evaluation of the students' performance should be much more objective.

Blind procedures may be of two sorts: **single-blind** procedures where *either* the subject or the person collecting the data is unaware of the hypothesis being tested, or alternatively, **double-blind** procedures where *neither* party knows what the aims of the study are. This sort of double-blind procedure is very common in medical research, particularly when carrying out drug trials (see the section on RCTs in the previous chapter). In these cases, one group of patients is given the drug being evaluated, while another group is given a placebo. Neither the doctors assessing the outcome nor the patients themselves know who has been given which. In this way, the results cannot be biased by expectations, or deliberate or unintentional manipulation.

Key Concepts

Sometimes experimenters unwittingly influence the outcome of their experiment by the way in which they behave, appear or interact with the subjects. This is known as **experimenter bias**. Subjects sometimes distort their responses too.

To overcome this sort of problem in your research, you should use a **blind** procedure, whereby you ask someone who is absolutely unaware of what your hypothesis is to collect your data from subjects who may also be unaware of your hypothesis. In this way, any bias due to expectations and predictions will be eliminated.

However, there are still other variables which may influence our results (apart from the manipulation of the IV), even if we control for order and experimenter bias effects. These are called **constant errors** and **random errors**. Let's look at constant errors first.

CONSTANT ERRORS

Constant errors are all the possible sources of bias and influence that will affect the results in a constant and predictable way.

If we go back to our example of comparing students' performance on two placements, we can identify a number of potential sources of constant error. Suppose the neurological ward had 50 patients, 2 qualified clinical therapists and 10 students, while the orthopaedic ward had 25 patients, 5 qualified staff and 10 students. Under such conditions, it is quite possible that students do less well on the neurological ward because (a) of greater patient-to-staff ratios, which would increase workload, pressure, tension, etc., and (b) they have fewer qualified clinical therapists available to teach and support them. Therefore, their poor performance may be the direct result of these variables and not to do with problems inherent to neurological work. Also, the hospital manager responsible for clinical therapies at the neurological hospital may dislike the disruption caused by students and so may be less facilitative in a number of ways. The neurological placement may also involve a more arduous journey to the hospital (students arrive feeling fatigued), or longer shifts, or any one of a number of other problems.

Note that each of these factors can be called a constant error because of the predictable way in which they would distort the results. For example, poor patient–staff ratios are more likely to depress students' performance than improve it and so the effect of this variable is constant; less tuition will also depress, not improve, performance, as will fatigue. Thus, each of these factors will have a similar effect on all the students and so will distort the results in a constant, predictable way.

It is your job as a researcher to try to identify all the possible sources of constant error in your experiment and either eliminate or control them. If you leave any constant error uncontrolled then your results may be explained by that, rather than by the manipulation of the IV. Taking the constant errors quoted as examples here, we can eliminate or control them as shown in Table 8.2. In other words, you must standardise all aspects of the experimental situation in each placement.

Thus, when designing an experiment you must try to highlight all the factors which will

Table 8.2 Control or elimination of constant errors

Constant error	Solution
Different patient/ staff ratios	Ensure both placements have comparable ratios
Different numbers of qualified staff to act as tutors	Ensure ratios of students/ qualified staff are the same in each placement
Different amounts of supervision times	Ensure students in each placement receive the same amounts of clinical instruction
Different journey lengths	Either select placements which are equidistant or arrange transport to hospitals such that travelling times and problems are similar
Different shift times/ lengths	Ensure students in each placement work the same number of hours at similar times of day

bias your results in a constant and predictable way, and then attempt to eliminate or control these factors by standardising the situation and procedures in each condition.

RANDOM ERRORS

Random errors are not as easy to deal with. As their name suggests, they are random: randomly occurring, randomly distributed and with a random and unpredictable impact on the results. If we look back to our example, we identified some factors that would influence our results in a very predictable way, but there are other factors, the random errors, which will obscure our results in a totally variable or chance way.

In the above example, the moods of the patients, staff and students will all have an effect on performance. If all the neurological patients were always in a bad mood and all the orthopaedic patients always in a good mood, then moods would influence the results in a predictable way and so would be classified as constant errors. But moods aren't like that: they fluctuate up and down and interact with other people's behaviour, moods and attitudes. As a result they cannot be eliminated or controlled. Transitory changes in health among the patients, staff and students, their personalities, attitudes, beliefs, motivations, etc. are all examples of random error factors which will affect the results in an unpredictable, chance way and about which we can do very little.

The only real precaution that we can take against random errors is to ensure as far as possible that the people involved in our research are drawn randomly from the population they represent. Therefore, our students in the placement illustration should be fairly typical of clinical therapy students as a whole and not particularly deviant, disturbed, problematic, good, able or anything else. The neurological patients should be fairly typical of neurology patients as a whole, and similarly with the orthopaedic patients and staff. In this way the random errors should be fairly evenly distributed across both the placements, and therefore should (at least theoretically) affect the students' performance in each setting in a similar, if random, way.

One other point is important here: your subjects should be randomly allocated to conditions if possible (e.g. to different treatments, or, in this case, allocating students to a particular order of placements), because the random errors will then be evenly distributed – at least theoretically.

Key Concepts

- **Constant errors** are those factors that distort the results in a constant or predictable way. They can be eliminated or controlled by ensuring the procedures, conditions and other essential factors are similar.
- **Random errors** are those factors which obscure the results in a random or unpredictable way. They cannot be eliminated, although random selection and allocation of subjects will distribute them evenly across conditions (at least theoretically).

Activity 8.1 (Answers on p. 364)

Look at the following hypotheses and identify the sources of constant and random error and their solutions:

H_1 Men are more likely to suffer respiratory complications following thoracic surgery than are women.

H_1 Chiropractic achieves recovery rates for lumbar spine injury patients that are different from those of physiotherapy.

PROBABILITIES

If we cannot get rid of random errors, how can we be sure that the results from our experiment are due to some real and significant relationship between the variables (i.e. the impact of the IV on the DV), as predicted in the hypothesis, and not to the obscuring effect of random errors? The answer to this lies in the use of statistical tests. At a general level, when we use a statistical test to analyse a set of results, we end up with a numerical value. This value is looked up in a set of probability tables, to give us a probability or p value, which is expressed either as a decimal (e.g. 0.01) or as a percentage (e.g. 1%). The p value tells us how probable it is that the results from our experiment are due to random errors. It is very important to understand and remember this, as it is the basis of all statistical analyses.

Because this p value tells us how likely it is that the results from the experiment are due to random error (and not to the real and consistent relationship predicted in your hypothesis), then the smaller the p value, the smaller the possibility that random error or chance factors can account for your results. Therefore, by implication, the smaller the possibility that your results are due to random error, then the greater the possibility that they are due to the relationship you predicted in your hypothesis. Thus, the smaller the p value, the greater the implied support for your experimental hypothesis.

Do bear in mind that it is highly unlikely that you will ever get 100% support for your hypothesis, and so p will always have a value greater than 0. If your p value is very low, then you can reject the null (no relationship) hypothesis and conclude the experimental hypothesis has been supported. [Remember! When we carry out an experiment we do not set out to support our experimental hypothesis directly, but instead, we try to reject the null (no relationship) hypothesis.]

Probability values can be expressed either as a percentage or as a decimal. Therefore, if our p value was 5% (or 0.05), then we could say that there is a 5% chance that the results are due to random error. A p value of 3% means that there is a 3/100 chance that your results are due to the effects of chance or random error factors. Put crudely, then, the smaller the p value you obtain for your results the less the probability that random error can explain your findings and, consequently, the better it is for your hypothesis.

Key Concepts

When you carry out a statistical analysis, you end up with a numerical value which you look up in a set of probability tables to give you a p value. The p value tells you how likely it is that the results from your experiment are due to random error or chance. The smaller the p value, the stronger the support for your hypothesis. The p values are expressed as percentages or decimals.

Activity 8.2 (Answers on pp. 364–365)

Look at the following p values and order them in terms of greatest implied support for your experimental hypothesis. (Greatest support on the left, to least support on the right.)

$p = 5\%$ $p = 19\%$ $p = 7\%$ $p = 0.01\%$ $p = 15\%$ $p = 3\%$

When you have done this, convert each p value to a decimal.

Activity 8.3 (Answers on p. 365)

Suppose you saw the following p values in some clinical therapy articles; what do they mean, in percentage terms, about the possibility of chance or random factors being responsible for the results? The probability that the results are due to chance:

$p = 0.01$
$p = 0.07$
$p = 0.03$
$p = 0.05$
$p = 0.50$

SIGNIFICANCE LEVELS

It was said earlier that if your p value was very small you could reject the null (no relationship) hypothesis and conclude that your experimental hypothesis had been supported by the results. When the null hypothesis is rejected in this way, the results are said to be **significant**. But how small must your p value be before you can conclude that your results are significant? There is no simple answer to this as it depends upon the nature of the experiment you've carried out.

For example, suppose you had hypothesised that surgery is more effective than conservative therapy for hallux valgus. In order to carry out this research you randomly allocate 20 patients to the conservative therapy and 20 to surgery, and after a month you compare their progress, using the appropriate statistical test. Let's assume the results support your hypothesis, with a resulting p value of 5%, which means that there is a 5% probability that your results are due to random or chance factors. You would probably be quite happy to recommend the surgery in future if the 5% probability of random error didn't cause any serious problems for your patients. On the other hand, if, for 5% of the patients, surgery produced nasty side-effects, such as gangrene and ultimate amputation, you would be very reluctant to use it. Under these circumstances, you would need to consider reducing the significance level to 1 in 100 (1%) or even 1 in 1000 (0.1%) before surgery was used more widely. In other words, the effect of the random errors determines how small your p value must be before you can conclude your results are significant.

We could compare this to placing a bet on Grand National Day. Supposing you've looked at the horses, and you've decided to place a bet on a particular horse; you've unwittingly formulated an hypothesis that there is a relationship between this horse and final placing. If you're only going to put 10 pence on this horse, you won't mind a fairly large probability (or p value) that random error will influence the outcome because losing 10 pence is not too disastrous. However, if you've placed all your life-savings and assets on this horse, then you want to be fairly certain that it's going to win. In other words, you will want to be sure there is only a very small chance that random error will influence the outcome before you bet, since, if you are wrong, the effects will be devastating.

The p value you decide upon in an experiment is called the **level of significance**. It is so-called because when you look up the results of your statistical analysis in a set of probability tables, you will find the p value for your results. If this p value is equal to or smaller than the significance level you have selected as being appropriate for your research, then your results are said to be **significant**. This means that you can reject the null (no relationship) hypothesis and accept that your experimental hypothesis has been supported. If the p value is larger than the significance level you have selected, your results are classed as not significant, which means you cannot reject the null hypothesis.

Therefore, it is up to you, the experimenter, to state what significance level you think is appropriate for a particular piece of research, and the significance level you finally select will reflect the nature of your experiment. All this seems to leave the field wide open for you. However, a good rule-of-thumb if you're not doing anything that may have a disastrous outcome if you're wrong, is to use a cut-off point or significance level of 5%. So if you obtain a p value of 5% or less, then you can conclude that your results are significant and that your experimental hypothesis has been supported. For most clinical therapy research, the 5% significance would be appropriate.

This point will be referred to again later.

Key Concepts

The **p value** states the probability of your results being due to chance or random error. If the p value is very small you can conclude that your results are significant. This means you can reject the null (no difference) hypothesis and conclude that your experimental hypothesis has been supported. The experimenter decides upon how small the error margin must be before the results are said to be significant. The size of the error margin is called the **significance level**. The decision about the size of the significance level is based on the effects of the error. If the error is likely to be disastrous, then the significance level is reduced. If the effects are not likely to be terrible, then the significance level can be increased. A good rule-of-thumb is to use a 5% significance level as long as you are not doing anything dangerous.

MAKING ERRORS IN YOUR CONCLUSIONS REGARDING SIGNIFICANCE

When you have analysed your results and looked these up in the probability tables, you will obtain a probability or p value which is a statement of how likely it is that your results are due to random error. Usually, if this p value is 5% or less, the results are said to be significant and therefore support your experimental hypothesis. On the basis of such a conclusion, you would be in a position to make predictions and recommendations based on your findings. Obviously, you want to be sure that when you conclude that there was a relationship between the variables in your hypothesis, that this is correct. This is known as a True Positive. Likewise, when you conclude there was no relationship between the variables, then you want to be sure that there wasn't. This is known as a True Negative.

However, it is possible to draw the wrong conclusions from your study and these errors are known as Type I and Type II errors.

TYPE I ERRORS

These refer to those situations when we conclude our experimental hypothesis has been supported when, in fact, it hasn't. They are sometimes referred to as False Positives. Such errors can be avoided by two safeguards:

1. Ensuring that the selected significance level is appropriate; in other words, do not use a significance level of more than 5% for most research, and reduce this to 1% in cases where any errors in your conclusions could be disastrous (see previous section and the section on sample size).
2. Replication of the study and its findings by independent researchers adds credibility to the original conclusions.

TYPE II ERRORS

These refer to situations when the experimental hypothesis is rejected in favour of the null (no relationship) hypothesis, when the data do, in reality, support the experimental hypothesis. In other words, we have concluded that there was no relationship between the variables, when, in fact, there was. This is known as a False Negative.

The chance of making this mistake can be reduced by:

1. Increasing the size of the sample.
2. Using a less stringent significance level. The reasons for these safeguards will be elaborated in the section on size of sample.

It is essential when selecting a significance level that all the implications of any errors deriving from decisions about the results are considered. If they are not, then patient wellbeing could be at risk.

These outcomes can also be expressed in Table 8.3 below:

Table 8.3 Type I & Type II errors and their implications

Decision	Relationship between the variables does exist	Relationship between the variables does not exist
Researcher concludes that relationship exists	True positive	False positive
Researcher concludes that relationship does not exist	False negative	True negative

True positives, true negatives, false positives and false negatives are all described in more detail in Chapter 22 on ROC analysis.

STATISTICAL AND CLINICAL SIGNIFICANCE OF RESEARCH FINDINGS

It should also be pointed out that results are sometimes statistically significant but yet have very little clinical meaning. For example, you might conduct a study of the relative strength of the pelvic floor muscles post-partum, dependent on the type of exercise regime the women undertook. One group of women might exercise for 30 minutes per day and the other group for 60 minutes. Let us imagine at the end of the study that this latter group was found to have pelvic floor muscles which were significantly stronger statistically, but yet the women still suffered a high level of stress incontinence. It could be said that these results were statistically significant but were clinically meaningless.

Therefore, while significance levels are essential guides to deciding whether or not your data support your hypothesis, it is important to remember that these results should be considered in conjunction with their therapeutic implications. The issue of clinical significance is of importance when calculating the size of your sample.

SIZE OF SAMPLE

The issue of sample size in relation to surveys was introduced in Chapter 3, but the whole problem of calculating an appropriate sample size for use in experimental work involves some different principles. These principles include many of the concepts that have already been introduced and so it might be worth re-reading them at the relevant point. When selecting a sample, the researcher tries to ensure that the sample's results will be as close as possible to those of the parent population from which it was drawn. In this way, the results from the sample can be more confidently assumed to be applicable to the wider population. The particular piece of information that is of relevance to inferential statistics when trying to establish the similarity between sample and population is the **mean** of any characteristic under investigation. The characteristic as it applies to the population is called the **population parameter**. So the researcher would want to ensure that the mean of, say, upper arm movement for a sample is as close as possible to the mean of the population parameter for upper arm movement. The closer the two means, the more generalisable the results. However, there will always be a difference between the means of the sample and the population and this is called **sampling error**. In general, the larger the sample, the smaller the sampling error, and hence the more generalisable the results. The researcher does not need to know the actual mean value for the population parameter when analysing a data set, because the sampling error is calculated by the statistical test from the degree of variance in the sample's results (see pp. 58–59 for a more detailed description of variance). So the sample must be sufficiently large to ensure that it reflects the larger group or population from which it is derived if we are going to be able to say that our results also apply to that wider population.

As sample size calculations are becoming increasingly important in health research, it is probably worth developing these ideas before going on to how the researcher should decide on an adequate sample size for his/her research. In essence, the size of the sample needs to take into account the size of the **effect** of the IV and the power of the statistical test to **detect** the effect of the IV.

EFFECT SIZE AND POWER LEVELS

When we undertake a piece of experimental research, we are interested in finding out whether manipulating the IV has any effect on the DV. So when we have collected our data, we apply a statistical test which will tell us whether or not the IV has had any impact or **effect** on the DV. For example, in an hypothesis that predicts a relationship between a complementary therapy and the reduction of hot flushes in menopausal women, the IV is the complementary therapy and the DV is the hot flush. We would test this hypothesis by comparing two groups of menopausal women (of which one receives the complementary therapy and the other doesn't) on their incidence of hot flushes. The results would be analysed using the appropriate statistical test, which would tell us whether or not the IV (complementary therapy) is having a significant effect on the DV (hot flushes). Statistical tests differ in their power to detect the effects of the IV, with some tests being more powerful than others. This means that significant results will be more likely to be picked up by certain tests. For example, parametric tests are more powerful than non-parametric tests (see pp. 124–125 for an explanation of these terms), although, even within these broad categories, there are differences in power levels. The power of a test is not constant, though, because the test's capacity to identify whether or not the IV has had an effect is also dependent on the size of the sample and how big we want the IV's effect to be before we conclude the results are significant. In general, the larger the sample size, the more likely it is that a test will be able to detect the effects of the IV and, conversely, the smaller the sample size, the less likely this will happen. Put another way, tests become more powerful with larger samples. In crude terms then, if you only have a small sample, your data need to be 'better' for the test to identify the effects of the IV as significant, because the power of the test to detect significance with small numbers is reduced. This also means that, if you use the standard significance level of 5% when you have a small sample, there will be occasions when you conclude that your results are not significant, when in fact they might be, but the statistical test is not sufficiently powerful to pick up the effects with such small sample sizes.

As has already been noted, if you have a large sample, the statistical test is more likely to be able to detect the effect of the IV. In general terms, the larger the sample, the more likely this is to happen. However, it is also the case that a *very small effect* of the IV could be deemed significant if the sample size is very large. While this effect may be statistically significant, it may be clinically meaningless. This point is discussed on p. 110, but in essence it means that sometimes a set of results might be very significant *statistically*, while having absolutely no practical relevance whatsoever. Let's take, as an example, a study that is concerned with looking at the effects of electrical stimulation of the feet on the mobility of stroke patients. The IV here is electrical stimulation and the DV is mobility (measured as distance walked). The researcher is interested in comparing the effect of electrical stimulation on mobility and so randomly allocates 1500 stroke patients to either the 'stimulation' or the 'no-stimulation' group. After 6 weeks the mobility of the two groups is compared. Statistical analysis of the data might reveal that the electrical stimulation group walks significantly further ($p < 0.001$) and so, because the IV is clearly having a significant effect on mobility, the researcher might then be keen to use the technique more widely. But closer analysis of the results might indicate that the electrical stimulation group walked on average 9.74 m, while the non-stimulation group walked an average of 9.15 m, i.e. a difference of only 0.59 m. In reality this is about half a normal walking step and would probably have little functional relevance for the patient. In other words, a large sample might produce statistically significant results which are clinically unimportant. Therefore, to counteract this, the researcher needs to decide in advance what size of clinical effect s/he wants to achieve in order to classify the results as clinically significant or meaningful. Effect size is classified as small, moderate or large, and the **power** of a test to detect these different effect sizes will be determined in part by the size of the sample used. The researcher's decision to focus on a small, medium or large effect will depend on the existing knowledge in the area being researched. Therefore, the size of the sample a researcher needs depends on:

- The size of the clinical impact or **effect** of the IV that the researcher requires.

- The **power** of the test to detect this size of effect.

Ideally, a power level of 0.8 (i.e. an 80% chance of detecting the effect) is required of a test; this means that:

- because tests differ in their inherent power to detect an effect of the IV, with different tests having different baseline power levels

and

- because a test's power level fluctuates with sample size

and

- because a test's power to detect the effect of the IV depends upon the researcher's desire to obtain a certain effect size before claiming that the IV has clinical significance

all these factors must be taken into account when determining how big the sample needs to be. Therefore, to achieve 80% power, and with a pre-decided effect size, an appropriate sample size can be calculated. If you need to calculate the effect size for the results from your study, it is important to note that the statistical formula you use will depend on the test that has been used to analyse the data. The reader is referred to the following websites for further information on this (all websites valid as of January 2009):

http://www.waisman.wisc.edu/~yu/statistics.html
http://www.leeds.ac.uk/educol/documents/00002182.htm
http://www.cemcentre.org/renderpage.asp?linkID=30325015

On the other hand, if the data are to be analysed using a computer, some packages, like SPSS, provide a statement of effect size in the printout of results for some of the tests. These (like the formulae referred to above) are really retrospective effect size calculations, in that, alongside the test results for a given database and the corresponding probability values, the size of the clinical effect is also shown. There are several statistics that are used in computer packages that provide a statement of effect size, one of the most common being eta squared. The value of eta squared ranges from 0 to 1.0. Cohen (1992) defines an eta squared value of 0.01 as indicating a small clinical effect, a value of 0.06 as a moderate effect and a value of 0.14 as a large effect. So if you use a computer package to analyse your data set which provides you with effect size, the above values give an index of the clinical significance of the results.

It might also be worth noting a slight difference in research traditions between the medical and social sciences. Medical researchers are more likely to ask the question: How many participants do I need in a study to get significant results? In this case, the foregoing principles about how to calculate sample size on the basis of statistical power and effect size are essential first stages in the research design. I, on the other hand, come from a social science tradition where the question is more likely to be: Given my sample size of X, are the results significant? In this case, a sample of participants is targeted first and their results are then analysed to establish whether significant differences exist in the data. In other words, the sequence of actions is reversed. A useful indicator for those who wish to adhere more closely to the medical position, but who do not want to complicate matters by referring to formal sample size calculations, comes from Stevens (1996) who notes that, with sample sizes over 100, the power of the test is not an issue. However, with smaller samples, it must be emphasised that the test's power may be reduced. In other words, there may be significant results in the data base, but the statistical test does not have sufficient power to pick these up. In such cases, Stevens recommends that the significance level is raised to 0.10 or even 0.15, so that we do not run the risk of concluding that there is no relationship between the variables in the hypothesis, when in fact there may be but the test we've used is insufficiently powerful to pick this up with small numbers. For those who feel more allied with the social science philosophy, Coolican (1992) suggests that samples of 25–30 may be adequate. Bear in mind, though, that, with sample sizes of this order, the impact of the IV will need to be more pronounced for the results to be classed as significant.

Key Concepts

Calculating the appropriate sample size for experimental research is based on some key concepts:

- When undertaking experimental research, the investigator is concerned to identify the effect of the IV on the DV.
- Statistical tests differ in their inherent power to detect any effect of the IV.
- It is easier to detect an effect with larger sample sizes.
- Statistical tests might identify an effect that is statistically significant, but which has little practical or clinical relevance.
- The researcher must decide on the size of the effect that is required for clinical significance.
- Therefore to calculate a suitable sample size, the researcher needs to know the power of a particular statistical test to detect the required effect size.
- This means that there is no single formula for calculating sample sizes.
- Some researchers suggest that, as a rule of thumb, 100 participants are sufficient, while others recommend 25–30.

CALCULATING SAMPLE SIZES

All these points notwithstanding, there is increasing pressure on even beginning researchers to ensure that they have got a sample of sufficient size, and this pressure is particularly great when the research is being conducted within hospital settings or with doctors. Therefore, an introduction to the mechanics of calculating sample sizes will be given here, with references provided at the end of the chapter for those who want something more complex or unusual.

As has already been mentioned, it is important to ensure that any research you do has an adequate number of participants – too big a sample and it will waste time, effort and resources, both of the researcher and the participants; too small a sample and the results may not be reliable. It is worth noting, too, that any study can generate statistically significant results if the sample is large enough; however, these results may not be clinically meaningful, and clinical meaning is essential to sample size calculations. Therefore, the required sample for any study is the minimum number of participants needed to answer your research question reliably and usefully. In other words, if the IV in your hypothesis is having a real and reliable effect on the DV, then the selected sample size will be able to ensure this effect is detected. If the effect of your IV on the DV is expected to be large, then smaller samples can be used; conversely, if the IV's effect is likely to be small, then larger samples are required to detect it. It should be noted that the sample size calculation is based on your study's main outcome measure (i.e. the principal DV). If your study has more than one outcome measure, then sample sizes must be calculated for each outcome; the one yielding the largest sample would be the one selected for your study. This section is a guide to making these calculations.

For undergraduate and even Master's projects, it is unlikely that you will need to undertake any sample size calculations (but check the course guidance). However, there will be occasions when it is important. As a rule of thumb, the following principles apply:

- Sample sizes do *not* have to be calculated for: qualitative research or quantitative pilot studies
- Sample sizes *do* have to be calculated for: funding applications
- Sample sizes *may* have to be calculated for some academic work, e.g. PhD studies.

I would always recommend that you consult a professional statistician when calculating your samples size, especially when putting in grant applications (hospitals and universities will typically have someone experienced in doing this). If you consider this to be unnecessary or too difficult then there are a number of statistical packages that can help (e.g. Hyperstat or Clinstat); alternatively there are many articles and books (e.g. Altman 1991) and ready-made sample size tables (e.g. Lwanga and Lemeshow 1989) and Altman's nomogram. All these (plus some additional ones) are included in the references at the end of this chapter.

To calculate an adequate sample size, you need four pieces of information:

1. Power

As we have already noted, power relates to the probability that your null hypothesis will be *cor-* *rectly* rejected, and therefore, by implication, that you can *correctly* accept your experimental hypothesis. The higher the power of the study, the lower the chance of drawing incorrect conclusions; i.e. concluding that there was no effect of your IV on the DV when, in fact, there was. For example, a correctly powered study would not lead you to conclude that there was no effect of electrical stimulation (IV) on the muscle tone (DV) of patients with muscular dystrophy, when, in fact, there had been an effect. This is a Type 2 error (a False Negative) and is described on p. 110. A study that is properly powered would offset the likelihood of this error. For most of the studies that clinical therapists are likely to undertake, 80% power is acceptable; this figure can be increased to 90% or 95%, depending on the nature of your study, but it should never be any lower than 80%. It should be noted that the higher the selected power, the bigger the sample needs to be.

2. The clinically important treatment effect

This is a measure of the *clinical* importance of the IV's effect on the DV. Note that importance here refers to the clinical significance of the results and not to the statistical significance. This point has already been covered (see p. 110), but to reiterate briefly, a study can generate results that are statistically significant but have little clinical relevance. To take a previous example, you might be interested in testing the effect of electrical stimulation on the feet of stroke patients, measured as the distance walked unaided. You might find that patients on electrical stimulation walked on average 9.74 m, while patients on the standard rehab programme walked an average of 9.15 m. This difference might be statistically significant, but it is unlikely to be *clinically* significant, since it represents around a half of a single step difference. Therefore, the clinically important effect is defined as the minimum difference between your groups that would be considered to be clinically relevant. As the researcher, you can define what this value is. In the above example, you might define clinical importance as a difference of 3 m between the groups. A good benchmark for making a decision about the clinically important treatment effect is the question:

What sort of difference would I want to see between the groups before I changed my clinical practice?

The decision will be influenced by your judgment and experience. However, the larger the clinical effect size you select, the larger your sample will need to be.

3. The standard deviation of the samples on the outcome measure or DV

If the standard deviation (see pp. 59–60) of the sample on the outcome measure (or DV) is large, then a larger sample will be needed; if the standard deviation is small, then the sample size will be smaller. In the above example, a large standard deviation would mean that the distances walked by your stroke patients following treatment would vary greatly around the mean distances walked, while a small standard deviation would mean that the distances walked clustered closely round the means. The standard deviation of your particular sample will need to be used in the calculations, but may not be readily available. If this is the case, then you can opt for one of the following methods of obtaining it:

- estimating the standard deviation from other studies undertaking similar work with similar samples
- conducting a small pilot study prior to undertaking your main study and using the standard deviation of the pilot group
- starting your main study and calculating the standard deviation from the first set of recruits to establish how many more you will need.

It is not acceptable to simply say you don't know what the standard deviation of your sample is – one of the above methods can readily be used.

4. The significance level

The significance level has already been covered, but in essence, it refers to the probability that random errors (as opposed to the IV) have produced your results, so that the lower the significance level, the less the chance that random errors are responsible. The usual significance level adopted for most therapy research is 0.05 or 5%; however, if a smaller significance level is selected, usually 0.01 (1%), or 0.001 (0.1%) the larger your sample will need to be. Whether you decide to reduce your significance level from the standard 5% will depend very much on the nature of your study.

Sample sizes can be calculated for just about every variety of study: i.e. every type of design, different types of data, equal sized groups, unequal sized groups, 1 or 2-tailed hypotheses, studies which anticipate finding no difference between the treatment groups (known as equivalence studies), etc. The methods for calculating all these are beyond the scope of this text, but can be found in the online packages, books, articles and tables listed at the end of the chapter. This section will cover sample size calculations for the two most frequently used designs:

- equal sized groups, 2-tailed hypotheses and nominal data
- equal sized groups, 2-tailed designs and ordinal or interval/ratio data.

Please note that the method for calculating sample sizes for surveys has already been described on pp. 32–35.

Remember that:

Power should be a minimum of 80%, but that the greater the power, the better the study.
Significance level should be no greater than 5%, and that the smaller the significance level the better the study.
For the **clinically important difference,** the bigger it is the better the study.
For the **standard deviation of the outcome variable,** the smaller it is the better the study.

The following table presents the values that you will need to use in these sample size calculations (note the number of decimal places used here. Always work to plenty when calculating sample sizes).

Table 8.4 Values for various significance levels and power

Significance level	Associated value	Power	Associated value
5% (0.05)	1.96	80%	0.8416
1% (0.01)	2.5758	90%	1.2816
0.1% (0.001)	3.2905	95%	1.6449

Sample size calculation 1: equal sized groups, 2-tailed hypotheses and nominal data

The following formula is for calculating sample sizes for studies using these sorts of designs. Some examples might be:

1. You are interested in increasing the number of patients with burns injuries to the hand and lower arm who return to work within 6 weeks of their injury. At the moment, the return rate is 50%, but you hope that an intensive rehabilitation and counselling programme will increase this to 70%. Therefore, you take two groups of patients, one of which receives standard rehab, while the other receives intensive rehab + counselling. The outcome data are simply whether or not they return to work within 6 weeks; this is a nominal classification.

2. The number of 'did not attends' at an outpatient clinic is running at around 40%. In order to try to reduce this to 25%, a telephone reminder service will be set up and the number of 'did attend/did not attends' will be recorded. Here there will be two groups (one without a telephone reminder service and one with a telephone reminder service) and the data collected will be nominal (did or did not attend).

3. The percentage of coronary by-pass patients complying with their exercise regime is relatively low. You decide to introduce additional leaflet information and a daily diary log, in order to increase the compliance rate to around 80%. Two groups will be used – one with additional information + a daily diary, and one without. The data collected will be nominal (did comply/did not comply).

In each of the above examples, two groups have been used (which we will assume were equal sized) and the data collected were nominal. The following steps outline what you would need to do to calculate the sample size. We will take the first example to illustrate this.

1. Convert the percentages to decimals or *proportions*
   This involves taking the existing return to work rate of 50% and the desired return-to-work rate of 70%. The difference of 20% constitutes what you, as the researcher, would consider to be a clinically significant

increase. Convert the percentages to decimals (referred to as *proportions*), i.e:

   existing return to work rate is 50% = 0.5

   desired return to work rate is 70% = 0.7

   the clinically effective difference is 20% = 0.2

2. Calculate the average of the two proportions (current and desired) to give $\bar{p}$

$$\bar{p} = \frac{p_1 + p_2}{2}$$

Where $p1$ = the desired proportion
   $p2$ = the current proportion

$$= \frac{0.7 + 0.5}{2}$$
$$\bar{p} = 0.6$$

3. Calculate the standardised difference or effect size, represented as Δ

$$\Delta = \frac{p_1 - p_2}{\sqrt{\bar{p} \times (1 - \bar{p})}}$$
$$= \frac{0.7 - 0.5}{\sqrt{0.6 \times 0.4}}$$
$$= \frac{0.2}{0.4899}$$
$$\Delta = 0.4082$$

4. Calculate the sample size (known as m) required for a significance level of 5% and 80% power, using the values from Table 8.4 and the formula:

$$m = \frac{2 \times (\text{significance level} + \text{power})^2}{\Delta^2}$$
$$m = \frac{2 \times (1.96 + 0.8416)^2}{0.4082^2}$$
$$m = \frac{2 \times 7.849}{0.1666}$$
$$m = \frac{15.698}{0.1666}$$
$$m = 94.2257 \text{ participants per treatment group}$$

Always round up to the next whole number, which means that you would need 95 participants in each of the two treatment groups in your study or 190 in total.

If you felt that you wanted to reduce your significance level to 1% with 90% power, then the relevant values would need to be inserted in the formula:

$$m = \frac{2 \times (2.5758 + 1.2816)^2}{0.4082^2}$$

$$m = \frac{2 \times 14.8795}{0.1666}$$

$$m = \frac{29.759}{0.1666}$$

$$m = 178.6254$$

Therefore, 179 participants would be needed in each group of your study (358 in total).

If your significance level was reduced to 0.1%, with 95% power, then the calculation becomes:

$$m = \frac{2 \times (3.2905 + 1.6449)^2}{0.4082^2}$$

$$m = \frac{2 \times 24.3582}{0.1666}$$

$$m = \frac{48.7164}{0.1666}$$

$$m = 292.4153$$

Therefore, 293 participants would be needed in each group (586 in total).

You can see from these calculations that reducing your significance level and increasing the power mean that larger samples would be needed for your study.

Sample size calculation 2: equal sized groups, 2–tailed hypotheses and ordinal or interval/ratio data

The sorts of studies that might use this design would be those where the focus of interest was a comparison of different treatments, with the outcome or DV being measured using an ordinal or interval/ratio scale. Some examples might be:

1. You want to compare the effect of two different dietary supplements on the weight gain of head and neck cancer patients. One group receives the standard dietary supplement, while a second group receives the standard supplement plus a complementary feed. The average weight gain on the standard feed is 2 kg at the end of 2 weeks. You want to try to increase this to an average 4 kg, which would be a clinically relevant gain. The outcome is measured as kilos and is therefore interval/ratio data.

2. At a back pain clinic, the standard treatment for non-specific back pain is osteopathy, which currently has the effect of reducing pain by an average of 2 points on a visual analogue scale. You want to see whether adding exercise to the osteopathy reduces reported pain levels by 4 points. Therefore, you use two groups, one with osteopathy alone, and the other with osteopathy + exercise. The outcome is measured on a visual analogue pain scale, and is therefore interval/ratio data.

3. In order to assess the effectiveness of a guided movement training programme on the extend and grasp action of children with cerebral palsy, you compare a group of children receiving this intervention with a group receiving a placebo. The outcome is measured in degrees of accuracy and is therefore an interval/ratio scale.

If we take the first example to illustrate the calculation, the average weight gain using the standard dietary supplement is 2 kg over 2 weeks; if this could be increased to an average 4 kg over 2 weeks, then you would change your clinical practice and use the standard supplement + the complementary feed, because a further increase of 2 kg would be clinically important. A pilot trial has indicated that the standard deviation for weight gain in this patient group is 2.7 kg. It has been decided that a 5% significance level and 80% power will be suitable for this study.

1. Calculating the effect size Δ.
   The effect size is calculated from the following formula:

$$\Delta = \frac{\text{clinically important difference}}{\text{standard deviation}}$$

   The clinically important difference has been set at 2 kg and the standard deviation is known to be 2.7 kg.
   Therefore

$$\Delta = \frac{2}{2.7}$$

$$= 0.7407$$

2. Calculate the sample size m using the values from Table 8.4.

$$m = \frac{2 \times (\text{significance level} + \text{power})^2}{\Delta^2}$$

$$m = \frac{2 \times (1.96 + 0.8416)^2}{0.7407^2}$$

$$m = \frac{2 \times 7.849}{0.5486}$$

$$m = \frac{15.698}{0.5486}$$

$$m = 28.6147$$

Rounding this figure up means that you would need 29 patients in each of your treatment groups (58 in total).

If you decided that you wanted to reduce your significance level and increase to power to 1% and 90% respectively, then the calculation becomes:

$$m = \frac{2 \times (2.5758 + 1.2816)^2}{0.7407^2}$$

$$m = \frac{2 \times 14.8795}{0.5486}$$

$$m = \frac{29.759}{0.5486}$$

$$m = 54.2454$$

This means that you would need 55 patients in each of your treatment groups (110 in total).

Adjusting the significance level and power to 0.1% and 95% respectively, the calculations become:

$$m = \frac{2 \times (3.2905 + 1.6449)^2}{0.7407^2}$$

$$m = \frac{2 \times 24.3582}{0.5486}$$

$$m = \frac{48.7164}{0.5486}$$

$$m = 88.8013$$

Therefore, rounding this figure up, you would need 89 patients in each of your treatment groups (178 in total).

Again, it is clear from this that by reducing the significance level and increasing the power, more participants will be needed. However, it should be reiterated that for most clinical therapy research, a 5% significance level, with 80% power is sufficient.

The figures and calculations outlined above all refer to the actual number of participants taking part in the study. If you anticipate that there will be, for example, a 30% drop-out rate, then the initial starting figures must be increased by 30% to accommodate the losses. So if your calculations suggest a sample size of 220, but you expect a 40% drop-out rate, then the initial sample will need to be 220 + 88 = 308.

Key Concepts

Sample size calculations always need to be completed for projects being submitted for research funding

The method of calculating sample size depends on various aspects of your design, such as the level of data, type of design, numbers in each group, 1 and 2-tailed hypotheses etc

You will need the following information to make a sample size calculation:

- the significance level (usually 5%)
- statistical power (usually 80%)
- the standard deviation of your sample
- the clinically important treatment effect – the size of the difference between interventions that would make you change your practice.

FURTHER READING

General

Cohen L, Holliday M 1996 Practical statistics for students. Paul Chapman Publishing, London

Coolican H 2004 research methods and statistics in psychology, 4th edition. Hodder and Stoughton, London

Field FA, Hole G 2004 How to design and report experiments. Sage, London

Greene J, D'Oliveira M 2005 Learning to statistical tests in psychology, 3rd edition. Buckingham, Open University Press

Greenhalgh T 1997 How to read a paper: statistics for the non-statistician II: 'significant' relations and their pitfalls. BMJ 315:422–425

Peat J 2001 Health science research: a handbook of quantitative methods. Sage Publishing, London

Pett M 1997 Non-parametric statistics in health care research. Sage Publishing, London

Polgar S, Thomas, S 2007 Introduction to research in the health sciences. Churchill Livingstone, Edinburgh

Robson C 2002 Real World Research; a resource for social scientists and practitioner-researchers. Blackwell Publishing, Oxford

Effect size calculations

University of Wisconsin http://www.waisman.wisc.edu/~yu/statistics.html

University of Leeds http://www.leeds.ac.uk/educol/documents/00002182.htm

Centre for Evaluation and Monitoring http://www.cemcentre.org/renderpage.asp?linkID=30325015

Sample size calculations

Altman DG 1991 Practical statistics for medical research. Chapman & Hall, London

Clinstat. Online. Available http://www-users.york.ac.uk/~mb55/soft/soft.htm

Devane D, Begley CM, Clarke M 2004 How many do I need? Basic principles of sample size estimation. Journal of Advanced Nursing 47(3): 297–302

Hyperstat. Online. Available www.davidmlane.com

Soft Software www.xlstat.com

Lwanga SK, Lemeshow S 1989 Sample size determination on health studies; a practical manual. World Health Organization, Geneva

Whitley E, Ball J 2002 Statistics review 4: sample size calculations. Critical Care 6(4):335–341

Chapter 9

Matching the research design to the statistical test

DECIDING WHICH STATISTICAL TEST TO USE

The previous chapters have all been concerned with how to design a piece of research to test an hypothesis. Once you have designed and carried out your research, you need to analyse your data to find out whether the results do, in fact, support your hypothesis. The analysis involves using statistical tests. Essentially, what this means is that you apply a particular formula to your data and then work through the formula to get the answer. This answer is then looked up in the probability tables to see whether it supports your hypothesis.

However, there is no single all-purpose test which you can use to analyse your results, since each experimental design has an appropriate statistical test. Therefore, one of your tasks as a researcher is to match up the appropriate statistical test with your research design. If you select the wrong test to analyse your data, then your conclusions will be vitiated – it's as critical as that. Unfortunately, many people become very worried about this matching task, but as long as you ask yourself some basic questions about your design, you shouldn't have too much trouble.

A word of warning first, though: when you are planning your research project, do ensure that you know which statistical test you will be using. All too often people carry out their experiment without doing this first and then find that they don't know how to analyse the results, or that they need a complicated computer program which they can't access. So, make sure at the planning stage that you know which statistical test you will need for your design.

Key Concepts

Each experimental design has its own statistical test which must be used when analysing the results. Thus, a key feature when planning your research is to match up the design with the appropriate statistical test.

To decide on which statistical test to use with an experimental design, the following questions must be asked:

1. Is the design experimental or correlational?
2. How many conditions are there?
3. If the design is experimental, is it same-, matched- or different-subject?

We will now look at these questions in more detail.

IS THE DESIGN EXPERIMENTAL OR CORRELATIONAL?

To answer this, it is usually easier to look back at your hypothesis and decide whether you were predicting differences in your results (e.g. between patient groups, types of treatment, males and females) or whether you were predicting associations or patterns between sets of data. If you were predicting differences, you will have used an experimental design, while if you were predicting patterns you will have used a correlational design.

Since this is often a focus of confusion for some people, it may be useful to go over the concepts again.

If you look back to Chapter 2, you will see that, in an experimental design, we manipulate one variable (the independent variable, IV) and measure the effect of this on the other variable (the dependent variable, DV). So, if you were hypothesising that counselling is effective in pro-

moting the psychological adjustment of patients recently diagnosed with multiple sclerosis, your IV would be counselling and the DV would be effectiveness in promoting psychological adjustment. Typically, you would design an experiment whereby you gave one group of multiple sclerosis patients counselling and another group no counselling (manipulation of the IV), and after a fixed period you would compare the psychological adjustment of the two groups. (You measure the effect on the DV of manipulating the IV.) Here then, you would be looking for differences between the two groups in terms of the effectiveness of the counselling vs. no counselling in aiding adjustment.

On the other hand, in some hypotheses you may predict patterns between the two variables (look back to pp. 80–85): these require a correlational design. In these hypotheses you are predicting either:

a. that as scores on one variable go up, so the scores on the other variable will also go up (positive correlation)

or

b. that as scores on one variable go up, so the scores on the other variable will go down (negative correlation).

For example, if you hypothesised that clinical therapy students who do well on theory exams also do well on their practical assessments, you would take a group of students and look at their performance in both situations, on the assumption that, the higher the theory mark, the higher the corresponding practical mark. This is called a positive correlation.

Alternatively, you may predict a link between low job satisfaction and severity of migraine, such that, the lower the job satisfaction, the more severe the migraines. This is called a negative correlation.

In these correlational designs you do not manipulate one variable to see what effect it has on the other; instead you take a whole range of scores on one variable and see whether they are related to a whole range of scores on the other variable. If you are still unclear about the differences between experimental and correlational designs, re-read Chapter 6.

HOW MANY CONDITIONS ARE THERE?

Number of conditions and correlational designs

If you have a correlational design, you need to ask whether you are comparing two sets of data, or more than two sets. Once you have answered this, you need only ask yourself about the levels of measurement you have on each variable. This point is dealt with in Chapter 17, which covers analysis of data deriving from correlational designs.

Number of conditions and experimental designs

If you have an experimental design, however, you need to decide how many conditions you have (see pp. 75–80) since designs with only two conditions in total require a different type of statistical test from those with more than two conditions. For example, if you compared two groups of patients, one of which had received some treatment (experimental condition) and the other had received no treatment (control condition), then you would have two conditions. If you had compared two types of treatment (i.e. two experimental conditions) you would again have two conditions. On the other hand, if you had compared the effectiveness of three treatment procedures, you would have three conditions.

Look back to pp. 75–80 to refresh your memory on this.

IF THE DESIGN IS EXPERIMENTAL, IS IT SAME-, MATCHED- OR DIFFERENT-SUBJECT?

What type of experimental design was used? For example, did you use just one group of subjects for all conditions (e.g. comparing the attitudes of one group of clinical therapists to tuberculosis vs. emphysema patients)? Or did you use two or more totally different groups of subjects and compare them in some way (e.g. comparison of attendance levels, at an osteopathy clinic, of Asian vs. African–Caribbean patients)? Or did you use two or more groups of subjects who were matched on certain key features (e.g. a comparison of the quality of newly qualified occupational therapists from three different training schools, which would necessitate matching the

subjects on such variables as 'A'-level grades, attendance levels, etc.)? (See Chapter 7.)

Remember, for the purposes of statistical analysis, matched- and same-subject designs are treated alike, so you only have to decide between:

same-/matched-subject design

or

different-subject design.

CHOOSING THE APPROPRIATE TEST

The above questions can be set out as a decision chart like those in Figures 9.1 and 9.2.

Note that the names of the appropriate statistical tests are given in the boxes on the charts. You can see from these charts that sometimes the names of two or three tests are given. This does not mean that any one of them can be selected, but that instead each requires slightly different conditions for use (e.g. a different level of measurement). These differences are outlined in the relevant chapter.

You will also notice that you are given the choice of 'non-parametric' or 'parametric' tests. The differences between these will be outlined in the next section.

Key Concepts

Every experimental design has its own statistical test(s) which must be used to analyse the data. In order to select the appropriate statistical test for your own design you must ask yourself a number of questions:

1. Were you looking for differences (i.e. an experimental design) or patterns (i.e. a correlational design)?
2. If you had a correlational design, you must also ask: how many sets of data did I have?
3. If you had an experimental design, then you must ask: How many conditions were there? (Two or more than two.)
4. If you did, did you use the same or matched subjects in each condition? Or did you use different subjects in each condition?

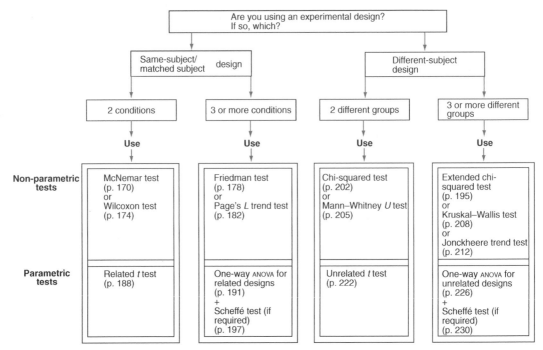

Figure 9.1   Choosing the correct test for an experimental design.

PARAMETRIC AND NON-PARAMETRIC TESTS

You will notice that the statistical tests in Figures 9.1 and 9.2 are classed as 'parametric tests' and 'non-parametric tests'. Essentially, for most of the designs you are likely to use, you have a choice of using a parametric test or a non-parametric test. What is the difference?

Basically, a parametric test is a much more sensitive tool of statistical analysis. If, for example, you are comparing responses to two different kinds of treatment, and there are differences in responsiveness, the parametric test is more likely to detect them than is the non-parametric test. In this sense they are more powerful than non-parametric tests for detecting any effect of the IV (see previous section on sample size calculations). Perhaps the point can be clarified by an analogy. Supposing you were making a cake and you wanted to weigh out the ingredients. You have two weighing machines in the house: the bathroom scales and the electronic kitchen scales. You could use your bathroom scales to weigh out your quarter kilo of sugar, but they will give you a less accurate and less sensitive reading than your kitchen scales. The non-parametric test is like the

bathroom scales as it will analyse your results but it will not be as fine or as sensitive as the analysis of the parametric test (the kitchen scales).

If parametric tests are so good, then why do we bother with non-parametric tests at all? Like most things that are good, there are prices to pay and conditions to fulfil, and so it is with parametric tests. Before you can use one to analyse your results, four conditions have to be satisfied.

The first of these is critical: your data must be of an interval/ratio level of measurement, since parametric tests cannot be used on nominal or ordinal data. This condition should never be violated. However, it should be noted that a number of statisticians have suggested that, if an ordinal scale has a reasonable number of points (I would suggest at least 7) and the intervals between them are assumed to be approximately equivalent, then parametric tests may be used. If you want to play safe, however, you should use a non-parametric test, because it is an error to caution.

At the risk of being challenged by pure statisticians, the other three conditions are not quite as important, and may be waived to some degree. The first of these is that your subjects should be randomly selected from the population they represent.

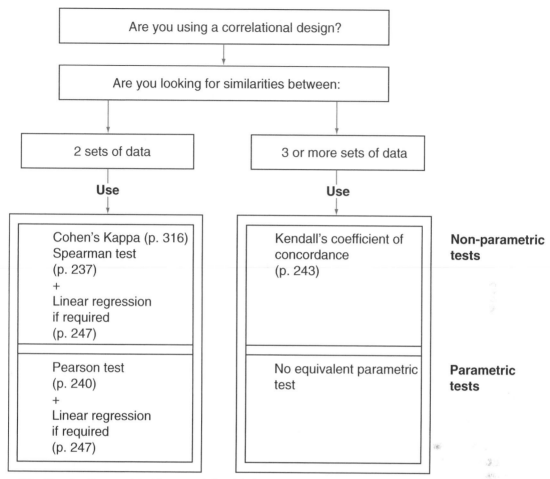

Figure 9.2   Choosing the correct test for a correlational design.

Second, your data should be normally distributed. As you will probably remember from Chapter 5, a normal distribution looks somewhat like an inverted-U shape and you can plot your data on a graph to find out whether it is (more or less) normally distributed. Unfortunately, in a lot of research that involves human subjects, many of the attributes we wish to measure are not normally distributed and therefore this condition cannot always be met.

Third, the variation in the results from each condition should be roughly the same. This means that the range of scores in each condition should be more or less similar. If, for instance, the scores in one condition ranged from 20 to 120, while for the other they ranged from 60 to 80, the degree of variation in each condition's scores would be too dissimilar for a parametric test to be used. On the other hand,

if they ranged from 50 to 100 in one condition and 60 to 90 in the other, this would be acceptable.

To each of the last three conditions we would add the caveat 'within reason', because parametric tests are said to be 'robust' in that they can tolerate minor violations of assumptions. Essentially, what this means is that it does not matter too much if you cannot fulfil perfectly the last three conditions; as long as your data are of an interval/ratio level (or an equivalent-interval ordinal scale), and there are no glaring deviations with respect to the other three conditions, you can use a parametric test.

Table 9.1 may help to clarify this point.

If you're ever not sure as to whether you've satisfied the conditions adequately, then use a non-parametric test. So, when in doubt, use the non-parametric equivalent.

ANOTHER WAY OF DECIDING WHICH TEST TO USE

Alternatively, some students prefer to make this decision by using diagrammatic representations of the design. These are set out with examples, in Tables 9.2–9.4 for experimental designs, and Tables 9.5 and 9.6 for correlational designs. You should note that in Examples 2, 4 and 6 you can use more than three groups or conditions and still apply the same test.

Table 9.1   Levels of measurement for parametric and non-parametric tests

Level of measurement	Type of test which can be used
Nominal	Non-parametric
Ordinal	Non-parametric
Interval	Parametric and non-parametric
Ratio	Parametric and non-parametric

Key Concepts

The results from any research design may usually be analysed either by a parametric or a non-parametric test. A parametric test is much more sensitive and will identify significant results more readily than a non-parametric test. However, before you can use a parametric test, four conditions must be fulfilled:
- The data must be on an interval/ratio level.
- The subjects should have been randomly selected.
- The data should be normally distributed.
- The variance in the results from each condition should be similar.
- The first condition is very important.
- The other three can be violated to some extent.
- Non-parametric tests do not require these conditions to be fulfilled and can be used with any level of measurement.

EXPERIMENTAL DESIGNS

Table 9.2   Same-subject designs

			Test	
			Non–parametric	Parametric
Example 1				
One group of Ss	takes part in Condition 1 / takes part in Condition 2	Compared for differences between conditions	McNemar test (if data are nominal) or Wilcoxon (if data are other than nominal)	Related *t*-test (if data are interval/ratio)

H$_1$ Elderly patients develop more rapport with uniformed podiatrists than with non-uniformed podiatrists.

Method   Select a group of elderly patients and measure rapport:
(1) with uniformed podiatrists and
(2) with non-uniformed podiatrists
i.e. one group of patients measured under both conditions.

			Non–parametric	Parametric
Example 2				
One group of Ss	takes part in Condition 1 / takes part in Condition 2 / takes part in Condition 3	Compared for differences between conditions	Friedman or Page's L trend (if data are other than nominal)	One-way ANOVA for related designs (if data are interval/ratio) + Scheffé test if required

H$_1$ The attitudes of a group of clinical therapists to 3 (or more) types of patient differ significantly.

Method   Select a group of clinical therapists and measure their attitudes to 3 types of patient, i.e. one group of clinical therapists measured under 3 different conditions.

(It can be seen that this design is an extension of Example 1.)

Table 9.3   Different-subject designs

			Test	
			Non–parametric	Parametric
Example 3				
Subject group 1	takes part in *Condition 1*	⎱ Compared for differences between conditions	Chi-squared test (if data are nominal)	Unrelated *t* test (if data are interval/ ratio)
Subject group 2	takes part in *Condition 2*	⎰	or Mann–Whitney *U* test (if data are other than nominal)	

H₁ Men are more likely to experience respiratory difficulties following cardiac surgery than are women.

Method Select a group of male cardiac patients and a group of female cardiac patients and compare degree of respiratory difficulty, i.e. two different groups of Ss compared.

Example 4				
Subject group 1	takes part in *Condition 1*	⎱ Compared for differences between conditions	Extended chi-squared test (if data are nominal)	One-way ANOVA for unrelated designs (if data are interval/ratio)
Subject group 2	takes part in *Condition 2*	⎰	or Kruskal–Wallis	
Subject group 3	takes part in *Condition 3*		or Jonckheere trend (if data are other than nominal)	+ Scheffé test if required

H₁ There is a difference in responsiveness to interferential treatment of middle-age stress incontinence in women with no children, 2 children or 4 children.

Method Select 3 groups of women: 1 with no children, 1 with 2 children and 1 with 4 or more children and compare their responsiveness to treatment, i.e. 3 different groups of Ss compared.

(This is an extension of Example 3.)

Table 9.4   Matched-subject designs

			Test	
			Non-parametric	Parametric
Example 5				
Subjects **matched** on key variables				
Subject group 1	takes part in *Condition 1*	Compared for differences between conditions	McNemar (if data are nominal)	Related *t* test (if data are interval/ratio)
Subject group 2	takes part in *Condition 2*		or	
			Wilcoxon (if data are other than nominal)	

H₁	Cast-bracing is more effective than traction in the treatment of leg fractures.
Method	Take two groups of leg fracture patients, matched on key variables such as age, sex, prior fractures and fitness and treat one group with traction and the other with cast-bracing. Compare their progress. i.e., two groups of Ss matched on certain factors and compared for progress.

			Non-parametric	Parametric
Example 6				
Subjects **matched** on key variables				
Subject group 1	takes part in *Condition 1*	Compared for differences between conditions	Friedman	One-way ANOVA for related designs (if data are interval/ratio)
Subject group 2	takes part in *Condition 2*		or	
Subject group 3	takes part in *Condition 3*		Page's *L* trend (if data are other than nominal)	+
				Scheffé test if required

H₁	To extend the hypothesis in Example 5, you add a further treatment group which uses plaster of Paris.
Method	You select a further group of leg fracture patients matched with groups 1 and 2 on age, sex, prior fractures and fitness and compare the progress of the 3 groups, i.e. 3 groups of Ss matched on certain critical factors, and compared for progress.

CORRELATIONAL DESIGNS

Table 9.5   A correlational design where two sets of scores are involved

	Test	
	Non-parametric	Parametric
Example 7 These may predict: a. Positive correlation, i.e. high scores on one variable are associated with high scores on the other (Fig. 9.3).	Cohen's Kappa (if data are nominal) Spearman (if data are other than nominal) + Linear regression if required	 Pearson (if data are interval/ratio) + Linear regression if required
$\quad$ H₁ $\quad$ There is a correlation between age and recovery time following total hip replacement, such that the older the patient, the longer the recovery time. Method $\quad$ Select a large age range of total hip replacement patients and note their recovery time from operation to discharge.		
b. Negative correlation, i.e. high scores on one variable are related to low scores on the other (Fig. 9.4).	Cohen's Kappa (if data are nominal) Spearman (if data are other than nominal) + Linear regression if required	 Pearson (if data are interval/ratio) + Linear regression if required
$\quad$ H₁ $\quad$ There is a correlation between degree of osteoporosis and number of cigarettes smoked, with high numbers of cigarettes being associated with low bone density. Method $\quad$ Select a whole range of smokers (e.g. non-smokers to 80+ per day) and measure their bone density.		

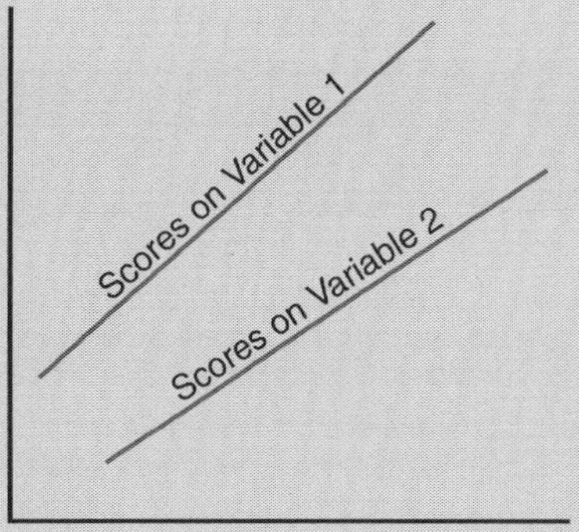

Figure 9.3

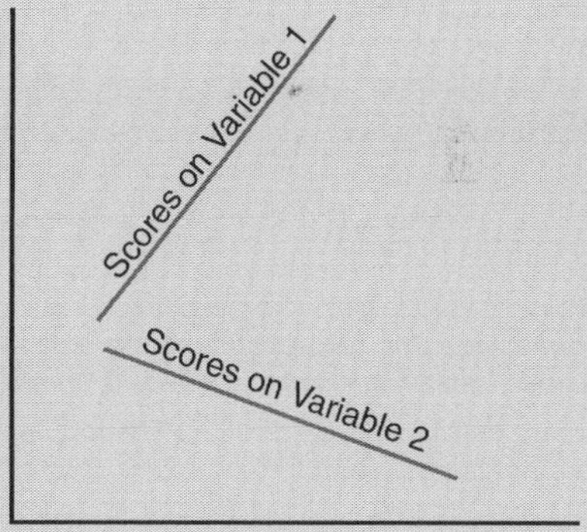

Figure 9.4

Table 9.6   A correlational design where more than two sets of scores are involved

	Test	
	Non-parametric	Parametric
Example 8 Here you are looking for the degree of similarity between 3 or more sets of scores (Fig. 9.5). (Here you can only predict a positive correlation; see Chapter 17 for the reason why.)	Kendall coefficient of concordance (if data are other than nominal)	There is no parametric test
H_1 There is a positive correlation among different clinical therapists' judgements of the handicapping nature of various clinical conditions. Method Select 4 different types of clinical therapist and ask them to rank order 6 clinical conditions (blindness, lower leg amputation, deafness, emphysema, osteoarthritis of the hip, carpal tunnel syndrome) for their assumed handicapping impact on the patient.	 Figure 9.5	

Activity 9.1 (Answers on p. 365)

Using the decision guidelines presented earlier, look at the following brief descriptions of some research projects, and decide which statistical tests you should use. (Quote both the parametric and non-parametric alternatives where relevant, since at this stage you would not know whether your data would allow you to use a parametric test.)

1 In order to compare the clinical speciality preferences of a group of newly qualified clinical therapists and a group of senior clinical therapists, you select two groups of 30 subjects to represent each group and ask them to state whether they prefer geriatric or paediatric work.

2 To find out whether leg fracture patients progress faster on hydrotherapy or suspension, you select two groups of 15 Ss, matched on certain key features such as age, sex, prior fractures, etc. and compare their progress after 4 weeks' treatment.

3 On the assumption that chiropractors' seniority is related to high absenteeism rates (the higher the grade, the greater the absenteeism), you look at

the number of days off taken by all grades of chiropractor in a large urban community.

4 To find out whether social class is related to compliance with exercise regimes for severe carpal tunnel syndrome, you select 30 patients from social classes 1 and 2, and 30 from social classes 4 and 5, and compare their reported compliance, on a 5-point scale.

5 To compare the effectiveness of three types of walking aid for hip replacement patients, you select three groups of Ss, matched on key variables, such as age, fitness, etc. and give one group Zimmer frames, the second group walking sticks and the third group crutches. Their mobility after 3 weeks is compared.

6 In order to compare the attitudes of three different grades of podiatrists to a new set of shift hours, you select a group of 15 senior grade podiatrists, 15 middle grade podiatrists and 15 basic grades and compare their attitudes, using a point scale.

LOOKING UP THE RESULTS OF YOUR ANALYSIS IN THE PROBABILITY TABLES

Let's suppose you have designed and carried out your experiments and have analysed the results using the correct statistical test. As you will remember, it was stated earlier that a statistical test will give you a result which you look up in a set of probability tables in order to find out whether your results are significant and support your hypothesis. This process will be described more fully in the chapters which deal with the particular statistical tests, but an outline of the general principles will be given here.

When you have worked through the appropriate statistical test or formula, you will end up with a number which you look up in a set of probability tables for that particular test. It is important to note that each statistical test has its own set of probability tables, which you will find at the back of this book. Thus, the Mann–Whitney U test will provide you with a numerical value which is looked up in the probability tables for the Mann–Whitney test (see Tables A2.7a–d). The Wilcoxon test provides you with a numerical value which is looked up in the probability tables for the Wilcoxon test, and so on.

More details on this will be given with the description for each statistical test.

DEGREES OF FREEDOM

Before you can look up the numerical value mentioned above, some tests require an additional value: either the number of Ss you used or a number called the **degrees of freedom (df)**. This concept, which is quite a complex one to understand, refers to the degree of potential variability in the data. However, although the concept is hard to understand, the df is very easy to calculate. The details of how to do this will be given in the description of the tests which require the df.

However, before you can conclude whether your numerical value represents a significant result from your experiment, you require one further piece of information: namely, whether you have a one- or a two-tailed hypothesis.

ONE- AND TWO-TAILED HYPOTHESES

The way in which you state your hypothesis has implications for how you look up your numerical value in the probability tables.

One-tailed hypotheses

Some hypotheses are stated very specifically in that they predict precisely what the outcomes will be. For example, if the hypothesis was 'elderly patients experience more rapport with uniformed rather than non-uniformed clinical therapists', we are predicting a very precise outcome in that we are saying that the patients will experience more rapport with uniformed clinical therapists. Again, if we hypothesised that 'leg fractures improve faster with traction than with cast-bracing', we are making a precise prediction, because we are assuming faster progress with traction. These are known as **one-tailed hypotheses** or tests because the results are expected to go in one particular direction. The following are all examples of one-tailed hypotheses:

1. Women are more likely than men to experience linguistic difficulties following cerebral embolism.
2. Ultrasound is more effective than megapulse for arthritic toe joints.
3. Social classes 4 and 5 are less likely to keep to exercise regimes than are social classes 1 and 2.
4. Children with lower leg amputations are less likely to suffer from negative body image than adolescents with lower leg amputations.
5. Male clinical therapy students are more likely to fail the clinical assessment than are females.

Two-tailed hypotheses

However, hypotheses can be stated much more vaguely, without any precise predictions. For example, it might have been hypothesised that elderly patients experience different degrees of rapport with uniformed and non-uniformed clinical therapists. In contrast to the one-tailed hypothesis, which predicted more rapport with uniformed clinical therapists, this hypothesis allows for the possibility that more rapport could be experienced either with uniformed or with non-uniformed clinical therapists, because it simply predicts differences in rapport, without specifying what these differences might be. Similarly, if we predict that leg fractures respond differently to traction and cast-bracing, we are not specifying how they respond, but simply that there is a difference in response, which could mean leg fractures improve more either with cast-bracing or with traction.

These hypotheses are known as **two-tailed hypotheses** or tests because the results could go in either of two directions. The following are examples of two-tailed hypotheses:

1. Senior and basic grade occupational therapists differ in their absenteeism rates as a result of stress.
2. Student clinical therapists with 'A'-level physics differ from students without 'A'-level physics, in terms of their theory exam marks.
3. Interferential and exercise techniques are differentially effective in treating stress incontinence.
4. Zimmer frames and walking sticks afford different degrees of mobility for patients with ankylosing spondylitis.
5. Patients who are given pre-operative respiratory exercises differ in their incidence of postoperative complications from patients who are given no pre-operative respiratory exercises.

Activity 9.2 (Answers on p. 365)

Look at the following hypotheses and identify which are one-tailed and which are two-tailed:

1 Praise is a more effective motivator for complying with exercise regimes when used in group rather than one-to-one situations.
2 Social modelling and social skills training are differentially effective in developing interaction skills of head injury patients.
3 Patients who attend for chiropractic in back schools have less pain following treatment than patients who attend for conventional traction treatment.

4 There is a difference in the strength of muscle contraction of a selected muscle group when preceded by 2 minutes of infrared radiation as opposed to 2 minutes of specific warm-up.
5 The elimination of lactose in the diet is more effective than pharmacological intervention in diminishing primary hypertension.

Look back at the examples of one-tailed hypotheses and convert them to two-tailed hypotheses. Then look at the example of two-tailed hypotheses and convert them to one-tailed hypotheses. (It does not matter in which direction you predict the results will go.)

One-tailed or two-tailed: why does it matter?

Why is this important? Supposing you had stated a one-tailed hypothesis (i.e. that your results will go in one specific direction) and, having done your experiment and statistics, had ended up with a p value of 1%. This means that there is a 1% chance that your results are due to random error. However, had your hypothesis been two-tailed instead, you would be predicting that your results could go in either of two directions. Therefore, because your results could go in either of two directions, there will be twice the possibility that random error could account for your results, and so, for exactly the same data, your p value would be doubled to 2%, i.e. a 2% chance that your results are due to random error.

Let's illustrate this with an example from the list above: the comparison of social modelling and social skills training in developing interaction skills in head injury patients. Suppose that, rather than the two-tailed hypothesis stated earlier, you had hypothesised instead that social skills training is more effective than social modelling for these patients (i.e. you have stated a one-tailed hypothesis). To test this you would probably have selected two groups of patients, one of which received social skills training and the other social modelling. You would expect that the interaction skills of the group receiving social skills training would be generally better. Suppose again that your results suggest this is the case, and you end up with a p value of 5%. This means that there is a 5/100 chance that your results are due to error.

However, had you simply hypothesised that social skills training and social modelling are differentially effective in improving interaction skills, then you would expect either the social skills group or the social modelling group to do better. This is now a two-tailed hypothesis, because you have allowed for the possibility that the results could go in either of two directions. You carry out exactly the same study and achieve exactly the same results, but your p value would now be 10% (i.e. doubled) because, if your results are expected to go in either of two directions, there must be twice the possibility that random error can account for the results.

Let's see how this works in practice by turning to Table A2.2 (Wilcoxon).

At the top of the table you will see two headings: 'Level of significance for one-tailed tests' and 'Level of significance for two-tailed tests'. You can see that every level of significance for a two-tailed test is twice the corresponding level for a one-tailed test, i.e. 0.10 is twice 0.05, 0.05 is twice 0.025, 0.02 is twice 0.01, 0.01 is twice 0.005.

Should an hypothesis be one–tailed or two–tailed?

Many students ask how they should decide on whether an hypothesis should be one- or two-tailed. The answer to this lies in the background theory associated with the research you are carrying out. For example, if you are concerned with the relationship between smoking and bronchitis, the background reading that you will have done, prior to embarking on this research, will probably have revealed that:

- Smoking is related to lung cancer.
- Bronchitis is associated with particular atmospheric pollution.

It would therefore be reasonable to predict that heavy smokers are more likely to get bronchitis (i.e. a specific one-tailed prediction). Thus, the existing research and literature will guide your prediction here.

If, however, you were interested in looking at patients' confidence in treatment when clinical therapists wear uniform, you may well have found background literature which suggests that some patients are more comfortable with uniformed therapists, while others prefer the infor-

mality of the therapist in 'civvies'. Thus, because the background research is less clear-cut here, you would probably not wish to make a specific prediction about patients' confidence when being treated either by uniformed or non-uniformed therapists. Therefore, in this case, you would formulate a two-tailed hypothesis. In other words, existing research knowledge and theory should guide you when making predictions in the hypothesis.

Key Concepts

When you use a statistical test to analyse the results from your research you will end up with a numerical value.

This value is looked up in the set of probability tables which are specific to the statistical test you have used. In order to look up the value you will also need to know either the **df** value or the **number of subjects** who participated in the experiment; each statistical test requires one or the other.

Additionally, you must decide whether your hypothesis is **one–tailed** (predicts that the results will go in one direction only) or **two–tailed** (predicts that the results will go in either of two directions). Hypotheses which are two–tailed have twice the probability that random error can account for the results, and so will affect the p value for your data.

Using these two values, you will end up with a p value, i.e. a decimal or percentage probability that your results are due to random error. According to the size of the p value you can either claim your results are **significant** (i.e. support your hypothesis) or **not significant** (do not support your hypothesis).

A CHECKLIST OF STAGES INVOLVED IN SETTING UP YOUR RESEARCH PROJECT

Let's recap on the essential guidelines that have been covered so far, and are involved in designing a piece of research. Please note that this checklist only applies to studies that are involved in hypothesis testing, and not to surveys, observational studies, etc.

1. Have you formulated an experimental hypothesis which clearly predicts a relation-

ship between two variables? Have you stated your null (no relationship) hypothesis?

2. Are you going to test this hypothesis using a correlational design (i.e. are you predicting that, as scores on one variable go up, so scores on the other variable go up or down accordingly)? Or are you going to use an experimental design which will test for differences between conditions or subject groups?

3. If you are using a correlational design, what level of data do you have on each variable?

4. If you are going to use an experimental design, have you sorted out what you are going to measure (i.e. what is the DV)? Have you decided when you will take the pre-test measures of the DV and the post-test measures? What level of measurement are you using?

5. Are you going to use a different- , same- or matched-subject design? Are you sure that this is the most appropriate design for your hypothesis? Why? If you are going to use a matched-subject design, have you identified the critical variables on which the Ss have to be matched?

6. Will you be using a control group? Is this ethically acceptable? If you are not using a control group, how many experimental conditions have you decided upon?

7. Who are your subjects going to be? Can you select them randomly? How many will you need?

8. Is there any need to counterbalance the conditions to overcome order effects?

9. Have you controlled for experimenter bias?

10. What are the sources of constant error? Have you controlled or eliminated them? Have you taken account of the random errors as far as you are able?

11. Is your experimental hypothesis one- or two-tailed?

12. What test will you need to analyse your results?

FURTHER READING

Cohen L, Holliday M 1996 Practical statistics for students. Paul Chapman Publishing, London

Coolican H 2004 Research methods and statistics in psychology, 4th edition. Hodder and Stoughton, London

Coolican H 2006 Introduction to research methods in psychology, 3rd edition. Hodder Arnold, London

Davies MB 2007 Doing a successful research project: using qualitative or quantitative methods. Palgrave Macmillan. London

Field A, Hole G 2004 How to design and report experiments. Sage, London

Greene J, D'Oliveira M 2006 Learning to use statistical tests in psychology, 3rd edition. Open University Press, Buckingham

Polgar S, Thomas S 2007 Introduction to research in the health sciences, 5th edition. Churchill Livingstone, Edinburgh

Chapter 10

Putting the theory into practice

Everything that has been said so far is theory. To carry out a piece of research, you need to put this theory into practice. This chapter is concerned with providing some practical guidelines to help you set up your research project.

STATING YOUR AIMS AND OBJECTIVES

It is essential that you clarify in your own mind what the object of your research is to be. All too often students say rather vaguely 'I'd like to do something on neck pain/patient satisfaction/clinical assessments/torticollis', etc. without having any idea what exactly they want to investigate. While a general topic area like this is a good starting point, since it defines your area of interest, you will need to develop a more precise idea of what you are trying to find out before you start your research. In some cases, this will involve collecting large amounts of data for a survey.

Alternatively, you may wish to test a specific hypothesis at the outset. If this is the case, ensure that the hypothesis conforms to the principles outlined on pp. 70–72, in that it makes a clear prediction of a relationship between two variables, and that it is a testable hypothesis. Some topics in which you are interested may simply not be researchable because the necessary skills, techniques, procedures, etc. are not available or ethically acceptable, or because the project would involve major policy changes, which are out of the control of the researcher or would take too long or involve too many people. So do ask yourself whether the hypothesis is testable and feasible.

Furthermore, do define the terms in your hypothesis clearly and unambiguously. Using terms like 'safe practice', or 'effective' or 'improvement' are too vague as they stand, and you must have a clear idea of what they mean in real terms.

Even if you are interested in a particular area and simply want to explore it fully without formulating any hypothesis (i.e. some form of survey technique) you will still need to clarify your aims and terms so that you can define the area to be studied precisely.

REVIEWING THE BACKGROUND RESEARCH

Once you have formulated your hypothesis or defined your survey area, you will have to review all the relevant literature relating to the area you want to investigate. The purposes of this activity are to:

- Acquaint yourself fully with the theoretical background to the topic, so that you have a full understanding of the issue.
- Familiarise yourself with all the existing research that has been carried out in the area, firstly to ensure that your own project has not been conducted before, and secondly to provide a context for your experiment. These points are particularly important if you want to write up your research project for publication in a journal.
- Consider the possible methods and techniques of conducting your research.

However, having just said that one of the purposes of reviewing the research literature is to ensure that your intended study has not been carried out before (i.e. it is an original piece of work), there will be occasions when you simply want to replicate someone else's experiment in order to see whether their results apply to your own professional setting. In such a case, the process is slightly different, in that your aim or hypothesis will be identical to that of the study you wish to replicate, and the entire experimen-

tal procedure will also be the same. You will still need to acquaint yourself with the background literature so that you are familiar with the theories and related studies, but its purpose is obviously not to ensure the originality of your project.

It should be pointed out that it is perfectly acceptable to replicate an existing study as long as this is your real intention and not just the result of your not being aware of what has already been done in the area!

Do not underestimate the importance of a really thorough search of the literature: there is nothing more infuriating than carrying out a superb piece of research with earth-shattering results, only to be told by a colleague that Bloggs et al performed an identical piece of research a year ago. A full search of the literature will prevent time wastage and disappointment. The following information is a basic guide to searching the existing published literature.

ELECTRONIC DATABASES

Undoubtedly, one of the most relevant developments in communication technology has been the CD-ROM (compact disc, read-only memory) mechanised information retrieval system. Many abstracts and indexes relating to health care are available in the form of CD-ROM databases, which allow a very fast computer search for specific topics, articles, keywords and author names to be carried out. For example, if the researcher is interested in chronic neck pain and its treatment, using these key words, a CD-ROM database can produce a list of citations, which the researcher can access and print off directly from the computer if they are deemed to be relevant. Accessing this information usually involves a reasonably user-friendly 'dialogue' between the user and the computer, which allows the identification of both individual and combined topics, authors, journal details, etc. This means that, within about an hour, a researcher can obtain a vast amount of relevant background literature on a given subject. If you are not familiar with electronic searching, there are many websites that can help you, such as http://www.netskills.ac.uk/onlinecourses/tonic

However, unless you are a student or your unit has some special arrangement with the library, you may have to pay for this facility and the cost may depend on the number of articles produced. Information about the availability and the precise method by which a database can be accessed can be obtained from your library. It should be noted that libraries have their own particular system of entering a database, so it is important to ask library staff for this information.

The following is a list of the main computer databases that are relevant to the clinical therapies. Only brief details have been provided; the speed of technology advances means that a comprehensive coverage of a database would be out of date very quickly. You will need to register your details in order to use some of them.

- **Medline**. This database covers the whole field of medicine and many allied health care professions. It is an international base, which includes editorials, letters and biographies, as well as journal articles and abstracts. Medline is the major computer database and is the CD-ROM version of the old Index Medicus. It has details of articles from over 3000 of the world's most important journals in the areas of nursing, professions allied to medicine, medicine and dentistry. Many medical libraries offer courses in how to use Medline fully; alternatively, you could seek help from library staff.
- **CINAHL**. This is the name of the Cumulative Index to Nursing and Allied Health Literature. It is updated monthly and, while its primary focus is nursing, it covers the allied professions. By using key words, authors or topic areas, the user can access details of books and journal articles.
- **AMED**. This is an online database for Allied and Complementary Medicine. Search the web for 'Allied and Alternative Medicine', as the web address may change.
- **Chartered Society of Physiotherapy**. This offers access to a range of documents and research. http://www.csp.org.uk/
- **Cochrane Library**. This is a comprehensive database of systematic reviews, RCTs etc providing a reliable source of information about effective healthcare interventions and research. http://www.thecochranelibrary. com

- **PEDro**. The physiotherapy evidence database. This covers systematic reviews and RCTs in physiotherapy. http://www.pedro. org.au/
- **SPORT Discus**. This is a comprehensive, international database of sports and fitness literature. It contains information from articles, books, theses, conference proceedings, etc., in the areas of sports medicine, exercise physiology and biomechanics.
- http://www.ex.ac.uk/library/guides/ comphealth.html is a useful resource for complementary therapies
- http://www.library.nhs.uk/CAM/. This covers a wealth of information for all health Care Professionals, with links to specialist libraries covering a host of topics.
- http://www.internethealthlibrary.com/ covers alternative and complemenatry therapies
- http://www.intute.ac.uk/ healthandlifesciences. This is an invaluable site with information relevant to an enormous range of specialisms, e.g. acupuncture, speech and language therapy, dietetics, podiatry, chiropractic, etc.
- **BNI – British Nursing Index**. Indexes British nursing journals from 1985 onwards.
- **DARE**. A compendium of free databases of interest to health care professionals. http:// www.shef.ac.uk/scharr/ir/trawling.html

All websites valid as of March 2009.

There is also an array of other databases that may have some relevance for the health researcher:

- **ASSIA** (Applied Social Sciences Indexes and Abstracts). http://www.csa.com
- **Science Citation Index**. This covers past and current abstracts and citations from over 3700 international journals http://www. thomsonreuters.com/products_services/ scientific/web-of-science. It can also be accessed by Web of Science, which also includes the Social Science Citation Index http://wok.mimas.ac.uk
- **PyscINFO** (for psychology research literature). This is a comprehensive database of psychology literature dating from 1800s. http://www.apa.org/psycinfo/

- **ERIC** (for educational research literature. This provides free access to 1.2 million bibliographic records of journal abstracts and articles relating to educational research). http://www.eric.ed.gov
- **EMBASE**. This specialises in biomedical and drug research.
- **COPAC**. A consortium of research libraries, providing access to merged online catalogues. http://www.copac.ac.uk

All websites valid as of March 2009.

And don't forget the internet search engines, which can often provide valuable information. There are also many online electronic journals and the reader is strongly advised to get advice from the librarian or information services personnel about how to access these. For further details on using the internet for accessing literature, see Chapter 25 on Systematic Reviews.

These systems, while an invaluable source of information on the available literature, are by no means exhaustive nor necessarily totally complete or accurate. There may be research projects on the fringe of conventional and complementary medical approaches which are not included or which are thought to be more appropriately classified elsewhere. It is a good idea, therefore, to browse through any professional journals which you think may contain relevant articles, as well as textbooks on the topic. And, at the risk of being accused of being a Luddite, I think there is a great deal to be gained from a serendipitous manual search of the journals.

OTHER SOURCES OF INFORMATION

An enormous amount of information is available on the internet and much of it is very useful. However, as there is no control over what is included on websites, the researcher should be cautious when using this information.

Statistics

Undoubtedly, the internet is probably the best and most up-to-date source of statistical information. As there is no control over website contents, do ensure that you use official government or health organisation websites. Some useful general addresses are:

- http://www.dh.gov.uk/en/Publication-sandstatistics/index.htm (UK health data)
- http://www.statistics.gov.uk/ (UK health statistics)
- http://www.lib.gla.ac.uk/Depts/MOPs/Stats/medstats.shtml (medical statistics for North and South America, Europe, the Commonwealth and the UK)
- http://who.int/research/en/ international health data from the World Health Organization
- http://www.opsi.gov.uk contains official statistical data

All websites valid as of March 2009.

REFERENCE INFORMATION

There are a number of computerised systems for managing references. These include Papyrus, Endnote, ProCite and Reference Manager. They enable the researcher to systematically organise, classify and manage references, as well as modifying them for various purposes. Many organisations have site licences for at least one of these packages and this might be worth pursuing if you feel that you will have a large number of references that you will need to use time and again.

If, on the other hand, you don't wish to involve computers or you are unlikely to pursue your research topic, then you might feel that a hard copy system would be preferable. In this case, you will need to keep a card index of all the references you think are useful.

For each relevant reference include, for journal articles:

- the full name of the author
- the publication date
- the precise title of the article
- the precise title of the journal where the article appears
- the volume (and part, if relevant) of the journal
- the first and last page numbers of the article
- a résumé of the article with all the relevant details.

For chapter references in a book, where the book has an editor, include:

- the full name of the author of the chapter
- the date of publication of the book
- the title of the chapter
- the full name of the editor
- the full title of the book
- where the book was published
- the name of the publisher
- a résumé of the chapter, with all the relevant details.

For references to a book which has an author rather than an editor, include:

- the full name of the author
- the date of publication of the book
- the full title of the book
- where the book was published
- the name of the publisher
- a résumé of the relevant information.

You may think this is rather fussy, but I can assure you that a fully detailed index system is worth its weight in gold. All too often researchers assume (and I have been amongst them) that, if they need a particular reference again, they'll know where to find it, and so then fail either to make a note of it at all or make an insufficiently detailed note of it. I can guarantee that, by the time you've completed your project and you're ready to write it up, your memory for references will have let you down, and you will consequently waste hours in libraries trying to track down a piece of information which you're sure you saw on the top right-hand page of a newish blue book!

Shortcutting references really isn't worth the time, frustration and energy so do keep a full record of all relevant references as you go along. And, in addition, if you continue to research a topic, such a fund of references will be used time and again.

DECIDING HOW YOU WILL CARRY OUT THE PROJECT

Once you have completed a thorough literature review and made sure that your proposed project has not been carried out before, you must then decide on the best method of proceeding with your research. Are you going to conduct a survey, whereby you collect a large quantity of data and then use some form of descriptive statistics to highlight important features of it (see Chapter 5)? Or are you going to use a correlational design whereby you measure two (or more) variables to see whether they co-vary in some predicted way (see Chapter 6)? Or is an experiment more appropriate for the particular project, which will involve manipulating one variable to see what effect it has on the other (see Chapter 6)?

There follows a brief re-cap on the salient issues involved in each approach.

Survey methods involve collecting a large quantity of data on a particular subject and using descriptive statistics to highlight the important aspects of the data. Surveys can be used for a number of purposes:

- To describe the topic area, e.g. how many patients suffer lower leg amputations as a result of circulatory defects, their ages, sex, social class, previous health, occupation, length of time in hospital, etc.
- To pinpoint problem areas. If, in the above example, you found that 50–60-year-old men who worked in the brewery trade were more likely to have lower leg amputation, this might point the way to further research on any possible causal links. This might then give rise to an experimental study where you tested this hypothesis.
- To identify trends, both past and present. Is there, for instance, an increased tendency towards these lower leg amputations over the last decade? If so, is it conceivable that this trend may continue? If it does, then this might point the way towards developing clinical therapy expertise in the area of lower limb amputation and rehabilitation.

Remember, though, that survey techniques may be unsuitable for testing specific hypotheses. For this, experimental and correlational designs are needed.

Experimental designs are used to test whether the relationship predicted between the two variables in the hypothesis actually exists. To do this, one of the variables must be manipulated and the effects of this on the other variable are then measured. Such an approach has to be carefully designed and controlled, which may involve the researcher in a considerable amount of effort. The results of this approach have to be analysed using statistical tests (see Chapters 13–17). If the experiment has been carried out properly, the results can provide very useful answers, by identifying causes and effects of certain events. The approach can also establish which of a number of treatment procedures is more effective, which types of patient respond best to particular therapies, etc., and so may be especially useful in streamlining and systematising professional practice.

However, it does, of course, have its disadvantages. Experiments can be complicated and time-consuming to carry out and they may be entirely unsuitable if any ethical issues are involved. For example, it would be of dubious ethical value to look at the effects of epidural analgesia during childbirth on length of labour by comparing a group who had been offered the pain relief with a group who had not been offered it. In such cases, alternative approaches must be considered. One such is the correlational design.

Correlational designs are used to test hypotheses where it would be unethical to manipulate deliberately the independent variable (in the latter case, epidural analgesia) to see what effect it had on the dependent variable (length of labour). In correlational designs, the researcher simply takes a range of measures on each variable to ascertain whether they vary together in an associated way. For example, are high scores on one variable associated with high scores on the other? Or alternatively, are high scores on one variable associated with low scores on the other? Because the technique does not involve any artificial manipulation of patients or treatments, it is easier to carry out than experimental procedures and can more easily be used in naturalistic settings. However, it is for the same reason that cause and effect cannot be established using a correlational design, and therefore cannot provide the same degree of conclusive evidence.

You must decide which of these approaches is most suited to the topic you wish to research.

PREPARATION FOR THE RESEARCH: WRITING A RESEARCH PROPOSAL

Once you have decided on your research topic, carried out a literature review and established which general approach to the project would be most appropriate, it is a good idea to write out a fairly detailed research proposal, so that you can plan the structure and specifics of the project. Many people consider a research proposal to be a waste of time unless they are trying to obtain financial support from some organisation, when a proposal is absolutely essential. However, in an era of rapidly expanding health care research, your proposal will almost certainly have to be presented to an ethics committee before you can proceed. It is absolutely critical that you check whether this is the case before starting your research, because you might compromise your participants and invite litigation if you don't. The research proposal is essential in these cases, since it not only provides the necessary details of the project so that the ethical issues can be fully evaluated, but also demonstrates the researcher's competence, expertise and understanding of the topic area, an important consideration when a patient's health and wellbeing may be affected. Details of how to submit a proposal to your relevant ethics committee will be available from the health care or educational organisation where you will be conducting your research and general guidelines are given in Chapter 6.

Besides the need to gain ethical approval, writing up a research proposal has two other important functions:

- It helps the researcher to plan the project and to focus attention on all the essential issues, such as aims, methods, analysis and relevance.
- On occasions, the research you wish to do will require more time, staff or equipment than is readily available and it may, therefore, be necessary to obtain financial support for your project (see next section). In order to apply for funding you will need to provide the potential sponsors with a fairly detailed research proposal, so that they can assess its value, viability and relevance.

Thus, for these reasons, it is good practice to prepare a research proposal prior to starting your project. No great detail about writing proposals will be given here, since a lot of the content will be similar to that contained in the next chapter on writing up research for publication.

Where this is the case, it will be indicated. Nonetheless, the following information should be included in a proposal in the order given:

1. The title of the research project (see next chapter), which should be clear and succinct.

2. Background theory and the research context for the project (similar to the 'Introduction' in the next chapter).

3. A clear statement of the aim or hypothesis under investigation.

4. The method of conducting the research should be clearly outlined. This is very similar in content to the 'Method' section of an article (see next chapter) and should include a statement of the design of the project, the subjects (type, number, etc.), materials, apparatus and actual procedure. In addition, any relevant information about how the public relations aspect will be handled should be included here (i.e. feedback of results to patients, anonymity of the subjects, security of the data, cooperation with other members of the hospital staff, etc.).

5. The type of statistical analysis to be used for the results should be included.

6. The implications, relevance and anticipated benefits of the study must be highlighted, particularly if the proposal is to go to an ethical committee or a funding body. It is pointless merely to outline an experiment without indicating its direct application and worth to the patients/hospital/staff/funding body, etc.

7. The estimated length of time required to carry out each section of the research, as well as the overall time involved, should be included, since this will obviously influence the feasibility and finances of the study; 500 Dupuytren's contracture patients might be difficult to find in a fortnight! Obviously, you cannot be exact in your time predictions because all sorts of unforeseen circumstances will crop up which will delay completion. Hence, it is better to be pessimistic rather than optimistic on this one. If you can draw some sort of chart showing the sequence and timing of the main events, this would be invaluable, both in setting an overall idea of the project and in guiding its execution.

8. If the proposal is to be presented to ethical or funding bodies, then it will be necessary to include details of any ethical implications for the participants (see pp. 86–89). Also, include information about the personnel (including yourself) who may be involved in the project, either existing personnel or staff recruited specifically for the purpose of the project. There are usually three types of personnel involved in research work:

– Research supervisor or director. This is the person who takes overall responsibility for the project's execution, directing and rescuing as necessary. If you are the person generating the ideas and submitting the proposal for consideration by ethical and financial committees, the odds are you will also be the research supervisor.

– Research workers. These people carry out the everyday running of the project, collecting data, administering the treatments, etc. They usually have some grounding in research methods or at least receive some training prior to the start of the project. Obviously, careful thought needs to be given to the qualifications and skills required of the research staff.

– Support staff. These are quite often the lynchpin on which the whole project depends. They include secretarial and clerical staff, computer operators, technicians, etc.

In a research proposal, you may need to name the personnel involved, together with their qualifications, work and research experience and particular expertise for the job. If you need to recruit anyone specially for the project, you will need to specify the sort of person you want, how long you want them for and what the cost will be. Always remember when you specify the salary range that the appointee will probably only be on a short-term contract and so should be paid slightly more than usual. In addition to the cost of the salary, you will need to add the employer's national insurance (NI) contributions, superannuation, additional costs and overheads.

Even if you are not applying for any funding, it is still a good idea to work out the cost of the project, even if only approximately. You may find that an outcome of limited impact may not justify the expense of new equipment, staff time, computing, etc. However, if you are applying for outside money then you should itemise the following costs (overall or per annum) if the project is to last longer than 12 months:

1. Salaries, superannuation, NI numbers of all staff to be employed on the project.
2. Any capital outlay on equipment, together with revenue expenditure on any apparatus, etc.
3. Travel and subsistence costs; if anybody needs to travel to other hospital departments, patients' homes, etc., these costs should be incorporated.
4. Stationery costs, postage, telephone, typing, computing, etc. must be estimated. If you are proposing to handle a large amount of data, your computing costs may be fairly high. It is worthwhile having a preliminary chat with the computing centre you intend to use about estimated costs and the types of statistical analysis available.

Two words of caution, though. First, don't forget to build in some allowance for inflation; too many promising projects have had to be abandoned before completion simply because the money ran out. Second, check out the sort of financial information your potential sponsors require and the format they wish to receive it in before you submit your proposal. A familiar layout and content can go a long way towards getting your proposal seriously considered. I would always suggest that you seek advice from your organisation's finance office before submitting any proposal (and indeed, most funding bodies and organisations would make this a requirement of submission).

Allied to this is the length of the proposal. Many funding agencies have specific criteria for proposal formats and length and it is always wise to find these out and stick to them. Skimpy, underworded proposals look superficial and ill-thought-out, while excessively verbose ones will lead to boredom and irritation in the readers. Consequently, you should pay close attention to any recommendations laid down by the appropriate body.

Before taking off on your research, do ensure that not only does it have the approval (if necessary) of the ethics committee, but that it has been discussed and given the go-ahead by all the necessary people. This may involve your senior and peer colleagues, the relevant consultant, etc. It does little for staff relations for a senior colleague to find suddenly that there is a major research programme starting tomorrow, which will involve a total reorganisation of the department. And in our compensation culture, any research that has not been granted ethics committee approval may be subject to litigation. So, do discuss your proposals with all the relevant personnel from the outset. This is a critical stage in any research project and should never be overlooked.

OBTAINING FINANCIAL SUPPORT

Some research projects can be extremely expensive in both time and money, and you may, therefore, need to apply for financial aid in order to carry out your research. Sources of financial support are many and various and all should be considered as possible sponsors at the outset. Undoubtedly, the easiest avenue through which to apply for money (though not necessarily to obtain it!) is your own professional body's or organisation's research fund. Many hospitals and health authorities have money available for research, although its existence is not always widely known. However, a relevant research programme carried out on home ground, with direct value to the sponsoring institution or organisation, is often a tempting cause and you may find the money forthcoming. Furthermore, there are often advertisements in the national press or professional journals, inviting bids or tenders for earmarked research funds. These may be worth pursuing. Do bear in mind though that, at the time of writing, multi-site, multi-disciplinary research is very much the flavour of the month and to stand a reasonable chance of getting sponsorship you may need to collaborate with other organisations and professional groups. There is undoubtedly great kudos to be gained from obtaining external funding, but to be successful requires a considerable amount of skill, hard work and persistence.

Beyond this immediate channel, there are outside sources, such as pharmaceutical companies, manufacturers of apparatus and the like, all of whom may be suitable targets for your application for money.

In order to decide which of these is likely to be most profitable, it is worth doing some homework. Some agencies obviously favour certain types of research and these inclinations will be indicated by the sort of projects they have supported in the past, as well as the nature of their own activities. Obviously, a manufacturer of traction beds is unlikely to sponsor research into the impact of wearing uniforms vs. civvies by clinical therapists, unless the project has some direct impact on their product. Some funding bodies even lay down specific guidelines as to the sort of project they will consider sponsoring.

Once you have decided who to approach, have an informal discussion with them about your ideas and, if they are interested, get the relevant application forms from them, together with any general information they might provide to guide intending applicants. These must be read thoroughly and completed in accordance with any regulations laid down by the organisation.

Some words of advice: the funding bodies are only likely to concern themselves with novel, useful and relevant pieces of work. Projects which are run-of-the-mill or contentious are usually avoided for obvious reasons. Therefore, before applying for money, do think carefully about the nature and implications of your research and how likely it is to fit in with the overall flavour of the sponsor's interest. Also, check the final presentation of your research proposal, ensuring that it is typed, and without errors. Omissions, incorrect spelling and poor syntax will do little to create a favourable impression of your professional competence!

If your proposal is turned down in the end, try to find out why and whether the sponsors would reconsider it if amendments were made. If, on the other hand, it is accepted, then you must keep your sponsor happy. This will involve you in three activities. First, do try to keep within your time and financial budget: funding agencies are rarely pleased with requests for more money or time extensions. Second, do send regular progress reports so that they can be satisfied that all is going according to plan (or if it isn't that they are informed about the problem and what you're doing about it). And third, do provide a detailed final report on time, with clear conclusions, implications and recommendations. (You should consider inviting someone from the sponsoring organisation to be on a steering committee for the project. In that way, the sponsors can be kept fully informed at all stages.)

All this may seem like a lot of time and effort which perhaps could be better spent on the actual research project itself. Undoubtedly, there are borderline cases where you're not sure whether it really is worth the trouble to make an application for money. I did some ballpark estimates of the cost of applying for funding. Taking into account all the preparation, development and time involved, I found that it may cost the organisation an additional £10 000–20 000 per bid of around £50 000. To ensure that your organisation doesn't lose out in this way, you might have to build these additional monies into the costings. This is something only you and the other researchers can decide. However, if you do decide to apply for funding, remember that the sponsors are being asked to invest a lot of money in you and they will obviously want to assure themselves that it will be money well spent.

PLANNING THE DETAILS OF THE STUDY

If you write a proper research proposal, many of the details of the study will have been considered and decided upon. Even if you don't need a formal research proposal, you must make a detailed outline of your plans and ideas for your own benefit, since when you come to write up the research report (probably a considerable time after the completion of the project) you will be surprised at how difficult it is to remember why you actually decided on one approach rather than another. So keep detailed notes for yourself, as you go along, about the reasons for choosing each methodological or design approach of your research.

At this juncture, if you are using an experimental design, you should also address, in detail, the following points:

- Any instructions you will be giving to your subjects during the course of the experiment should be prepared verbatim, and typed up.
- Prepare sufficient score sheets on which to record the data; if your subjects are to be

asked to make written replies during the experiment, ensure that you prepare enough response sheets for them.

- If you are going to randomise the order of presentation of the experimental conditions, or the order of subjects' participation, make sure this is done in advance.
- If you are keeping the subjects' identity anonymous and just assigning them numbers, do keep a record of any relevant details of all the subjects (age, health, sex, experimental condition) on a separate sheet with the appropriate number attached.
- How you will select your subjects and who they will be.
- Prepare for yourself, and for any other researchers who will be working with you, a worksheet which outlines detailed instructions of what should happen and when and how it should be carried out.
- Make sure that you know how to analyse the data and, if it requires a computer, where and how you can obtain appropriate computing facilities.
- If you are going to use someone else to run the experiment, because you suspect there will be some experimenter bias if you carry it out, make absolutely sure that the substitute experimenter has only the relevant details (i.e. exactly how to carry out the project) and not what the predicted outcome will be, otherwise the possibility of experimenter bias will remain.
- If you have to write to people to ask them to participate as subjects, do enclose a stamped, addressed envelope for their reply, and do check just before the start of the project that they are still able and willing to come.
- Do run a pilot study, before carrying out the experiment proper, to iron out any problems in advance.

If you are conducting a survey, you must decide:

- How you will collect your data, e.g. by using a questionnaire, by post, in person, etc.
- How to design your measuring instrument, i.e. your attitude scale or questionnaire. This

must be piloted before you run the full survey.
- What instructions for completion you will append to the questionnaire.
- How you are going to select your subjects.
- How you will ensure an adequate response rate if you are using a postal survey.
- How you are going to analyse your data.

CARRYING OUT THE STUDY

A number of points are important here:

1. If you are using any apparatus do double-check before you start that it works properly. It is extremely irritating to collect your subject sample from far and wide only to discover when they arrive that the necessary equipment is out of order and they have to go away again. This is the way in which you lose subjects, time, patience and motivation. Also, do make sure you know how to use the equipment properly. While this may seem a ludicrously obvious point to make, it has been known for experimenters to spend a considerable time fiddling about with the apparatus, attempting to find the necessary switches. Trying to convince the subjects of your competence thereafter becomes a major task.

2. Always, always, always run some pilot trials before you begin the experiment proper. Pilot trials simply mean running through the experimental procedure with a few subjects to see whether there are any practical hitches. By doing this, you can establish:
   (i)   Whether your procedure is appropriate.
   (ii) Whether the tasks you've set your subjects are of the right level; if they're too hard or too easy, they can be adjusted.
   (iii) Whether you've allocated a reasonable amount of time for the tasks.
   (iv) Whether your instructions can be clearly understood by the subjects.
   (v)   Whether there are any practical problems in the project.
   If you do find any hitches or difficulties at this stage, you can iron them out before beginning the real experiment.

3. Do familiarise yourself totally with the experimental procedure, and what should be done when. It does not inspire the confidence of subjects to see the experimenter scrabbling around for scraps of paper or trying to find out what to do next. So make the running of the experiment as smooth and automatic as possible. The pilot trials should help in this.

4. Treat your subjects well. They are the cornerstone of your study and must be looked after. This means keeping them informed (as far as is reasonable) of the purpose of the study and of the outcome. Should it ever be necessary to keep your subjects in the dark over the aim of a study, because their knowledge of this would bias the results, do debrief them when the project is over. Also tell them in advance, if possible, what is required of them and how long it will take. Do not do anything which will cause distress or embarrassment. People are understandably apprehensive about any form of research, so it is in their, and your, best interest, to try to achieve some rapport with them and an easy, pleasant atmosphere. Lastly, try to minimise the amount of inconvenience subjects experience during the course of the study. If they have to make lengthy and expensive journeys at unsociable hours of the day or night, they are unlikely to turn up. Quite simply, try to keep your subjects happy, particularly if they are patients, when not only their psychological, but also their physical, wellbeing may be at stake.

INTERPRETING AND DISSEMINATING THE RESULTS OF YOUR RESEARCH

There is no value in simply analysing your results and then forgetting all about them: they must be interpreted fully in terms of their relevance to the profession. What is the meaning of the outcome? How does it relate to current clinical therapy practice? What are the implications for policy changes/therapeutic procedures?

However, even this is not enough. If you are the only one who is aware of the nature and implications of your results then they are of limited value. The information must be disseminated to other members of the profession. The easiest way to do this is by writing up the research, either as an article for publication in a professional journal or as a report produced within your department for circulation. While the former method will reach a greater audience, both require the same sort of format and approach.

With the increasing emphasis on research-based clinical practice within the health care professions, together with reductions in resources, it is essential that the results of sound research projects are published. Without this knowledge, clinicians will not be able to make informed decisions, practice will not be accountable on objective grounds and patients' welfare will not be optimised through the best intervention procedures. Publication of results is an essential final stage of research, and is a moral obligation for any clinical therapists who have conducted good research with potentially useful findings. Guidelines for writing up research are given in the next chapter.

Finally, remember that there is no such thing as a perfect piece of applied research. In designing any study involving human subjects, compromises will have to be made in the design. However, these considerations must be informed and well judged. As long as the researcher can make reasoned, judicious adjustments to the design in order to accommodate the practical problems surrounding their study, the research will still be valid.

FURTHER READING

Besides the websites recommended in this chapter, the following may be useful:

Bell J 2005 Doing your research project: a guide for first-time researchers in education, health and social sciences, 4th edition. Open University Press, Buckingham

Berry R 2004 The research project: how to write it. 5th edition. Routledge, London

Blaxter L, Hughes C, Tight M 2006 How to research. 3rd edition. Open University Press, Buckingham

College of Emergency Medicine UK http://www.collemergencymed.ac.uk/ Click on 'Search' and type in 'Writing Research Proposal'

Davies MB 2007 Doing a successful research project: using qualitative or quantitative methods. Palgrave Macmillan, London

Denscombe M 2002 Ground rules for good research. Open University Press, Buckingham

Denscombe M 2003 The good research guide: for small scale research projects. Open University Press, Buckingham

Fink A 2005 Conducting research literature reviews: from paper to the internet. Sage, London

Gitlin L, Lyons KJ 2008 Successful grant writing strategies for health and human service professionals. Springer, New York

Greenhalgh T 1997. How to read a paper: papers that summarise other papers. BMJ 315:672–675

Khan KS, Kunz R, Kleijnen J, Antes G 2003 Systematic reviews to support evidence-based medicine: how to review and apply findings of healthcare research. Royal Society of Medicine, London

Robson C 2006 How to do a research project; a guide for undergraduate students. Blackwell, London

The Leads Teaching Hospitals UK http://www.leedsth.nhs.uk/sites/research_and_development/sections3.php

Watson R, McKenna H, Cowman S, Keady J 2008 Nursing research: designs and methods. Churchill Livingstone, Edinburgh

Chapter 11

Writing up the research for publication

Sometimes you will want to carry out a piece of research just for your own satisfaction or to resolve some issue that exists in your own work. However, there will be occasions when your experiment produces such an interesting and useful outcome that you will want to publish it so that the results can be disseminated to other related professionals. Hence you will need to prepare an article for publication in a suitable journal. I would urge you always to consider publishing your research, however, for two main reasons. First, if you have some interesting findings there is a moral obligation to share these with other clinical therapists so that they can integrate them in their practice. Second, if patient care is to be improved through the use of research results then it is essential that these are widely disseminated to other practitioners.

A word of caution, though. Good scientific journalese comes with practice. Even if you follow the guidelines provided here you will probably not be terribly satisfied with your first attempt at writing up a piece of research. I would recommend that you don't despair and throw it in the bin, but instead put the first draft away for a week or two and forget about it. When you re-read it afresh you will probably find a number of points that could be expressed more clearly or succinctly. If you're still not satisfied after doing this, repeat the process. You will soon find that you are able to produce a written style which is suitable for scientific journals at the first attempt.

GENERAL GUIDELINES FOR WRITING UP RESEARCH

1. Always bear in mind that the aims of writing up research for publication are to inform readers of: (a) the purpose of your study (i.e. the aims or hypothesis); (b) the results; (c) how you came by them (i.e. the procedure you adopted for your experiment); and (d) what the implications of your results are. More details of the basic structure of a report are given in the next section.

2. Unless you are reporting a first-hand, phenomenological study (outside the realms of this text), always write in the third person, not in the first or second person. In other words, use phrases such as 'The subjects were required to …' rather than 'I asked the subjects to …'

   While this is easy enough when describing the experimental procedure, many students find it more difficult when discussing the implications of their results, tending to write phrases such as: 'I think the results can be explained by …' The 'I think' would be better replaced by phrases such as 'it is suggested/posited/hypothesised that the results, etc. …' or 'One possible explanation for the results is …' or 'The results can be explained by …', etc. If you have difficulty in writing in the third person, it's often a good idea to take a passage from a book which is written in the first person and simply rewrite it in the third person, for practice.

   If all this sounds unnecessarily pedantic, remember that any research should be objective and disinterested. If you start 'I', 'me', 'my', 'personally', etc. the report begins to look highly subjective and consequently not very scientific. Use of the third person is a much better style for journal articles (and gives you a greater chance of publication).

3. Keep your sentences clear and simple and try to convey just one idea per sentence. Remember that your report may well be read by someone unfamiliar with the field, so confronting them with complex grammar or sentences with several adjectival clauses will keep them unfamiliar with it! Clarity of style is easier to attain if you do not assume your reader had any prior knowledge of the specific area. (However, don't fall into the trap of writing as though the reader is a halfwit!) And finally, if you are going to use abbreviations, give their meaning in full at the first mention. For example:

   Two National Health Service (NHS) community podiatry services were compared on a range of patient satisfaction and clinical outcome measures.

4. Do not include any anecdotal evidence in the report, however relevant and interesting it may appear. Science is too formal, theoretical and empirical for personal experience to be introduced.

5. Try to make your article clear, logical, succinct and free of irrelevancies. Remember always that the purpose of any article is to provide information. Therefore, if someone unfamiliar with your area of research is to understand the article, it is essential that it is clear and logical. Similarly, in order to get the essential points across to the reader, it is important not to wrap them up in irrelevant information. The colour of the subject's pyjamas is rarely apposite, although I have seen it included in one student's report!

6. It is important to quote relevant research in your article for a number of reasons. First, it shows the reader that you are familiar with the research area and that you have a number of important facts at your fingertips. Second, it adds weight to any argument you produce: if you simply say that 'the administration of lumbar traction relieves back pain' the reader may think 'who says?'. On the other hand, if you state that 'Bloggs & Smith (2008) found that back pain patients commonly report less pain following lumbar traction', your argument carries more credibility. (You will note that I have quoted the surnames of the researchers here, together with the date of their publication on back pain. Some journals specify different formats when quoting research; do check what is required by your intended publisher.) And third, you need to refer to some plausible theory when explaining your results. As you might imagine, theories by identifiable authors carry more weight than

anonymous theories which cannot be checked out.

7. There is no one correct way of writing up a report, since each journal tends to have its own format and requirements. It is therefore important to look at the journal's specifications (usually inside the front or back cover) and to read a couple of articles produced in it before starting your own. That having been said, the following subheadings should provide you with a structure for presenting the essential information from your experiment; you can leave out the subheadings when a particular journal does not use them. Further reading on how to write for publication is provided at the end of this chapter.

DETAILED GUIDELINES FOR STRUCTURING AN ARTICLE

THE TITLE

This should convey succinctly to the reader the essential point of your experiment. For an experimental report it is often easier to construct your title from the relationship predicted in your experimental hypothesis.

For example, if your experimental hypothesis had been: 'Vital capacity is diminished during administration of lumbar traction for back pain', then the predicted relationship would be between lumbar traction and vital capacity. Your title could then be:

An investigation into the relationship between lumbar traction and vital capacity in back pain patients.

To practise producing pithy and clear titles, you could turn back to the hypotheses on pp. 70–71 and construct titles from them.

ABSTRACT OR SUMMARY

The abstract or summary is a short précis of the experiment or study. Usually around 10 lines or 100–150 words long, the abstract includes:

- The aim or hypothesis of the study
- A brief summary of the procedure

- The results, stating their level of significance if appropriate
- A brief, general statement of the implications of the results.

Therefore, the abstract for an experiment testing the previous hypothesis might be:

In order to investigate the relationship between lumbar traction and vital capacity in back pain patients [aim and hypothesis], 20 subjects between the ages of 40 and 55 were measured for vital capacity before receiving lumbar traction and again during the receipt of lumbar traction, over a number of treatments [brief experimental procedure]. Using the related t test to analyse the data, the results were found to be significant ($t = 2.912, p < 0.01$) [brief results].

The implications of the findings are discussed with respect to the treatment of patients with reduced vital capacity [implications].

Obviously, though, you do not include the words in square brackets, and for some journals you would continue from one section to the next, without starting a new line. (You should also note that all the illustrations are fictitious and not derived from any actual research evidence!)

While not all journals require abstracts, they are very useful, not only to the reader who can find out whether the article will be worth reading in full by simply looking at the abstract, but also to the writer who is forced to summarise the critical points of the research in a few lines. This usually focuses the author's mind on the basic structure of the article.

INTRODUCTION

The point of the introduction is to put your study into a context. There are five main topics you should include:

1. It should start off with a general description about the background to the research area. This might involve some national or local policy changes that gave rise to the study or to a general health problem, etc. In the above example some reference could be made to any relevant work which has been carried out on vital capacity and back exercises/ general traction. You might start off by stating something like:

Over the last few years there has been increasing evidence of links between vital capacity and degree of shrinkage in the vertebral column.

In other words, you have defined the topic area.

2. The next stage is to review the relevant literature which relates to this, by briefly quoting appropriate research work. So, you might continue with, for example:

Brown & Green (2007), in a study of osteoarthritis patients, found that vital capacity increased following back extension exercises. Similarly, Black & White (2008) compared the vital capacity of cervical spondylosis patients and patients with prolapsed intervertebral discs during traction and found vital capacity was smaller in the latter group than in the former.

3. The third stage involves providing the reader with some theoretical explanation for these findings. Thus:

One possible explanation for these results comes from the work of Bloggs (2007) who suggested that the effects of the mechanical restriction by the traction harness reduce vital capacity.

4. The next part of the introduction provides a rationale for your own research, so the previous two stages of the introduction should be structured in such a way as to highlight the need for your study. Most

reported research is original; that is to say, the study has usually investigated previously unexplored areas. Therefore, the initial part of your introduction should present any relevant work which has been carried out, and should involve some statement as to where there was a gap in the research. For example, you may find that a particular treatment has not been tried out with a specific patient group, or that a variation on a treatment procedure has not been evaluated. This gap provides you with the rationale for your experiment. Therefore, you might conclude the previous section with:

However, while numerous studies have looked at the effects of exercise or cervical traction on vital capacity, to date no work has specifically looked at the effects of lumbar traction on vital capacity during treatment. This provided the focus for the present research.

5. Finally, you need to state clearly what your experimental hypothesis was, i.e.

The hypothesis under investigation, therefore, was that there is a relationship between vital capacity and lumbar traction in back pain patients.

If you now read just the parts in smaller type, you can get the overall idea of what the introduction should look like. Think of the introduction as an inverted triangle, working from the general background or context area, through the specific research findings, down to your own particular study, as illustrated in Figure 11.1.

Figure 11.1 Suggested structure for an introduction to a research report.

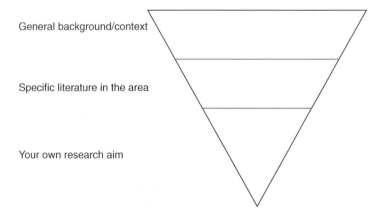

General background/context

Specific literature in the area

Your own research aim

Bear in mind that the literature you quote in the introduction should be comprehensive, up-to-date and critically evaluated if appropriate. An elderly literature review suggests that the author knowledge of the area is out of date, and this does not inspire confidence. However, you will need to include any seminal works in the area, which may not always be very recent. Do not present the literature review like a shopping list by simply recounting who did what. The information must be criticised and synthesised in order to make a coherent case for your own piece of research.

METHOD

The aim of the method section is to tell the reader exactly how the study was carried out. It has to be so clear that anyone reading your method section would be able to replicate your research exactly, without having to ask for clarification on any point.

It is usually subdivided into the following sections (but, once again, you should check the journal first).

Design

The independent and dependent variables in your experiment are usually defined here (if appropriate), together with a statement of whether you used a same- , matched- or different-subject design (again, if appropriate). Furthermore, if you have eliminated any sources of error by counterbalancing, randomising the allocation of subjects to conditions, using a double-blind procedure, etc., you should say so in this section. If you have conducted a survey, you might include here any essential decisions concerning your questionnaire design, how the questionnaires were distributed and why you chose this method. Whatever design you have chosen, you must provide justifications for your choice. This usually means that you must demonstrate your awareness of the strengths and weaknesses of the design and why the one chosen was preferable to any alternatives. You might state, then, for this section:

> The independent variable was traction, while the dependent variable was vital capacity. A same-subject design was used, with subjects being measured on vital capacity before and

during traction. Because of the possible contaminating effect of individual differences that would result from a different-subject design, a same-subject design was selected, where the subjects could act as their own controls. Each subject's vital capacity was measured by three different clinical therapists on nine separate occasions, in order to eliminate any bias in procedure.

Subjects

You should describe your subjects succinctly, giving all the relevant details, e.g. age, sex, medical condition, mean length of time ill, previous treatment, occupation and how they were selected. The specific inclusion and exclusion criteria should be stipulated. If you just asked the first 20 patients who required treatment for back pain, say so. However, it is important to specify whether they volunteered, were press-ganged, paid, etc., since it makes a difference to the way in which they react. Therefore, in the above example, the subject section might read:

> Twenty subjects, 10 male and 10 female, were randomly selected from a back pain clinic. All were aged between 40 and 55; they had been experiencing back pain for at least 6 months and all had been diagnosed as having non-specific back problems. There were no smokers among the subject sample. None of the subjects had received any previous treatment for their complaint and all took part in the experiment on a voluntary basis.

Apparatus

Any apparatus used should be referred to in sufficient detail so that anyone wanting to replicate your experiment can obtain the same equipment. Thus, manufacturer's name, make and type of apparatus, plus a brief description of its capacities should be included. If the equipment has been made specially for you, it should be described in detail and should be accompanied by a diagram showing its main features.

In the above example, then, the apparatus section might be:

> Two pieces of apparatus were used in the experiment. The first was an Akron traction-bed and the second piece of equipment was an electrical spirometer used for measuring vital capacity (Vitalograph).

Materials

Any non-mechanical equipment used should be included in this section, e.g. score sheets, record cards, etc. If a questionnaire or attitude scale was used, you should describe the measure in detail, together with the details of how it was developed and tested. In addition, it is often appropriate to include a copy of it in an appendix at the end of the article. Here, the section would read something like:

> The materials used in the current experiment included patient record cards to keep records of the treatment and graphs from which vital capacity could be calculated.

Procedure

This subsection of the method is very important and should include a detailed description of what you did when you actually carried out the study. It should be clear and logical and should provide the reader with something akin to the method part of a recipe, i.e. a step-by-step account of what was done in the appropriate order. Remember that, although this part, like the rest of the report, should be relevant and succinct, it should also be sufficiently detailed that anyone who reads the procedure could go away and replicate what you did, to the letter.

The word 'relevant' is important as well: you should only include those details which might have some influence on the outcome of the experiment. For example, the height of a chair a patient sat in to carry out the experiment would not be relevant unless you were carrying out research into an area which related to ergonomics or the ability to get in and out of chairs. It is not always easy at first to include just the right amount of detail, but it is a skill which develops over time.

Details that should be included here are things like order of presentation of tasks, and standardised instructions to the subject (which should be reproduced verbatim), how the dependent variable was measured and at what time intervals, number of treatment sessions, etc. Therefore, the procedure section here might be:

> Each subject's vital capacity was measured in the standard way prior to beginning treatment using the spirometer. The results were noted on the appropriate graph. Each patient then received 15 minutes traction three times a week

for 3 weeks (nine treatment sessions in total). Constant traction was given for a period of 15 minutes and was identical for every subject. During the last 5 minutes of every treatment session, vital capacity was measured. Pound weights on the traction bed were increased in relation to body weight in the usual way. The treatment sessions all took place during the morning and were carried out by one of three senior physiotherapists. The subjects were randomly assigned to therapists in a pre-arranged order, such that every patient was treated three times by each therapist. At the end of the 3 weeks, the nine vital capacity scores for each patient were averaged.

Ethics

You must state clearly which ethical procedures were followed and how approval was sought, and when.

RESULTS

The actual scores derived from your study do not need to be presented in this section, but may be included in an appendix, if this is appropriate. However, it is necessary to include the mean scores for each group or condition. If you present a graph, ensure that it conforms to the guidelines outlined in Chapter 5.

Perhaps the most important part of this section, though, are the results of the statistical analysis performed on the scores. While it is unnecessary to include the working-out you do need to say:

1. What statistical analysis you used.
2. What the result was.
3. What the level of significance was (if inferential techniques were used).
4. (A point many people forget) a brief statement of what these results actually mean. It is insufficient to just say: 'The results are significant at the 0.01 level'. You must interpret this for the reader.

So, in the above example, the results section might be (the numbered points refer to the list above).

> The mean pre-test score for the subjects was 4.21 litres, while the mean vital capacity score during treatment was 3.13 litres. The results were analysed using the related t test [1] and

were found to be significant ($t = 2.912$, df $= 19$ [2], $p < 0.01$ (two-tailed [3]). These results suggest that there is a significant decrease in vital capacity during traction [4].

DISCUSSION

1. This section starts off with a re-statement of the outcome of your statistical analysis (usually a variant on the last sentence in the results section), and may add a comment as to whether or not they support the experimental hypothesis (if this is appropriate). For example:

   The results of the present experiment indicate that the vital capacity of the patients diminished significantly during traction, thereby supporting the experimental hypothesis.

2. You should then go on to make some statement about how your results fit in with the findings from other related research. This can incorporate studies which produced contradictory as well as corroborative findings, as long as you provide some plausible explanation for the discrepancy. Here, then you might say:

   These results accord with those of Brown & Green (ibid), Black & White (ibid) as well as those of Grey (2008). Grey found in a study of patients wearing lumbar surgical supports that vital capacity was reduced by 20% due to limitations of diaphragmatic movement. However, work by Gold & Silver (2007) provided contradictory findings. Their results indicated that traction had a negligible effect on vital capacity. However, all the subjects in their sample were smokers and it is conceivable that the existing limitations in vital capacity as a result of smoking minimised the effect of the traction.

3. You must produce a cogent theoretical explanation for your results and also some comment about their practical implications. It is absolutely insufficient simply to describe the findings without explaining them. For instance:

   The results of the present experiment can be explained by Bloggs' Mechanical Restriction Theory (ibid). However, the work of Barnes &

Bridges (2006) is also relevant. They suggest that when the thoracic cavity is elongated, even marginally, then the lung capacity is restricted. Given that lumbar traction alters the length of the spinal column, it is conceivable that there is a consequent elongation of the thoracic cavity, thereby accounting for the present results.

Furthermore, Gold & Silver (2007) have convincingly demonstrated that any fear-inducing treatment procedure, such as that involving large mechanical apparatus, causes shallow respiration and a consequent reduction in vital capacity. Taken together these two theories could account for the present results. These findings, however, have important implications for the treatment of back pain patients who also suffer from chronic respiratory conditions in which the vital capacity is already low. In such cases, alternative therapeutic procedures should be considered.

4. Next you should include any additional analysis which you carried out and which produced some interesting results, together with some comment on these (ideally their theoretical and practical relevance). For example, you might compare male vs. female subjects, older vs. younger subjects, social class or occupational groups, etc. In the present example:

   Further analysis of the results suggested that the vital capacity differences were greater for men than for women ($t = 2.103$, df $=18$, $p < 0.05$, two-tailed). This finding may be interpreted in terms of the generally larger physique of males, thus accounting for the relatively greater difference in vital capacity.

5. You should then acknowledge any limitations of your study, design flaws, unforeseen practical problems that you encountered (e.g. patients not turning up, apparatus breaking down, etc.), variables which you failed to control for, etc. While this may look as though it is condemning your experiment to the waste bin, it isn't, as long as there are no major methodological flaws which would totally vitiate your results. Most research (especially applied research like clinical therapy) will have some minor faults since the perfect experiment is all but a fantasy. However, if you acknowledge the problems and recommend ways of overcoming them were the study to

be repeated in future, then your work will not be dismissed as nonsense. The researcher who thinks his/her study is perfect is the one who is more likely to be rejected. For example:

> The experiment highlighted a procedural flaw, in that traction weights were not identical, but related to body weight instead. While this may have only limited impact on the results since a same-subject design was used, it might have been better to use patients with similar body weights and standardised traction weights.

6. Finally, if your study throws up any ideas for future research, say so. Here you might suggest:

> While the study has demonstrated that vital capacity diminishes during traction, it would be interesting to ascertain whether this is a continuous process or whether there is a point in the treatment when there is a sudden reduction. In addition, the permanency of the reduced capacity needs investigating. These areas could form the basis of a future research project.

REFERENCES

Every bit of research that you have quoted in your report must be included in the reference section in order that the reader can follow up ideas and theories in the area by going back to the original source.

While many journals have their own formats (which you should check first), there are standard ways of presenting references for books and journal articles. There are two main systems of referencing. The first is the Harvard system and is often referred to as the author–date approach, because this style presents the surnames of the authors and the dates of their work in the body of the text (as I have done above), e.g. Smith & Jones (2007). The full reference list is provided in alphabetical order at the end. This is the style most commonly found in social science research. The second style is the Vancouver system, often known as the footnote/endnote approach, because only a reference number is provided in the body of the text, with the full reference provided in numerical order at the end. Vancouver is often favoured by medical journals. Each system will be described in detail.

Harvard

In the text, the reference is presented as the surnames followed by the date of the citation in brackets, e.g. Adam & Eve (2008). If there are more than two authors, the convention is to provide the name of the first author, followed by et al, when the citation is made in the text. The full references are provided in alphabetical order in the reference list. The format varies slightly according to the nature of the reference.

For books, the author's surname is quoted first followed by initials, date of publication, title of the book (underlined or italicised), where it was published and by whom.

Therefore, the reference would look like:

> Bloggs A.B. (2007) Mechanical Restriction Theory, 2nd edition. Camford: Camford University Press.

However, you must check the journal's requirements first, because, if the above reference was listed in a book published by Churchill Livingstone, it would appear as follows:

> Bloggs AB 2007 Mechanical restriction theory, 2nd edition. Camford University Press, Camford.

Book chapters would be referenced thus:

> Barnes F and Bridges H (2006) Therapy and the back pain sufferer. In: Bridges H (ed) Back Pain. London, Chiropractic Press, pp 25–37.

That is, initials, date, chapter title, In: surname and initials of the book's author(s) (ed), title of the book, place of publication, publisher and page numbers of the chapter.

For journal articles, the format is similar: surname, initials, date of article, title of article, title of journal (underlined or italicised), volume of journal and first and last page numbers of the article. Therefore, a journal article would be:

> Black, C. & White, R. (2008) A comparison of the vital capacities of cervical spondylosis and prolapsed intervertebral disc patients. Therapeutic Medicine 14, 15–22.

In the example quoted throughout, all the cited research would have to be referenced in alphabetical order, using the correct format. You would therefore have:

Barnes, M. & Bridges, P. (2006) etc.
Black, C. & White, R. (2008) etc.
Bloggs, A.B. (2007) etc.
Brown, D. & Green, F.A. (2007) etc.
Gold, E. & Silver, S. (2007) etc.

Note in the above examples where the italics are used and the format. While this is a typical layout, many journals have their own variations on the theme and you must ensure that your style is exactly the same as that required by the receiving journal. There are, of course, many other sources of information that would need to be cited in the reference list according to the Harvard convention (e.g. conference abstracts, unpublished PhD theses, newpaper articles and the like). Further guidance is presented in the reading lists at the end of this chapter.

Vancouver

The Vancouver style is more economical in terms of space, because the authors' names only appear in the references, rather than in the references and the text. Thus the text citation might look like this: 'The number of working days lost through back pain has increased significantly over the last decade (1,2)'. The numbers can also be presented in superscript[1,2], but check the notes for authors in your intended journal. In the reference section, the citations are presented in the numerical order in which they appeared in the text.

Books are usually referenced in the following way: surname, initials, book title, edition, place of publication, publisher and year:

Bloggs A.B. Mechanical restriction theory, 2nd edition. Camford, Camford University Press 2007.

For chapters in books, the order is chapter author(s) and initials, chapter title, In: the name(s) of the authors of the main text, book title, edition, place of publication, publisher, year and pages of the chapter:

Barnes F and Bridges H. Therapy and the back pain sufferer. In: Bridges H (ed) Back Pain, 2nd edition. London, Chiropractic Press 2006 pp 25–37.

For journal articles, the format is surname, initials, article title, journal title, year, month, volume (part) and pages:

Black C and White R A comparison of the vital capacities of cervical spondylosis and prolapsed intervertebral disc patients. Therapeutic Medicine, 2008. 14(1) 15–22

Note where the dates come in this format compared with the Harvard system.

In the reference section, the references would be referred to in the numerical order in which they appeared in the article:

1. Bloggs and Smith etc.
2. Jones and Davies etc.

I must reiterate that you should check the journal's notes for authors for any subtle requirements and changes to the punctuation systems compared with the above. And again, further information can be found in the references at the end of this chapter.

General points

There are some other points to note:

- If you provide a direct quote from a reference, you must indicate the page(s) from which it was taken.
- Website addresses should be presented as an author and date where possible in the text, with the full website address in the reference list. Again, the notes to authors will tell you exactly how the journal wants this information presented. A useful website that details how to reference electronic information is: www.shef.ac.uk/library/useful/refs.html

As you may have gathered, the cardinal rule is: check the journal's requirements on format of article and reference presentation.

If you go back and read just the sections in smaller type you should get an idea about the style and format of a journal article, although I should emphasise that the 'article' provided above is a very short one for the purposes of illustration only; obviously, for a full article, the points would be developed in more detail. I would stress again that, prior to writing up your research, you should select a journal which specialises in your research area and check the details of presentation it requires.

SUBMITTING ARTICLES FOR PUBLICATION

Finally, just a few tips on submitting articles for publication:

- Do not submit the article to more than one journal at a time. If the journal of your choice turns it down, then send it off to another one, but never submit simultaneously. (And always keep a copy!)
- If you carried out the research with colleagues, then it may be appropriate to include their names as authors. Where there is multiple authorship of an article, the person quoted first is usually assumed either to be the most senior contributor (in terms of professional status) or alternatively to have carried out the bulk of the work. However, there is no fixed precedent for the order of names, and trouble frequently arises when the most senior author has done least work but still wants to take first place. So, sort out the issue in advance.
- Throughout the course of any research project many individuals will have helped, e.g. by sponsoring the research or helping with any computing. Those people who have made significant contributions should be acknowledged at the end of the article.
- You might consider checking that the article will be refereed 'blind' since there is some evidence that this produces a fairer and more objective evaluation. Remember that getting research published may be something of a game (if you're interested to know just what sort of game, you might like to read Peters & Ceci 1982). However, if you observe the rules of the game as outlined above you should be successful in having your article accepted for publication.

SOME MORALE BOOSTERS

- Don't be disheartened if your article is rejected: even the most seasoned researchers regularly experience rejection. Try to use the referees' comments to improve your article before sending it off to another journal. In other words, use the rejection as a learning exercise.
- Bear in mind that getting something published takes a long time. It may be months before the editor comes back to you with the referees' views, and, if adjustments have to be made, the referees may need to see the article again, which will add to the time it takes for your report to be accepted formally. Added to this is the time lag before the article appears in print once it has been accepted, and this can run into months or sometimes years.
- Seeing your article in print is always gratifying, however many times you have experienced it before. It makes all the effort in its production worthwhile.
- Don't ever lose sight of the fact that a sound piece of research, however small, may have the power to influence patient care radically. You have a moral imperative to put up with the problems of publication, given the potential benefits to clinical therapy practice at all levels.

PREPARING POSTERS FOR PRESENTATION

Presenting your study in poster format is a very good way of disseminating your findings in a more informal setting. A poster involves summarising your research on a large sheet (or several smaller ones), which is attached to a display board. The researcher is usually present for most of the time the poster is on display, so that s/he can discuss the research with people who wander round, asking questions and showing an interest. A poster also offers a more permanent record of your research than an actual conference presentation. For these reasons, posters are a valuable way of presenting your research work, enabling it to reach a wide audience. They are also increasingly being used as a means of course assessment, in order to simulate conference conditions, and in so doing, encouraging students to disseminate their work.

Poster presentations can be used as a first stage in the publication process; because it is a less formal process than presenting a conference paper, it is a good way of getting started along the publishing route. They are also particularly suitable for small-scale and pilot studies, and for presenting work in progress, but not yet completed. And because they offer an opportunity for informal discussion with people interested in the work, they provide an opportunity to get valuable feedback and suggestions, which can be incorporated into a subsequent paper.

Whether your poster is for a course assessment or for a conference, specific guidelines for presentation will be provided and it is important that you stick to these. Therefore, a first rule of poster presentations is *follow the instructions*. This means, then, that the guidance given below is for general purposes only, and must be adapted to comply with the conference or assessment rules.

General principles – some dos and don'ts

For layout and appearance

Do ensure that you:

- Make your poster attract people's attention
- Make the poster a suitable size, e.g. around 80 cm × 110 cm
- Use a mix of colour and white space
- Use bright primary colours, because they are more effective than pale pastels
- Use one main colour, with one or two subsidiary colours
- Use colours that complement each other, i.e. are opposite each other in the colour wheel; this means blue + orange; purple + yellow; red + green – see 'Further reading' for details
- Use warm colours as accent colours, and cool colours as background
- Make about ⅔–¾ of the poster coloured and keep the rest white.
- Use a suitable font size – too big or too small makes the poster difficult to read. As a guide, font size 18–20 for the text, 36 for subheadings and 72 for the main title would be appropriate for a poster of around 80 cm × 110 cm
- Use a simple sans serif font like Tahoma or Ariel, rather than a serif font such as Times New Roman or Gothic
- Use lower case letters for the main body of the text
- Break up the text into small, bite-sized stand-alone boxes or sections
- Include lots of space around the sections

- Illustrate your work, if appropriate, with photos, graphs and diagrams to break up the text; ensure they are labelled
- Consider using 'sound-bites' to highlight important points or findings, by selecting key phrases from the text and presenting them in a larger font.
- Check your grammar and spelling thoroughly
- Make the sections of the poster flow logically and clearly, perhaps by numbering the boxes or by using directional arrows
- Make your poster readable from a distance of about 1 metre
- Consider the use of bullet points to reduce the amount of text
- Have made the most of your space in terms of layout, content and design
- Consider laminating the poster.

Do not:

- Use too many colours
- Change the font style
- Present dense passages of text.

For content

Do ensure that you:

- Are focused – keep the material to the key points
- Remember that most people who read your poster will only take away a few key points – typically the title, aims, the reasons for conducting the study and the conclusions/implications; everything else is likely to be overlooked
- Have made the research question crystal clear
- Have pitched the level and content of your poster appropriately for the audience – practitioners will want a different style and message than academic researchers
- Are clear about the message you want to convey
- Keep to the recommended headings, e.g. **Title, Background, Research question, Sample, Method, Results, Discussion, Conclusions**
- Have included a clear title, author details and affiliation

- Focus on the WHAT of your research – the purpose, aim, research question or hypothesis must be plain
- Explain the WHY of your research – the background, reasons, relevance and justification for your study
- Describe the HOW of your research – the design, sample and methods must be presented
- Present the RESULTS of your research – what has been found so far and what the findings mean
- Discuss the MEANING and IMPLICATIONS of your findings – what can you conclude, what implications do the findings have for policy and practice, what does your study add?
- Admit to the limitations of the study.

Do not

- Have superfluous words – be brutal
- Use abbreviations or jargon
- Use complicated concepts and arguments
- Use too much material
- Use material that lacks cohesion and coherence.

Some final tips

- Prepare handouts to give to anyone who's interested; these can be extended versions of your poster, a reduced version, or just the abstract
- Ensure you go equipped with something to attach your poster to the display board
- Be on time; if you can't be there at some point, ensure that someone suitable can cover for you

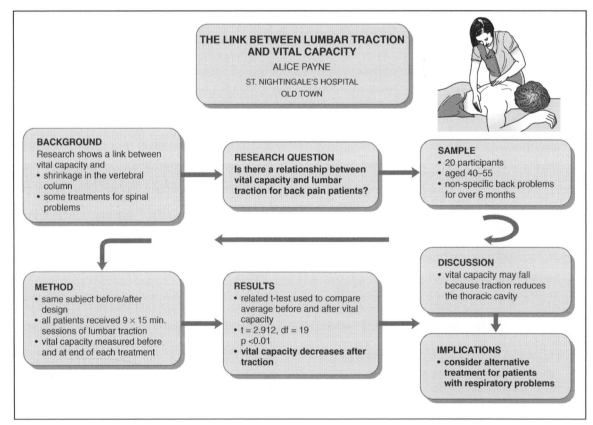

Figure 11.2   Possible presentation of the hypothetical lumbar traction study in poster form. As indicated in the chapter text, it would be better to use a contrasting background/border colour, which can't be shown here because of the colour printing limitations of this book. Remember that if you insert any borrowed illustrations, such as the one used in this poster, you need to check their copyright status and obtain permission to use them if necessary.

- Be prepared to answer questions
- Know your study – prepare yourself as you might for an exam
- Provide details of where you can be contacted
- Follow to the letter the presentation instructions provided by the conference or course.

The skill in preparing a poster is in managing the information in a way that is appealing, informative and focused, with a clear message and a clear layout. It often takes several drafts to get the poster right and I would suggest that you make a small-scale mock-up first, i.e.

- Decide on the key points for each section
- Type them up in their relevant boxes
- Cut the boxes out
- Place them on the background sheet and move them around until the appearance, flow and content are suitable.
- In this way, you can vary the background colours, the font style and size, etc. until you are satisfied with the overall impression.

Figure 11.2 shows how the hypothetical study reported earlier in this chapter could be presented as a poster. Bear in mind, though, that the example is very simple and unsophisticated because of space and layout restrictions.

FURTHER READING

All websites valid as of March 2009

Referencing

http://www.bma.org.uk/ap.nsf/Content/LIBReferenceStyles
http://www.southampton.ac.uk/library/infoskills/references/vancouver.html
www.shef.ac.uk/library/libdocs/hsl-dvc1.pdf
www.shef.ac.uk/library/useful/refs.html

Writing for publication

Berry R 2004 The research project: how to write it, 5th edition. Routledge, London
Cormack DFS 1994 Writing for health care professions. Blackwell, London

Crème P, Lea MR 2006 Writing at university: a guide for students, 2nd edition. Open University Press, Buckingham
Domholdt EA, Malone TR 1985 Evaluating research literature: the educated clinician. Physical Therapy 65(4):487–491
Field FA, Hole G 2004 how to design and report experiments. Sage, London
French S, Sim J 1993 Writing: a guide for therapists. Butterworth Heinemann, London
Hall GM (ed.) 1998 How to write a paper. BMJ Publishing, London
Happell B 2005 Disseminating nursing knowledge. International Journal of Psychiatric Nursing Research 10(3):1147–1155
Kallett RH 2004 How to write the methods section of a research paper. Respiratory Care 49(10):1229–1232
Lester JD, Lester JD 2004 Writing research papers: a complete guide, 4th edition. Longman, New York
Pamir MN 2002 How to write an experimental research paper. Acta Neurochirugica Supplement 83: 109–113
Skelton J 1994 Analysis of the structure of original research papers: an aid to writing original papers for publication. British Journal of General Practice 44(387):455–459
Skelton JR, Edwards SJL 2000 The function of the discussion section in academic medical writing. BMJ 320(7244):1269
Watson R, McKenna H, Cowman S, Keady J 2008 Nursing research: designs and methods. Churchill Livingstone, Edinburgh
Witt P 1980 Research writing tips: the introduction section and research hypothesis. Physical Therapy 60(2):209–210
Witt P 1980 Research writing tips: the methods section. Physical Therapy 60(6):805–806

Preparing posters

Colourwheel. http://images.google.com/images?q=colour+wheel&hl=en&rls=com.
microsoft:en-US&um=1&ie=UTF-8&sa=X&oi=images&ct
http://educ.queensu.ca/~ar/poster.htm
Lowcay B, McIntyre E 2005 Research posters – the way to display. BMJ Career Focus 331:251–252
Lyratzopoulos G 2003 Stand and deliver. BMJ Career Focus 327:35

General

Peters DP, Ceci S 1982 Peer review practices of psychological journals: the fate of accepted, published articles submitted again. Behavioural and Brain Sciences 5(2):187–195

Chapter 12

Reading published research critically

If clinical therapy practice is to become increasingly research-based, then three essential requirements must be fulfilled. First, clinical therapists must carry out sound research which has the capacity to influence service delivery; second, this research must be published; and third, the published reports must be read and evaluated prior to any findings being implemented into clinical practice.

While it is neither appropriate nor realistic to expect that all clinical therapists will become research-active, it is imperative that they become research-minded. This means (a) that well-carried out research is universally acknowledged to be of value to the clinical therapy professions and to the patients they serve, and (b) as a consequence of this, that clinical therapists keep themselves updated on relevant research findings, with a view to modifying their practice if it is appropriate to do so in the light of those findings. This, of course, means that they should be in a position to assess the quality of the research they read and the validity of its conclusions before implementation into service delivery.

Many clinical therapists express concern at the prospect of evaluating published research, particularly if it has appeared in a reputable journal. Such diffidence may in part be a function of our society's traditional belief that anything that appears in print must be true, but it is often also the result of clinical therapists' lack of confidence about how to go about evaluating published research. Clearly, where patients' physical and psychological wellbeing may be adversely affected by unquestioningly implementing the results of a poorly conducted study, it is self-evident that clinical therapists should have a working knowledge of how to assess what they read. This will also mean that they will need to be familiar with some of the concepts outlined earlier in this section of the book, since, without this information, their judgements may not be fully informed.

This chapter is concerned with providing general guidelines on how to make informed assessments of published research. It may be useful to read Chapter 11, on presenting research for publication, prior to reading this one, since it gives a fairly detailed account of what should normally go in a research report. There is also a chapter on systematic reviews (Chapter 24), which provides guidance on how to evaluate research literature by making rigorous quality appraisals and synthesising the results into a manageable review.

ASSESSING PUBLISHED RESEARCH

THE TITLE

When you first look through a journal, you need an at-a-glance knowledge of what the contents are, to see if they have any relevance for you. Consequently, the title of the article will be your first point of contact. Therefore, the title should be a clear statement of what the research project was about so the first question you need to ask is:

1. Is the title a clear and succinct statement of the research study?

ABSTRACT OR SUMMARY

The abstract is a short statement of the aims, methods, findings and conclusions of a research project. While not all journals use abstracts as a means of providing a summarised overview of the research, where they do, you should ask:

2. Does the abstract provide a clear statement of the aims, methods, results and conclusions/implications of the study?

3. After reading the abstract, are you clear in your mind about the nature of the study?

A negative answer to either question may constitute a flaw. Certainly if no clear aim is stated then it may be impossible to evaluate the rest of the abstract, since it would not be obvious whether the method adequately tests the aims, nor whether the results and conclusions support them.

INTRODUCTION

The introduction to a piece of research should give a clear statement of the context and general background to the study, since this will give the reader an idea as to the importance and relevance of the project; it should provide a comprehensive and up-to-date critical review of the research literature, since this will demonstrate the researcher's knowledge of the topic area and enhance the credibility of the project as a whole; it should provide a rationale for why a further piece of research was necessary, since the project should plug a gap in existing clinical therapy knowledge; and it must give an unambiguous statement of the aims, or hypothesis to be tested. Without this, it will be impossible to assess whether the study is a proper test of the aims. Therefore, the questions concerning the introduction are as follows:

4. Is there an adequate description of the general context for the study?
5. Is the literature review thorough, relevant, recent and properly used to provide a structured argument leading to the reason for conducting the reported piece of research?
6. Is the hypothesis (if appropriate) clearly stated, and the predicted relationship between the variables apparent?
7. If the research does not test the hypothesis, are the aims of the study clear?
8. Are the aims or hypothesis useful to clinical therapy?
9. Is the project likely to be of value to clinical therapy?

If the answers to these questions are 'no' then doubt must be cast on the quality of the project.

METHOD

The general format of the method section varies from journal to journal. However, the actual content is usually very similar. The method section should tell the reader exactly what was done, how it was done, the order in which it was done, why this approach was chosen, and with whom the project was conducted.

After reading this section, you should know all the relevant details and be in a position to replicate the study exactly if you so wish. If you have to ask any questions or you need clarification on anything at all, then this section is not adequate, and the report must be considered flawed.

So the questions concerning the method section are:

10. Has the design of the study been properly described?
11. Has the researcher made it clear why this design was chosen?
12. Is the design appropriate for the aims/hypothesis stated in the introduction?
13. Are sources of error acknowledged and controlled?
14. Is the sample suitable? Of an appropriate size? Fully described? Properly selected?
15. Were any sources of bias or error evident in the sample and/or in the process by which they were chosen?
16. Would this impact upon the study's outcome?
17. Was any mechanical apparatus used in the study and, if so, was it properly described? Was it suitable for the project?
18. Were any other materials used, such as questionnaires, score sheets, attitude scales, etc.?
19. Were these described fully and/or included in the appendix, if appropriate?
20. Were any questionnaires or scales which were used properly constructed and adequately tested before using them in the study? Were they suitable for their purpose?
21. Is the description of what was done absolutely clear?
22. Does it state the order in which things were done?
23. Does it provide a verbatim report of any instructions given to the subjects? Were the instructions clear?
24. Were the sources of error dealt with appropriately?
25. Was the method of data collection clearly described and appropriate?
26. Were the data a suitable measure of the dependent variable (if the study tested an hypothesis) or of the information required by the survey's aims?
27. Were the subjects treated well, their rights and confidentiality protected?
28. Was the study ethical?
29. Could you repeat this study to the letter if it was considered necessary?

If the answer to the last question in particular was 'no' then the method section does not fulfil its purpose. Other negative answers in this section would suggest not only a report beset by omissions and obscurities, but might also reflect a poorly conducted piece of research.

RESULTS

The results section should summarise what was actually found in the project. While it does not typically include raw data or the working-out of any statistical analysis, both these elements can be summarised. Raw data can be presented by tabulating means, standard deviations, etc. and the results of any statistical analysis by the numerical value obtained as a result of performing the correct statistical test. This should be accompanied by a p value and an interpretation of this.

Whatever the nature of the study, the meaning of the results should be made clear to the reader.

The questions relating to this section then are:

30. Are the graphs (if provided) clear, self-explanatory and useful?
31. Are the tables (if used) clearly labelled and constructed and with an obvious relevance to the study?
32. Are the statistical tests used the correct ones for the project's design?

33. Is the selected level of significance appropriate for the topic area?
34. Is the p value clearly stated and correct for the hypothesis as stated (i.e. one- or two-tailed)?

If the analysis at any level is incorrect this will invalidate the study and conclusions. Therefore, positive answers to every question in this section are critical.

DISCUSSION

The discussion section of a research report should do just as it says: it should discuss the findings from the project in relation to other research work in the area, thus providing a broader context for the project's results.

In addition, some theoretical explanation for the results should be provided, as theory and practice should go together. Sometimes results do not tie in with findings of existing research and some convincing reason for this discrepancy must be put forward, otherwise doubts must inevitably be cast on the methodology and analysis used in the study.

The conclusions drawn in the discussion should reflect the results. They should not be extravagant and extend beyond what was actually found. Neither should the conclusions be incomplete and refer only to those parts of the data that confirm the researcher's original aims while ignoring results which oppose those aims. Such selective discussion has the potential to be every bit as misleading as incorrect analysis and interpretation.

In addition, the discussion section offers the researcher an opportunity to acknowledge flaws in the study, together with suggestions for how these may be rectified in the future. Unconditional acceptance of the design of a research project may mean that the results are given more credence than they are due. Field research is never perfect and it is essential that the researcher recognises that, in order that the results can be interpreted with due caution.

Lastly, a good research project should spawn ideas for other studies. If it doesn't, then it is possible that the original project was too narrow and limited to be of much real value.

So the questions relating to this section are:

35. Are the results and conclusions clearly stated?
36. Are they related to other studies in the area, thereby putting them into a broader research framework?
37. Is a cogent theoretical explanation for the findings provided?
38. Are the results interpreted fully and correctly, or selectively and/or extravagantly?
39. Are any flaws in the study's design highlighted, together with recommendations for improvement?
40. Are the results interpreted with these limitations in mind?
41. Are any practical ramifications of the results discussed?
42. Do any ideas for future projects emerge?

The answer 'no' to any of the questions must produce reservations about the overall quality of the project.

REFERENCES

Every piece of work or research quoted in the report must be fully acknowledged and properly recorded in the reference section. These references should give the full name of the author, the date of the work, its title and where it was published (see section on references, pp. 154–155).

Omissions in the references are suggestive of sloppiness, and may then reflect adversely on the rest of the study.

Therefore:

43. Is every article, study, research report and book quoted in the reference section?
44. Do these references give all the required information?

OVERALL CONSIDERATIONS

Finally, there are some general questions that need to be asked:

45. Was the project a worthwhile one, contributing to the knowledge base of clinical therapy?

46. Was it clearly written, so that the content was easily accessible to the reader?
47. Is the report scientific and objective both in the way in which it was conducted as well as the way in which it was analysed and written up?
48. Is the article devoid of jargon?
49. Has the research project advanced clinical therapy in any way?

These questions may seem pedantic and tedious, but a poorly reported project may suggest a poorly conducted project. Remember, that no research project is perfect. What is important, though, is that the researcher recognises this, justifies why design and analysis decisions were taken, and interprets the results in the light of these. Asking the above questions of an article means that patient well being will be safeguarded to some degree, since the reader will be in a position to make sound assessments of a research project before deciding whether to implement the findings into his/her practice.

These guidelines for critically evaluating published articles are applied to an actual paper in Appendix 4 and further guidance for reading research critically is provided at the end of this chapter.

FURTHER READING

Ajetunmobi O 2002 Making sense of critical appraisal. Hodder Arnold, London

Centre for Dissemination and Reviews report 4 2001, 2nd edition, – Phase 5. Undertaking systematic reviews of research on effectiveness. York, York Publishing Services Ltd

Critical Appraisal Skills Programme (CASP). Online. Available http://www.phru.nhs.uk/Pages/PHD/resources.htm December 17 2008

Greenhalgh T 1997 How to read a paper: getting your bearings (deciding what the paper is about). BMJ 315: 243–246

Greenhalgh T 1997 How to read a paper: assessing the methodological quality of published papers. BMJ 315: 305–308

Greenhalgh T 1997 How to read a paper: the Medline database. BMJ 315:180–183

Greenhalgh T 1997 How to read a paper: papers that report drug trials. BMJ 315:480–483

Greenhalgh T 1997 How to read a paper: statistics for the non-statistician I. Different types of data need different statistical tests. BMJ 315:364–366

Greenhalgh T 1997 How to read a paper: statistics for the non-statistician II.'Significant' relations and their pitfalls. BMJ 315:422–425

Greenhalgh T 1997 How to read a paper: papers that summarise other papers (systematic reviews and meta-analyses). BMJ 315:672–675

Greenhalgh T 1997 How to read a paper: papers that go beyond numbers (qualitative research). BMJ 315:740–743

Greenhalgh T 1997 How to read a paper: papers that tell you what things cost (economic analyses). BMJ 315:596–599

Guyatt GH, Sackett DL, Cook DJ 1993 Users' guides to the medical literature.I. JAMA 270(21):2598–2601

Guyatt GH, Sackett DL, Cook DJ 1993 Users' guides to the medical literature.II. JAMA 271(1):59–63

PEDro. Online. Available http://www.pedro.fhs.usyd.edu.au December 17 2008

Wood M 2003 making sense of statistics: a non-mathematical approach. Palgrave, London

SECTION 2

Statistical tests

It is essential that the data from any research project are properly analysed. Where research involves testing an hypothesis, through the use of either an experimental or correlational design, it is critical that the correct statistical test is used to find out whether the results support the prediction made in the hypothesis. Using the wrong test gives invalid results and conclusions, which is potentially very damaging in an area such as clinical therapy where patient wellbeing is involved. Ways of choosing the correct test were outlined in Chapter 9. This section is concerned with how to carry out those tests.

Chapter **13**

Non-parametric tests for same- and matched-subject designs

INTRODUCTION

As was mentioned in Chapter 9, the results from most of the designs you are likely to use can be analysed using either a non-parametric or a parametric statistical test. Each test does essentially the same job, but the parametric test is rather more sensitive. However, in order to use a parametric test, certain conditions have to be fulfilled (see Chapter 9). If you cannot fulfil these or if you have any doubts then you should use the equivalent non-parametric test. All the tests in this chapter are **non-parametric for same- and matched-subject designs**. In the next chapter, the equivalent parametric tests for the same designs will be covered.

So, the statistical tests covered in this chapter are appropriate for any experimental design that involves either: one group of subjects which is used in two or more conditions (same-subject design); or alternatively two or more groups of subjects, each of which is used in one condition only, but who are matched on certain key variables (matched-subject design). (Have a look back to the examples given on pp. 126 and 128 in Chapter 9.) Therefore, the sort of designs we are talking about are:

1. **Same-subject design**: one group of subjects used in two or more conditions.
    a. Two conditions (Figure 13.1).
    b. Three or more conditions (Figure 13.2).

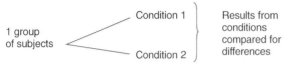

Figure 13.1 Same-subject design: one group of subjects and two conditions.

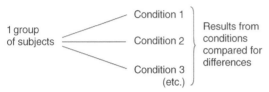

Figure 13.2 Same-subject design: one group of subjects and three or more conditions.

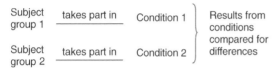

Figure 13.3 Matched-subject design: two groups of matched subjects each taking part in one condition.

Subject group 1 — takes part in — Condition 1
Subject group 2 — takes part in — Condition 2
Subject group 3 (and so on) — takes part in — Condition 3
Results from conditions compared for differences

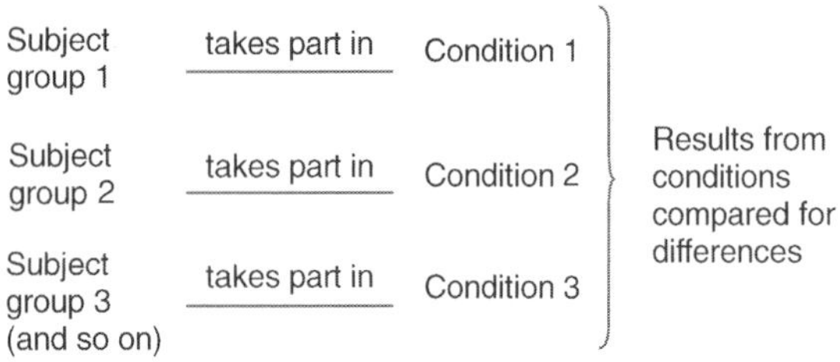

Figure 13.4 Matched-subject design: three or more groups of matched subjects each taking part in one condition only.

2. **Matched-subject designs**: two or more groups of matched subjects, each of which is used in one condition only.
   a. Two matched groups only (Figure 13.3).
   b. Three or more matched groups (Figure 13.4).

The designs which involve one group doing two conditions (Design 1a), or two matched groups doing one condition each (Design 2a) are analysed using the **McNemar test** if the data are only nominal, or the **Wilcoxon test** if the data are ordinal or interval/ratio.

Table 13.1 Non-parametric tests for related- and matched-subject designs

Design	Non-parametric test
1a. One group of Ss taking part in two conditions	McNemar test if the data are nominal
Results from conditions compared for differences	or Wilcoxon test if the data are ordinal or interval/ratio
2a. Two groups of matched Ss each taking part in one condition only	McNemar test if the data are nominal
	or Wilcoxon test if the data are ordinal or interval/ratio
Results from conditions compared for differences	
1b. One group of Ss taking part in three or more conditions	Friedman test or Page's *L* trend test (see pp. 178–185 for which one to use)
Results from conditions compared for differences	Both of these can be used with ordinal or interval/ratio data
2b. Three or more groups of matched Ss each taking part in one condition only	Friedman test or Page's L trend test (see pp. 178–185 for which one to use)
	Both of these can be used with ordinal or interval/ratio data
Results from conditions compared for differences	

The designs which involve one group doing three or more conditions (Design 1b) or three (or more) matched groups doing one condition each (Design 2b), are analysed using either the Friedman test or the **Page's *L* trend test**. Pages 178–185 will explain which of those two you should select, since each one requires slightly different conditions. This is summarised in Table 13.1.

NON-PARAMETRIC TEST: SAME- AND MATCHED-SUBJECT DESIGNS, TWO CONDITIONS AND NOMINAL DATA

MCNEMAR TEST FOR THE SIGNIFICANCE OF CHANGES

Just to remind you, this test is used when you either have one group of subjects which is measured or tested on two conditions (a same-subject design) and the two sets of results are then compared for any differences between them; or when you compare two groups of subjects who are matched on all the critical variables which might influence the results (i.e. a matched-group design). Each group is tested in one condition and the results are compared for differences between them. In other words you would use this test if you had either experimental Design 1a or 2a.

The McNemar test is particularly suitable for 'before and after' type situations. However, there is one very important feature of this test: it is used with nominal data, i.e. a level of measurement which simply allows you to allocate people or responses to named categories. Essentially what the McNemar test does is to record the changes from one category to the other, across the two conditions, to see if these changes are significant. When you calculate the McNemar test, you find a numerical value called 'chi-squared', written as χ^2, which you then look up in Table A2.1 (p. 341) to see if this figure represents significant differences between the two conditions or the two matched groups.

Example

Let's imagine you've noticed over the years the high degree of fear most patients experience prior to laryngectomy. It occurs to you that a talk prior to the operation to explain what will happen, and the type of postoperative treatment available, may go some way towards reducing their tension. You decide to try this and see whether your hunch is correct.

Your experimental hypothesis is:

H₁   A preoperative talk will reduce anxiety levels in patients referred for laryngectomy.

What would your null hypothesis be?
Is this a one-tailed or two-tailed hypothesis?
You select 20 patients referred for laryngectomy and note whether or not they are frightened about the procedure. You classify them as either:

1. little or no anxiety or
2. high anxiety.

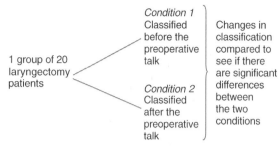

Figure 13.5   Design for experiment to assess effectiveness of preoperative talk for patients referred for laryngectomy.

This is nominal data because you are simply allocating patients' responses to a named category. You then spend some time explaining to the patients what will happen, discussing any issues and problems they have, etc. Following this session, the patients are asked whether their anxiety levels have reduced. According to their response, you again allocate them to one of the categories, as before.

You therefore have the design shown in Figure 13.5.

You have all the conditions required by the McNemar test, that is, a same-subject design and nominal data.

You obtain the results shown in Table 13.2.

Calculating the McNemar test

1. You must first of all record the changes that occurred from one testing to the other. In other words you must count up:
   (a) How many patients changed from 'little or no anxiety' to 'high anxiety' as a result of the talk, i.e. from 'ø' before the talk to 'X' after. In the above example there are no changes of this kind.
   (b) How many patients had very little or no anxiety both before and after the talk, i.e. were 'ø' before the talk and 'ø' afterwards. In this example, there are 6 such patients.
   (c) How many patients had high anxiety both before and after the talk, i.e. were 'X' before and 'X' after. Here there were 4 such patients.
   (d) How many patients changed from feeling high anxiety before the talk to feeling little or no anxiety after, i.e. changed

Table 13.2 Patient anxiety about laryngectomy;
ø = little or no anxiety, X = high anxiety

Patient	Before talk	After talk
1	ø	ø
2	X	ø
3	X	ø
4	ø	ø
5	X	X
6	X	ø
7	X	X
8	ø	ø
9	X	ø
10	X	ø
11	X	X
12	X	ø
13	ø	ø
14	ø	ø
15	ø	ø
16	X	X
17	X	ø
18	X	ø
19	X	ø
20	X	ø

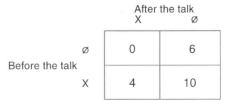

		After the talk	
		X	ø
Before the talk	ø	Cell A	Cell B
	X	Cell C	Cell D

Figure 13.6   Table used in calculating the McNemar test.

from 'X' before the talk to 'ø' afterwards. Here there are 10.

2. These figures now have to be put in a table like Figure 13.6.

Cell A represents those patients who changed from ø to X (little anxiety to high anxiety, i.e. 0). This is calculation (a) above.

Cell B represents those patients who had little or no anxiety before and after the talk (stayed at ø, i.e. 6). This is calculation (b) above.

Cell C represents those patients who had high anxiety before and after the talk (stayed at X, i.e. 4). This is calculation (c) above.

		After the talk	
		X	ø
Before the talk	ø	0	6
	X	4	10

Figure 13.7   Table of Figure 13.6 with data entered.

Cell D represents those patients who changed from high anxiety to low anxiety (changed from X to ø, i.e. 10). This is calculation (d) above. So, if we enter these figures into the cells, the table looks like Figure 13.7.

Remember! You must organise your cells in the way indicated above, otherwise your calculations will be incorrect. In other words, whichever category is on the left-hand cell for the 'After' condition, the other category should be at the top for the 'Before' condition. The numbers in the cells should add up to the same as the number of patients tested. In this case, the number is 20.

3. Find the value of χ^2 from the formula:

$$\chi^2 = \frac{([A-D]-1)^2}{A+D}$$

where
   A = the value in cell A (i.e. 0)
   D = the value in cell D (i.e. 10)
If we substitute our figures we get:

$$\chi^2 = \frac{([0-10^*]-1)^2}{10}$$

$$= \frac{(9)^2}{10}$$

$$= \frac{81}{10}$$

Therefore $\chi^2 = 8.1$

(*If you get a minus figure in the square brackets, ignore the minus and treat the figure as a plus; i.e. −10 becomes 10.)

4. Before looking up the results to see if they represent a significant change in fear levels, you need a further value: the df value. In the McNemar test, it is always 1.

Looking up the value of χ^2 for significance

To see whether this value of 8.1 represents a significant difference in fear levels, turn to Table A2.1, which is the probability table associated with the McNemar test (and the chi-squared or χ^2 test, see later). Down the left-hand column you will see df values from 1 to 30. To their right are five numbers, called **critical values of χ^2**.

To find out whether our χ^2 value is significant, look down the df column until you find our df value of 1. To the right you will see five critical values:

$$2.71 \quad 3.84 \quad 5.41 \quad 6.64 \quad 10.83$$

Each of these figures is associated with the probability value at the top of its column. For example, the critical value of 2.71 is associated with a probability value of 0.10, for a two-tailed test. You will notice that this table only refers to two-tailed hypotheses. Where you have a one-tailed hypothesis, look up the results in the way outlined, and simply halve the p value (see pp. 132–133).

For our χ^2 value to be significant, it has to be *equal to or larger than* one of the critical values to the right of df = 1. Our χ^2 value of 8.1 is larger than 2.71, 3.84, 5.41 and 6.64. Because convention dictates that we must always say that p is *less* than a given value (never *more* than), we therefore take the value of 6.64 which is associated with a probability value of 0.01 for a two-tailed hypothesis, and therefore 0.005 for a one-tailed hypothesis (i.e. half 0.01). (If you look back to our hypothesis, you will see that we are predicting a specific direction to our results, i.e. that a preoperative talk will reduce fear levels; therefore, our hypothesis is one-tailed.)

Now to be significant *exactly* at the 0.005 level, our χ^2 value must *equal* 6.64. Our χ^2 value is larger than 6.64, so that means that the probability of our results being due to random error is even less than 0.005. This is expressed as

$$p < 0.005 \ (< \text{means 'less than'})$$

Had our χ^2 value been exactly 6.64 we would have expressed this as

$$p = 0.005$$

Interpreting the results

Our results are associated with a probability of less than 0.005 or 0.5%. This means there is less than 0.5% chance of the results being due to random error. If you remember, a p value of 5% or less was a standard cut-off point for claiming results to be significant. As 0.5% is less than 5% our results are significant.

However, before going on to explain what this means, you must check that the changes in fear are in the direction you predicted, i.e.

| high fear before the talk | changed to | low fear after the talk |

It is possible to get significant results which are in the opposite direction to those predicted. In this case it would mean

| low fear before the talk | changed to | high fear after the talk |

These results, while significant, would not support your hypothesis.

If you look at the data in the table, you will see that the changes are in the predicted direction, and we can reject the null (no relationship) hypothesis and accept the experimental hypothesis.

We can state this in the following way:

Using a McNemar test on the data ($\chi^2 = 8.1$, df = 1), the results were found to be significant at $p < .005$ for a one-tailed test. This suggests that preoperative talks significantly reduce the levels of fear of patients referred for laryngectomy.

It is very important to note, though, that there should be sufficient numbers involved to compute the McNemar test. If (Cell A + Cell D) ÷ 2 comes to less than 5, you cannot use the McNemar. In such a case, it would be worth your while to collect sufficient data to satisfy the above requirement.

Activity 13.1 (Answers on p. 366)

1 To practise looking up χ^2 values for the McNemar test, look up the following and say whether you would classify them as significant.

(i) $\chi^2 = 3.98$ df $= 1$ one-tailed p
(ii) $\chi^2 = 6.71$ df $= 1$ one-tailed p
(iii) $\chi^2 = 5.41$ df $= 1$ two-tailed p
(iv) $\chi^2 = 2.59$ df $= 1$ one-tailed p
(v) $\chi^2 = 10.96$ df $= 1$ two-tailed p
(vi) $\chi^2 = 4.82$ df $= 1$ two-tailed p

2 Calculate a McNemar test on the following data: As a clinical therapist responsible for the management of clinical services, you wish to alter the 'on-call' duty rotas, but have so far met with opposition from the other clinical therapists in the clinic in which you work. In fact, on the last poll, only 5 out of 30 were prepared to alter their duties. You decide to send round an explanatory fact sheet, in the hope that presenting the reasons for your change might alter their views. At the end of the fact sheet you simply ask the clinical therapists to indicate whether or not they would accommodate the altered duties. Your hypothesis is:

H$_1$ Providing extra information about the reasons for changing on-call duty hours will modify the opinions of the clinical therapists involved.

Is this a one- or two-tailed hypothesis?
You obtain the results shown in Table 13.3.
State what your χ^2 value is and what your p value is. Write this out in a similar format to that given on p. 173.

Table 13.3 Effect of extra information on opinions of physiotherapists: ✔ for the change; ✗ against the change

Clinical therapist	Opinions prior to receipt of fact sheet	Opinions after the receipt of fact sheet
1	✗	✔
2	✗	✔
3	✗	✗
4	✗	✔
5	✔	✔
6	✗	✗
7	✗	✔
8	✗	✗
9	✗	✔
10	✗	✗
11	✗	✔
12	✗	✔
13	✗	✗
14	✗	✗
15	✗	✔
16	✔	✔
17	✗	✔
18	✔	✔
19	✗	✗
20	✗	✔
21	✗	✗
22	✗	✔
23	✗	✗
24	✔	✔
25	✗	✗
26	✗	✗
27	✔	✗
28	✗	✔
29	✗	✔
30	✗	✔

NON-PARAMETRIC TEST: SAME- AND MATCHED-SUBJECT DESIGNS, TWO CONDITIONS AND ORDINAL OR INTERVAL/RATIO DATA

WILCOXON SIGNED-RANKS TEST

To recap, this test is used when you have two conditions (either one control condition and one experimental condition or two experimental conditions) and you have either one group of subjects doing both conditions, or two groups of matched subjects, one group doing one condition and the other group the other condition (see Designs 1a and 2a on pp. 169–170). The data for this test must be ordinal or interval/ratio.

Essentially what the Wilcoxon test does is to compare the performance of each S (or pairs of matched Ss) in each condition to see if there is a significant difference between them. When you calculate this test, you end up with a numerical value called 'T', which you then look up in the probability tables for the Wilcoxon test, to see if this value represents a significant difference between the conditions.

Example

Let's take an example. The issue regarding the wearing of uniform by clinical therapists seems unresolved. Some clinical therapists are of the opinion that uniforms increase the psychological distance between the patient and therapist and thus discourage the development of rapport. Others feel that the nature of the clinical therapist's job can be very stressful and intimate; the uniform sanctions such activities and makes the patient feel more comfortable. Obviously central to this issue is the patient–therapist relationship, a factor of major importance in long-stay patients. You decide you will assess the effects of clinical therapists wearing uniform on the degree of confidence experienced by a group of long-stay patients. Therefore you decide to test the following hypothesis:

H₁ Long-stay patients experience different levels of confidence when being treated by uniformed clinical therapists than when treated by non-uniformed clinical therapists.

What would your null hypothesis be?
Is this a one- or two-tailed hypothesis?
You devise a questionnaire which simply asks the subject to indicate on a 5-point scale (ordinal data) how confident they feel when being treated (a) by a uniformed clinical therapist, and (b) by a non-uniformed clinical therapist. On your

scale, a score of 1 means 'not at all confident' while 5 means 'very confident'. You give this questionnaire to 15 long-stay patients. Thus, you have the design shown in Figure 13.8.

You have all the conditions required by the Wilcoxon, i.e. a same-subject design and ordinal data.

You administer your questionnaire to the 15 Ss (having, of course, included all the essential prerequisites for such a design; see Chapters 7 and 8) and you end up with the results shown in Table 13.4.

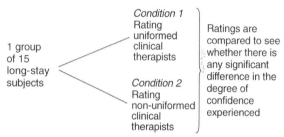

Figure 13.8 Design to test effect of clinical therapists wearing uniform on patient confidence.

Table 13.4   Results of questionnaire and calculation of Wilcoxon test

	Results			Calculations		
	1	2	3	4	5	6
	Condition A	Condition B*				
Subject	Uniform	Non-uniform	d = A − B	Rank order of d	Rank of + differences	Rank of − differences
1	5	3	+2	(+) 5.5	+5.5	
2	4	3	+1	(+) 1.5	+1.5	
3	5	2	+3	(+) 9.5	+9.5	
4	2	5	−3	(−) 9.5		−9.5
5	4	4	0	exclude		
6	3	3	0	exclude		
7	5	4	+1	(+) 1.5	+1.5	
8	5	3	+2	(+) 5.5	+5.5	
9	4	2	+2	(+) 5.5	+5.5	
10	4	2	+2	(+) 5.5	+5.5	
11	2	2	0	exclude		
12	3	1	+2	(+) 5.5	+5.5	
13	5	1	+4	(+) 11.5	+11.5	
14	4	2	+2	(+) 5.5	+5.5	
15	5	1	+4	(+) 11.5	+11.5	
Σ	60	38			+68.5	−9.5
x̄	4	2.533				

*It does not matter which condition is called A and which B.

Calculating the Wilcoxon test

In order to find out whether these ratings differ significantly for each condition, you must take the following steps.

1. Add up the total (Σ) for Condition A (uniformed):

$$\Sigma A = 60$$

2. Add up the total (Σ) for Condition B (non-uniformed):

$$\Sigma B = 38$$

3. Find the mean ($\bar{x}$) for each condition:

$$\bar{x}_A = 4 \quad \bar{x}_B = 2.533$$

4. Calculate the difference (d) for each pair of scores by taking A − B, remembering to put in the + and − signs. Therefore for Subject 1 (S1) you would have 5 − 3 = +2 and so on. Put the results in column 3 (d = A − B).

5. You must then rank order these differences, in column 4, by giving a rank of 1 to the smallest difference, 2 to the next smallest and so on. When you do this, you must ignore the plus and minus signs. However, where the difference between a pair of scores is 0, you omit this pair altogether from any further analysis. Therefore, in this example, Ss 5, 6 and 11 are now excluded from any further analysis and we are reduced to 12 subjects.

You will also note that there are a number of d values which are identical, e.g. Ss 2 and 7 both have a d of +1, Ss 1, 8, 9, 10, 12 and 14 all have a d value of +2. Where this happens a special procedure is used – the 'tied rank' procedure.

Tied rank procedure

To carry out the tied rank procedure, rank the scores as usual, giving a rank of 1 to the smallest, 2 to the next smallest (remember: we omit the 0s and ignore the + and − values).

Continue this procedure until you come to the tied scores. Here, Ss 2 and 7 both have d values of 1. These two scores are the lowest and should therefore occupy the two lowest ranks, i.e. ranks 1 and 2. So we add up these two ranks (1 + 2) and divide this by the number of d values that are the same score (i.e. two d values of 1):

$$\frac{1+2}{2} = 1.5$$

Therefore, the d values of 1 are both given the ranks of 1.5 (see column entitled 'Rank order of d').

We now find there are six d values of 2. These values occupy the next lowest ranks, i.e. 3, 4, 5, 6, 7 and 8, because ranks 1 and 2 have already been used up.

Therefore we add these ranks together:

$$3+4+5+6+7+8 = 33$$

and divide this by the number of d values which have the value of 2 (i.e. six d values of 2):

$$33 \div 6 = 5.5$$

Thus, all the d values of 2 are assigned the rank 5.5.

We now find there are two d values of 3 (Ss 3 and 4). These are the next two lowest scores and they would occupy the next two lowest ranks, i.e. 9 and 10, because ranks 1–8 have now been used up.

Therefore, we add these ranks together:

$$9+10 = 19$$

and divide this by the number of d values which have the same value of 3 (i.e. two d values of 3) which is:

$$19 \div 2 = 9.5$$

So, both the d values of 3 are given the rank of 9.5.

Now there are only two remaining d values, each of which is 4. These d values occupy the next two ranks, i.e. 11 and 12, because ranks 1–10 have now been used up. Therefore we add these ranks together:

$$11+12 = 23$$

and divide this by the number of d values which have the same value of 4 (i.e. two d values of 4):

$$23 \div 2 = 11.5$$

Thus, the d values of 4 are each given the rank of 11.5.

Many people get very irritated by this ranking procedure, especially when calculating tied ranks, because a slip of just one figure can throw everything out. To avoid this, you may wish to write out all the ranks you will be using (which will be the same as the number of difference values to be ranked) and cross them off as you use them. Here, then, we would write out the following ranks: 1, 2, 3, 4, 5, 6, 7, 8, 9, 10, 11, 12, and strike them off as we go along.

Remember, the highest rank you write down should be the same as the number of differences between scores you are ranking. Here we are ranking 12 d values, so the highest rank will be 12.

6. Now write in by each rank the plus or minus sign of the corresponding d value. Therefore, the first rank of 5.5 is given a plus sign because it has a corresponding d value of +2.

7. Put all the ranks with a + sign into column 5, 'Rank of + differences'. Put all the ranks with a – sign into column 6, 'Rank of minus differences'.

8. Add up the ranks for column 5, 'Rank of + differences', to give the total (Σ) for the + ranks, i.e. +68.5. Add up the ranks for column 6, 'Rank of – differences', to give the total (Σ) for the – ranks, i.e. –9.5.

9. Take the smaller of the two rank totals, ignoring the plus or minus sign, as your value of T (i.e. $T = 9.5$).

10. Find N by counting up the number of subjects (or in the case of matched groups, pairs of Ss) omitting those who had d values of 0, i.e. $15 - 3 = 12$.

Looking up the value of T for significance

To see whether this T value of 9.5 represents a significant difference in the confidence levels experienced with uniformed and non-uniformed clinical therapists, it must be looked up in the probability tables for the Wilcoxon test (Table A2.2, p. 342).

Down the left-hand column you will see values of N, while across the top you will see 'Levels of significance' for one- and two-tailed tests. Under each of these are columns of figures which are called critical values of T.

To find out whether our T value is significant at one of the levels indicated, we must first locate our N value of 12 down the left-hand column. To the right of this you will see four numbers which represent the critical values of T for this number of Ss. These values are:

$$17 \quad 14 \quad 10 \quad 7$$

Each of these figures is associated with the corresponding p value indicated at the top of the column.

For example, a critical value of 14 is associated with a probability of 0.05 for a two-tailed test, and 0.025 for a one-tailed test.

In order for your T value to be significant at a given level, it has to be *equal to or smaller than* one of these four figures. So, taking our T value of 9.5, look at the first figure to the right of $N = 12$, i.e. 17. Our T value is smaller than 17, so look at the next figure: 14. Our T value is smaller than 14, so look at the next figure: 10. Our T value is smaller than 10, so look at the next figure: 7. Our T value is larger than 7. Therefore our T value comes somewhere between the critical values of 7 and 10 in the table.

Because we have a two-tailed hypothesis (we have simply predicted that there will be a difference in confidence levels) this means our results are significant between the 0.02 and 0.01 (or between 2% and 1%) levels. Now, to be significant at a given level, the T value must be equal to or smaller than the critical value of T. Because it is smaller than 10 but larger than 7, we must comply with convention and select the value of 10, which is associated with a significance level of 2%. Had our T value equalled 10 exactly, we would say that our results are significant at p equals 0.01. However, our T value is smaller than 10, which means that its significance is actually less than 0.02. Therefore we express this as

$$p < 0.02 \, (< \text{means 'less than'})$$

This means that the probability of our results being due to random error is less than 2%.

Interpreting the results

Our T value is associated with a p value of <0.02 level (i.e. <2% level), which means that there is less than a 2% chance that our results are due to random error. If you remember, we said a good rule of thumb for claiming support for your hypothesis is a probability of 5% (or 0.05) or less. Because our T has a smaller p value than 5%, we can say that our results are significant. But, it is very important to note that you must check the averages for each set of data ($\bar{x}_A = 4$, $\bar{x}_B = 2.533$) to see whether the results are in the direction you predicted (i.e. larger on the uniform condition), since occasionally, you may get significant results which are actually the reverse of what you predicted and therefore would not support your hypothesis.

Here, the results are in the direction you predicted and therefore we can say that your hypothesis has been supported (i.e. we can reject the null hypothesis).

We can state this in the following way:

Using a Wilcoxon test on the data ($T = 9.5$, $N = 12$), the results were found to be significant at $p < 0.02$ level for a two-tailed test. The means of 4 and 2.533 suggest that long-stay patients experience greater degrees of confidence when being treated by a uniformed clinical therapist than by a non-uniformed clinical therapist.

(At what level would the results have been significant had the hypothesis been one-tailed?)

Activity 13.2 (Answers on p. 366)

1 To practise ranking, rank order the results in Table 13.5 using the guidelines above. Remember to rank from smallest to biggest, omitting any zero scores,

Table 13.5

Subject	Condition A	Condition B	d	Rank
1	10	9	+1	
2	8	9	−1	
3	9	7	+2	
4	6	7	−1	
5	5	4	+1	
6	8	3	+5	
7	7	6	+1	
8	9	9	0	
9	9	6	+3	
10	5	6	−1	
11	7	3	+4	
12	8	4	+4	

ignoring the plus and minus signs of the d values, and giving the average rank for tied d values.

2 To practise looking up T values, look up the following and say whether you would classify them as significant

(i) $T = 7$	$N = 9$	one-tailed
(ii) $T = 7$	$N = 15$	two-tailed
(iii) $T = 15$	$N = 13$	one-tailed
(iv) $T = 20$	$N = 16$	one-tailed
(v) $T = 16$	$N = 12$	two-tailed
(vi) $T = 32$	$N = 16$	one-tailed
(vii) $T = 7$	$N = 12$	two-tailed
(viii) $T = 12$	$N = 13$	one-tailed

3 Calculate a Wilcoxon on the following data:

H_1 Traction is more effective than surgical collars for patients with cervical spondylosis.

Is this a one- or two-tailed hypothesis? Brief method: Select two groups of 12 cervical spondylosis patients, matched on sex, age, length and severity of condition, and previous treatments, and treat Group 1 with traction and Group 2 with surgical collars. After 3 weeks, compare the movement regained on a 7-point scale (1 = no improvement, 7 = greatly improved). Table 13.6 shows some possible results.

Table 13.6

Subject pair	Condition A Traction	Condition B Collar
1	3	3
2	4	3
3	5	4
4	4	3
5	7	3
6	4	4
7	4	4
8	6	5
9	5	3
10	3	2
11	6	3
12	4	3

NON-PARAMETRIC TESTS: SAME- AND MATCHED-SUBJECT DESIGNS, THREE OR MORE CONDITIONS AND ORDINAL OR INTERVAL/RATIO DATA

FRIEDMAN TEST

This test is similar to the Wilcoxon in that it is used for related and matched-subject designs. However, the Friedman is used when either

- *one group* of subjects is tested under *three or more conditions*; the results from the conditions are compared for differences.

or

- *three or more groups* of matched subjects are each tested in *one condition*; the results from the groups are compared for differences.

You would use this test if you had either Design 1b or 2b on pp. 169 and 170 and ordinal or interval/ratio data.

However, the Friedman test only tells you whether the results from each condition differ and not whether the results from one condition are better. For this reason, any hypothesis which relates to the Friedman must predict general differences and not a specific direction to the results. In other words, it must be two-tailed. When calculating this test, you end up with a numerical value χr^2, which you then look up in the probability tables associated with the Friedman test to see whether this represents a significant difference between your conditions.

Example

To illustrate this, let's suppose that you are a teacher in a large school of clinical therapy. You've noticed that over the last 2 or 3 years students seem to do consistently worse on the geriatric and neurology clinical placements than on orthopaedic and cardiothoracic placements. This may be due to a number of factors, such as the quality of the theoretical preparation or clinical supervision. However, before moving on to find the cause, you must first establish whether or not your observation is correct. Your hypothesis is:

H$_1$ Third-year clinical therapy students perform differently in various clinical settings.

This is a two-tailed hypothesis, as it predicts no direction to the differences.

To test this hypothesis, you randomly select 17 students in the final year of their training and compare their marks (on a 10-point scale; 1 = disastrous, 10 = excellent) in four clinical settings:

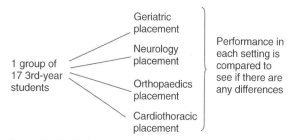

Figure 13.9 Design to test whether clinical therapy students perform differently in various clinical settings.

geriatric, neurology, orthopaedics and cardiothoracic.

Your design, then, looks like Figure 13.9.
Your data are as shown in Table 13.7.

Calculating the Friedman test

In order to calculate the Friedman you must take the following steps.

1. First, add up the scores for each condition, i.e.

$$\Sigma A = 85 \quad \Sigma B = 110 \quad \Sigma C = 138 \quad \Sigma D = 116$$

2. Calculate the means for each condition

$$\bar{x}_A = 5 \quad \bar{x}_B = 6.471 \quad \bar{x}_C = 8.118 \quad \bar{x}_D = 6.824$$

3. Rank the scores for each subject (i.e. across the row) giving the rank of 1 to the smallest score, a rank of 2 to the next smallest and so on. You will only need ranks 1–4 as there are only four scores for each subject. Where you have tied scores, use the tied rank procedure (see pp. 176–177), i.e. add up the ranks these scores would have had if they had been different, and divide by the number of scores which are the same. Therefore, if we look at subject 2, she scored 5 in cardiothoracic, 6 in geriatric, 6 in neurology and 7 in orthopaedics. Thus 5 gets a rank of 1; the two 6s, had they been different would have had ranks of 2 and 3 (because rank 1 has now been used up); so we add 2 and 3 to get 5, and divide this by the total number of scores which are the same (i.e. 2, because there are two scores of 6), giving 2.5. This, then is the rank we give the 6s. The score of 7 in orthopaedics gets a rank of 4 because ranks 1–3 have been used up.

4. Now add up the ranks for each condition (i.e. for each clinical setting). This is called T_c.

Table 13.7

Subject	Condition A Geriatric		Condition B Neurology		Condition C Orthopaedics		Condition D Cardiothoracic	
	Score	Rank	Score	Rank	Score	Rank	Score	Rank
1	5	1	6	2	8	4	7	3
2	6	2.5	6	2.5	7	4	5	1
3	3	1	7	3.5	7	3.5	6	2
4	8	2	9	3	10	4	7	1
5	7	1.5	9	3.5	9	3.5	7	1.5
6	6	1.5	8	3	9	4	6	1.5
7	5	1	8	3	9	4	7	2
8	5	1	8	2.5	10	4	8	2.5
9	4	1	6	2	8	3	9	4
10	3	1	5	2	8	4	7	3
11	6	2	5	1	8	4	7	3
12	6	2.5	4	1	7	4	6	2.5
13	7	2	5	1	9	4	8	3
14	3	1	7	3	8	4	6	2
15	2	1	5	2	7	3.5	7	3.5
16	5	1	6	2.5	7	4	6	2.5
17	4	1	6	2	7	3.5	7	3.5
	$\Sigma = 85$	$T_c = 24$	$\Sigma = 110$	$T_c = 39.5$	$\Sigma = 138$	$T_c = 65$	$\Sigma = 116$	$T_c = 41.5$
	$\bar{x} = 5$		$\bar{x} = 6.471$		$\bar{x} = 8.118$		$\bar{x} = 6.824$	

T_c for A = 24 T_c for B = 39.5

T_c for C = 65 T_c for D = 41.5

5. You now have to find the value of χr^2 from the following formula:

$$\chi r^2 = \left[\left(\frac{12}{NC(C+1)} \right) \left(\Sigma T_c^2 \right) \right] - 3N(C+1)$$

where
N = number of Ss in the group (or in the case of matched designs, the number of sets of subjects), i.e. 17
C = number of conditions, i.e. 4
T_c = total of the ranks for each condition
$\quad T_c$ for Condition A = 24
$\quad T_c$ for Condition B = 39.5
$\quad T_c$ for Condition C = 65
$\quad T_c$ for Condition D = 41.5
T_c^2 = each rank total squared
$\quad$ i.e. 24^2; 39.5^2; 65^2; 41.5^2
$\quad = 576$; 1560.25; 4225; 1722.25

Σ = sum or total of all the calculations following it

ΣT_c^2 = the sum of the squared ranks for each condition
$\quad$ i.e. $576 + 1560.25 + 4225 + 1722.25$
$= 8083.5$

Remember! Do all the calculations in brackets first, starting with divisions and multiplications and finally additions and subtractions.

Thus, if we substitute some values in the formula, then:

$$\chi r^2 = \left[\left(\frac{12}{17 \times 4(4+1)} \right) \times 8083.5 \right] - 3 \times 17(4+1)$$

$$= \left[\left(\frac{12}{68 \times 5} \right) \times 8083.5 \right] - 255$$

$$= [0.035 \times 8083.5] - 255$$

$$= 282.923 - 255$$

$$\chi r^2 = 27.923$$

Looking up the value of χr^2

To look up χr^2 in the tables, you also need the degrees of freedom value. This is the number of conditions minus 1, i.e. $4 - 1 = 3$. As you will see, there are three main tables for the Friedman test: Tables A2.3a, A2.3b (pp. 343–344) and A2.1 (p. 341). Table A2.3a is used where there are three conditions and only 2–9 subjects in each condition; Table A2.3b is for four conditions, with 2–4 Ss in each; and Table A2.1 is for anything larger, i.e. more conditions or more subjects.

Because we have four conditions and 17 subjects, we must use Table A2.1. (This table is also for use with the χ^2 test.) You will see that in the left-hand column, entitled 'df', there are various degrees of freedom values. Look down this column until you have found the df for this example, i.e. 3. You will see five numbers, called critical values, to the right:

$$6.25 \quad 7.82 \quad 9.84 \quad 11.34 \quad 16.27$$

Each of these values is associated with the level of probability shown at the top of its column, e.g. 11.34 is associated with a p value of 0.01. To be significant at a given level, our χr^2 value must be equal to or larger than the values here. So, if we take the first value 6.25, our χr^2 value is larger; it is also larger than 7.82, 9.84, 11.34 and 16.27. Therefore we take the value 16.27 and look up the column to see what the associated level of significance is, i.e. 0.001 or the 0.1% level. Because our χr^2 value of 27.923 is larger than the critical value of 16.27, this means that our results are significant at less than (<) the 0.001 level. (Had our χr^2 value been 16.27 exactly, we would say our p value equals 0.001.)

This means that there is less than a 0.1% chance that our results are due to random error.

Note that because the Friedman only allows you to predict differences and not specific directions to the results, your hypothesis must be two-tailed and so this level of significance represents the level for a two-tailed hypothesis. Because our usual cut-off point is 5% and our p value is less than that, i.e. 0.1%, we can say that our results are significant at the $p < 0.1\%$ level.

Interpreting the results

The results are associated with a p value of less than 0.1%. This means that there is less than a 0.1% probability of our results being due to random error. As the standard cut-off point is 5%, we can reject our null hypothesis and say that our results are significant. In other words,

students do perform differently in a variety of clinical settings. We can express this in the following way:

> Using a Friedman test on the data ($\chi r^2 = 27.923$, $N = 17$), the results were found to be significant at $p < 0.001$, for a two-tailed test. This suggests that third-year clinical therapy students perform significantly differently in four clinical settings, and so supports the experimental hypothesis. The null hypothesis can therefore be rejected.

Do note, however, that the Friedman only allows us to identify differences and not to say in which setting they performed better. If, however, you do expect a trend in the results of a related or matched-subject design (e.g. that students do worst in geriatrics, followed by cardio-thoracic, followed by neurology and best in orthopaedics) you would need the Page's L trend test (see next section).

If you had only three conditions and fewer subjects then you would use Table A2.3a. For example, supposing you had three conditions and seven subjects, and a χr^2 value of 7.5, you would look to find your value of N across the top of the table, (remember N = the number of Ss or subject pairs). Under this you will see a column for the χr^2 value, and to the right the corresponding p value or significance level. So taking the column for $N = 7$, look down the χr^2 value to find 7.5. Since our χr^2 value must be equal to or larger than those given to be significant at a particular level, we find that our value of 7.5 is larger than 7.143, but smaller than 7.714. We must take the critical value of 7.143 (because our χr^2 value must be equal to or larger than the critical value given) which gives us a corresponding p value of 0.027 or 2.7%.

However, because our χr^2 value of 7.5 is larger than 7.143, this means our p value is much less than (<) 0.027. Had our χr^2 value equalled the critical value of 7.143, we would say that our p value equals 0.027. So, our results have a p value of <0.027. Using the standard cut-off of 0.05, we can say our results are significant. We can therefore reject the null hypothesis, and accept the experimental hypothesis.

Supposing, however, we had four conditions, and four subjects or pairs of subjects and a χr^2 value of 2.6, we would need to use Table A2.3b which is for use with four conditions and 2–4 Ss. Here we would find the column corresponding to our N value, and look down the χr^2 values to find our own of 2.6. Because our value has to be equal to or larger than the values given to be significant at a given level, we can see that our χr^2 value of 2.6 is larger than 2.4 but smaller than 2.7. Therefore we have to take the value next smallest to our own, i.e. 2.4, which gives us a p value of 0.524 or 52.4%. Because of our standard 5% cut-off point, this p value cannot be classified as significant because it is larger. Therefore we would have to conclude that our results were not significant, our hypothesis was not supported and we would have to accept the null (no relationship) hypothesis.

Activity 13.3 (Answers on p. 366)

1 To practise looking up χr^2 values, look up the following and say whether they are significant.

 (i) $C = 4$ $N = 3$ $\chi r^2 = 7.4$ p
 (ii) $C = 4$ $N = 10$ $\chi r^2 = 9.92$ p
 (iii) $C = 3$ $N = 6$ $\chi r^2 = 5.72$ p
 (iv) $C = 3$ $N = 12$ $\chi r^2 = 35.7$ p
 (v) $C = 3$ $N = 8$ $\chi r^2 = 9.3$ p

2 Calculate a Friedman on the following data:

H_1 The muscle tone of the quadriceps differs for Asian, Caucasian and African-Caribbean children.

Method Select seven children in each ethnic group, matched for age, sex, fitness, activity levels and compare their muscle tone, using a 5-point scale: 5 = very high tone and 1 = very poor tone. You might obtain the results shown in Table 13.8.

Table 13.8

Subject	Condition A Asian	Condition B Caucasian	Condition C African–Caribbean
1	3	4	5
2	2	2	5
3	2	3	4
4	1	2	3
5	3	2	2
6	1	2	1
7	3	3	3

Write down the χr^2 value and the p value. State whether or not your results are significant, and what they mean, using the example given on p. 181.

PAGE'S L TREND TEST

This test is an extension of the Friedman test, in that it is used when

 a. the design is a same- or matched-subject one
 b. the data are ordinal or interval/ratio
 c. there are three or more conditions (i.e. one group of Ss doing three or more conditions, or three or more matched groups of Ss each doing one condition).

However, there is one salient difference: whereas the Friedman test can only be used to discover whether there are differences between the conditions without saying which condition is significantly better or worse than the others, the Page's L trend test is used when the experimenter had predicted a trend in the results. For example, when comparing the quality of three schools of chiropractic, the experimenter, in the hypothesis, predicts that School A is better than School B, which in turn is better than School C. This contrasts with the sort of hypothesis which must be used with the Friedman test, which would simply predict differences in quality between the three schools. Thus we might have the following types of design with the Page's L trend test.

1. In a comparison of a group of students' attitudes to three types of teaching method, it is predicted that the seminar method will be most popular, followed by the lecture method, with tutorials least popular. The design in Figure 13.10 could be used.

2. In a comparison of three types of exercise techniques for ankylosing spondylitis, it is predicted that Exercise A will be more effective than Exercise B which will be more effective than Exercise C. Three groups of patients, matched for age, duration and severity of condition, etc., are

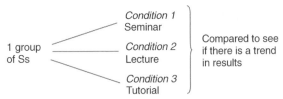

Figure 13.10 Design for assessing popularity of teaching methods.

given one of the exercise regimes and compared for progress after 1 month. The design shown in Figure 13.11 is used.

The Page's L trend test then essentially assesses whether there is a significant trend in the results. When calculating it you derive the value of L, which is then looked up in the probability tables associated with the Page's test to see whether this value represents a significant trend in your results.

Because you are predicting a specific direction to the results when you use a Page's L trend test, the hypothesis must be one-tailed.

Example

Let's take the first hypothesis that, in order to evaluate students' preferences for three types of teaching approach, you predict that the seminar method will be more popular than the lecture method, with the tutorial being least popular; a trend is predicted, i.e. seminar > lecture > tutorial (> means 'greater than').

You select a group of 10 students and ask them to rate the three methods on a 5-point scale (5 = most preferred, 1 = least preferred). In order to analyse the results you must set out your data such that the scores you predict will be the smallest (i.e. tutorial) are placed on the left, and the scores you predict to be the largest are placed on the right as in Table 13.9.

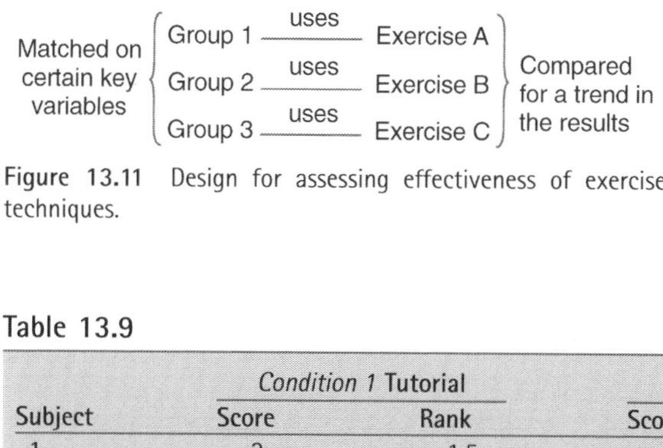

Calculating the Page's L trend test

1. In order to calculate the value of L you must take the following steps:

First, find the total scores for each condition:

$$\Sigma_1 = 20 \quad \Sigma_2 = 32 \quad \Sigma_3 = 38$$

Then find the mean score for each condition

$$\bar{x}_1 = 2 \quad \bar{x}_2 = 3.2 \quad \bar{x}_3 = 3.8$$

2. Rank the scores for each subject (or sets of matched Ss) across the row, as for the Friedman, giving the rank of 1 to the lowest score, the rank of 2 to the next lowest, etc. If you have two or more scores which are the same, you must give these the average rank (see p. •• on how to deal with tied scores), i.e. you add up the value of the ranks they would have obtained had they been different and divide by the number of scores that are the same. For example, S1 has two scores of 3. Had these scores been the two lowest but different scores they would have had the ranks 1 and 2. These rank values are added together (3) and divided by 2 (because there are two scores of 3) to give the average rank, 1.5, which is entered alongside the scores of 3.

3. Add up the ranks for each condition, i.e.

$$T_{c1} = 12 \quad T_{c2} = 22.5 \quad T_{c3} = 25.5$$

Matched on certain key variables { Group 1 —uses— Exercise A, Group 2 —uses— Exercise B, Group 3 —uses— Exercise C } Compared for a trend in the results

Figure 13.11 Design for assessing effectiveness of exercise techniques.

Table 13.9

Subject	Condition 1 Tutorial		Condition 2 Lecture		Condition 3 seminar	
	Score	Rank	Score	Rank	Score	Rank
1	3	1.5	4	3	3	1.5
2	2	1.5	2	1.5	4	3
3	3	1.5	3	1.5	5	3
4	1	1	3	3	2	2
5	2	1.5	3	3	2	1.5
6	2	1	4	2	5	3
7	1	1	2	2	4	3
8	3	1	4	2.5	4	2.5
9	2	1	4	2	5	3
10	1	1	3	2	4	3
	$\Sigma_1 = 20$	$T_{c1} = 12$	$\Sigma_2 = 32$	$T_{c2} = 22.5$	$\Sigma_3 = 38$	$T_{c3} = 25.5$

4. Find the value of L from the formula

$$L = \Sigma(T_{C1} \times C_1) + \Sigma(T_{C2} \times C_2) + \Sigma(T_{C3} \times C_3)$$

where

Σ = the total or sum of any symbols that follow it

Tc = total of ranks for each condition, i.e. $T_{c1} = 12$; $T_{c2} = 22.5$; $T_{c3} = 25.5$

C_1, C_2, C_3 = numbers allotted to the conditions from left to right i.e. 1, 2 and 3

$(T_c \times C)$ = total of the ranks for each condition multiplied by the number assigned to the condition

i.e. $Tc_1 \times C_1 = 12 \times 1$

$Tc_2 \times C_2 = 22.5 \times 2$

$Tc_3 \times C_3 = 25.5 \times 3$

Substituting our values in the formula:

$$L = (12 \times 1)(22.5 \times 2)(25.5 \times 3)$$
$$= 12 + 45 + 76.5$$
$$= 133.5$$

5. To look up your value of L, you also need two further values: C, the number of conditions, i.e. 3; and N, the number of Ss in the group or the number of sets of matched Ss, i.e. 10.

Looking up the value of L for significance

Turn to Table A2.4 (p. 345). Across the top you will see values of C (i.e. number of conditions) from 3 to 6, and down the left-hand column, values of N (i.e. number of Ss or sets of matched Ss) from 2 to 12. Look across the C values to find

---

Activity 13.4 (Answers on p. 366)

1. To practise looking up L values, look up the following and decide at what level (if any) they are significant:

   (i) $N = 5$ $C = 4$ $L = 142.5$ p

   (ii) $N = 8$ $C = 5$ $L = 384$ p

   (iii) $N = 7$ $C = 3$ $L = 92$ p

   (iv) $N = 12$ $C = 6$ $L = 971$ p

   (v) $N = 10$ $C = 5$ $L = 455.5$ p

2. Calculate a Page's L trend test on the following data:

   H_1 It is hypothesised that hydrotherapy is more effective than exercise which in turn is more effective than massage for mobilising lower limbs paralysed following a stroke.

   Method   Take three groups, each of eight subjects, matched for severity of paralysis, age, sex, previous health, length of time since stroke and other treatments, and give each group one of the three treatment procedures. After 1 month compare the percentage range of movement regained. The results are as shown in Table 13.10.

   State your L and p values, using the sample format given on this page.

   Remember! Put the scores which are predicted to be the lowest in the left-hand column and those predicted to be the highest in the right-hand column. In other words, you will need to rearrange the table.

   Remember, too, that the data in this example are of an interval/ratio type, which can be used with both non-parametric and parametric tests.

Table 13.10

Subject trio	Condition 1 Hydrotherapy Score	Rank	Condition 2 Massage Score	Rank	Condition 3 Exercise Score	Rank
1	40		25		30	
2	55		30		40	
3	35		35		45	
4	20		30		40	
5	30		20		30	
6	50		45		50	
7	55		45		55	
8	60		50		60	

our value of $C = 3$ and down the N values to find our $N = 10$ value.

At their intersection point you will see three numbers:

134

131

128

These are called critical values of L. If you look across these rows to the right-hand column, you will see that 134 represents a p value of 0.001; 131 represents a p value of 0.01 and 128 represents a p value of 0.05. To be significant at one of these levels, your L value must be *equal to or larger than* one of the numbers 134, 131 and 128. The obtained value of L in our example is 133.5. This is larger than 131, but smaller than 134. Therefore we must take the value of 131, which represents a significance level of 0.01 or 1%. But because our L value is larger than the critical value of 131, this means that the corresponding p value is less than (<) 0.01. This is expressed as $p < 0.01$. This means that there is less than a 1% chance of the results being caused by random error. Because you must be predicting a specific direction to your results in order to be using a trend test, your hypothesis, by definition, must be one-tailed. Therefore, all the values in this table are values for a one-tailed hypothesis.

Using our usual cut-off point of 5%, because the p value in our study is smaller, we can conclude that our results are significant at the <0.01 level. Thus we can reject the null hypothesis and conclude that there is a significant trend in results as predicted in our hypothesis.

Interpreting the results

Our results have a probability value of <0.01 which means that there is less than a 1% chance

of their being due to random error. Because this p value is smaller than the usual cut-off point of 0.05, we can say that our results are significant. This means we can reject the null hypothesis and accept the experimental hypothesis.

This can be expressed in the following way:

> Using a Page's L trend test on the data ($L = 133.5$, $N = 10$, $C = 3$), the results were found to be significant at $p < 0.01$ for a one-tailed hypothesis. This suggests that the experimental hypothesis has been supported, and that students prefer seminar teaching methods to lectures, with tutorials being the least preferred approach. The null hypothesis can therefore be rejected.

FURTHER READING

Cohen L, Halliday M 1996 Practical statistics for students. Paul Chapman Publishing, London

Coolican H 2004 Research methods and statistics in psychology, 4th edition. Hodder and Stoughton, London

Coolican H 2006 Introduction to research methods in psychology, 3rd edition. Hodder Arnold, London

Field A, Hole G 2004 How to design and report experiments. Sage, London

Greene J, D'Oliveira M 2005 Learning to use statistical tests in psychology, 3rd edition. Open University Press, Buckingham,

Pett M 1997 Non-parametric statistics in health care research. Sage, London

Polgar S, Thomas S 2007 Introduction to research in the health sciences. Churchill Livingstone, Edinburgh

Robson C 1994 Experiment, design and statistics in psychology, 3rd edition. Penguin, Harmondsworth

Siegel S 1956 Non-parametric statistics for the behavioural sciences. McGraw-Hill Kogakusha, Tokyo

Chapter 14

Parametric tests for same- and matched-subject designs

INTRODUCTION

All the statistical tests described in this chapter, like those in the previous one, are used to analyse the results from same-subject or matched-subject designs; in other words, those designs which either use one group of subjects for all the conditions, or alternatively, two or more groups of matched subjects who do one condition each (see pp. 95–98 for the designs).

There is one major difference, however; all the tests in this chapter are parametric, which means that they require certain conditions to be fulfilled before they can be used, in particular that the data should be of an interval/ratio level. This requirement concerning the level of data should never be violated, unless you have a good basis for claiming that the intervals along an ordinal scale are equivalent (see pp 42–43). Parametric tests are also rather more difficult to calculate than non-parametric tests. You should always remember that, for any given design, the relevant parametric and non-parametric tests do the same job: they assess whether there are significant differences (or in the case of correlations, similarities) between the conditions, but the parametric tests are more sensitive to these differences.

The designs we are interested in, then, are as follows:

1. **Same-subject design:** one group of subjects used in all the conditions.

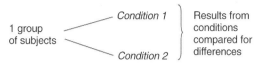

Figure 14.1 One group of subjects tested under two conditions.

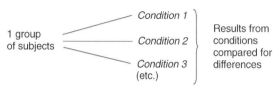

Figure 14.2 One group of subjects tested under three or more conditions.

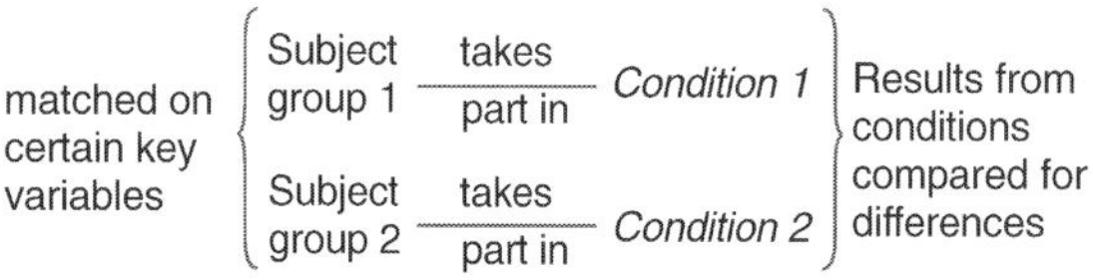

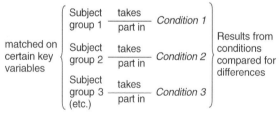

Figure 14.3 Two groups of matched subjects each tested under one condition.

Figure 14.4 Three or more groups of matched subjects, each tested under one condition.

a. Two conditions only (Figure 14.1).
b. Three or more conditions (Figure 14.2).
2. **Matched-subject design:** two or more groups of matched subjects, each of which is used in one condition only.
a. Two matched groups only (Figure 14.3).
b. Three or more matched groups (Figure 14.4).

Results from designs which use one group of subjects in both of two conditions (Design 1a) or two groups of matched subjects, each doing one condition (Design 2a) are analysed using the **related t-test.**

Table 14.1 Parametric tests for related- and matched-subject designs

Design	Parametric test
1a. One group of Ss tested in two conditions	Related t-test
2a. Two groups of matched Ss, each tested in one condition only	Related t-test
1b. One group of Ss tested under three or more conditions	One-way ANOVA for related designs, to be used with the Scheffé multiple range test
2b. Three or more groups of matched Ss, each tested in one condition only	One-way ANOVA for related designs, to be used with the Scheffé multiple range test

Results from designs using one group of subjects who take part in all three (or more) conditions (Design 1b) or three or more groups of matched subjects each doing one condition (Design 2b) are analysed using the **one-way analysis** of variance, or ANOVA as it is usually known, for related designs.

In addition we shall look at the **Scheffé multiple range test** which is used in conjunction with the ANOVA (see the relevant section).

These are summarised in Table 14.1.

It should be noted that the t-test is sometimes referred to as 'Student's t' in some texts.

PARAMETRIC TEST: ONE GROUP OF SUBJECTS AND TWO CONDITIONS, OR TWO GROUPS OF MATCHED SUBJECTS DOING ONE CONDITION EACH

RELATED T-TEST

Just to recap, this test is used for exactly the same designs as the Wilcoxon, in other words, where one group of subjects takes part in both of two conditions (a same-subjects design), and the results from the two conditions are then compared for differences. Alternatively, the related t-test is used where you have two groups of matched subjects, who do one condition each (a matched-subject design) and again the results from the two conditions are compared to see if there are differences between them.

The related t-test is especially suitable for 'before and after' type designs, for instance, when you wish to compare the effects of a treatment on one group of subjects.

When calculating the t-test, you find a value for 't', which you then look up in the probability tables for the t-test to see whether this value represents significant differences between the results from each condition. Remember that parametric tests are more difficult to calculate than non-parametric tests, so don't panic when you look at the formula. As long as you work through the stages systematically, you will have no difficulty.

Example

Let's suppose you are in charge of a large physiotherapy department and it has been brought to your notice that the eight basic-grade physiotherapists seem to show a distinct preference for treating young male sports injury leg fracture patients as opposed to elderly male leg fracture patients. You have challenged them about this but they deny it, so you want to produce some empirical support for your assertion.

Your experimental hypothesis, then, is:

H₁   Young male leg fracture patients receive more attention from basic-grade physiotherapists than do elderly leg fracture patients.

This is a one-tailed hypothesis as it predicts a specific direction to the results.

(Note: In case this appears to be an unlikely hypothesis, there is a huge literature on the ways in which physical appearance can affect how we behave towards one another. Darbyshire (1986) and Hicks (1993) both provide overviews of some of this research as it applies to health care situations.)

To test your hypothesis, you measure the length of time each physiotherapist spends with her three sports injury fracture patients in the course of 1 day and total this up in minutes. You do the same for the period spent with her three elderly leg fracture patients. Because time is an interval/ratio measurement the most necessary condition for using a parametric test can be fulfilled.

Therefore you have the design shown in Figure 14.5.

Your results are as shown in Table 14.2.

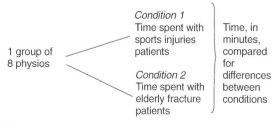

Figure 14.5   Design of experiment to assess whether physiotherapists spend more time with sports injury patients than with elderly fracture patients.

Table 14.2

1 Subject	Results from experiment		Calculations	
	2 Condition* A Sports injury	3 Condition* B Elderly patients	4 d (A – B)	5 d²
1	49	42	+7	49
2	57	45	+12	144
3	72	65	+7	49
4	64	65	−1	1
5	50	60	−10	100
6	45	35	+10	100
7	59	40	+19	361
8	65	49	+16	256
Σ	461	401	Σd = 60	Σd² = 1060
x̄	57.625	50.125		

*It does not matter which group of patients is called Condition A and which Condition B.

Calculating the related t-test

To calculate the related t-test, you must:

1. Add up the scores for each condition to give the total (Σ), i.e.

$$\Sigma A = 461 \quad \Sigma B = 401$$

2. Calculate the mean score ($\bar{x}$) for each condition, i.e.

$$\bar{x}_A = 57.625 \quad \bar{x}_B = 50.125$$

3. Calculate the difference (d) between each subject's pair of scores and enter this in column 4; i.e. for each subject take the score of Condition B away from the score of Condition A (e.g. for S1, 49 – 42 = 7). Remember to put in the plus and minus signs for each d value.

4. Add these differences up to give Σd, remembering to take account of the plus and minus values, i.e.

$$\Sigma d = 60$$

5. Square each difference to give d^2, e.g. $7^2 = 49$, and enter these in column 5 (d^2).
6. Add up the d^2 values to give Σd^2, i.e.

$$\Sigma d^2 = 1060$$

7. Square the total of the differences, i.e.

$$60^2 = 3600 = (\Sigma d)^2$$

It is important to recognise the difference in meaning between

Σd^2 (stage 6) which means to add up all the squared differences and $(\Sigma d)^2$ (stage 7) which means to add up all the differences and square the total.

8. Find t from the following formula:

$$t = \frac{\sum d}{\sqrt{\dfrac{N \sum d^2 - \left(\sum d\right)^2}{N-1}}}$$

where
Σd = the total of the differences (i.e. 60)
$(\Sigma d)^2$ = the total of the differences, squared (i.e. 3600)
Σd^2 = the total of the squared differences (i.e. 1060)
N = number of subjects, or pairs of matched subjects (i.e. 8)
$\sqrt{}$ = the square root of the final calculation of everything under the square root sign.
If we substitute some values, then:

$$t = \frac{60}{\sqrt{\dfrac{8 \times 1060 - 3600}{8 - 1}}}$$

$$= \frac{60}{\sqrt{\dfrac{8480 - 3600}{7}}}$$

$$= \frac{60}{\sqrt{697.143}}$$

$$= \frac{60}{26.404}$$

$$t = 2.272$$

Looking up the value of t

To see whether this t value is significant you need one further value, the degrees of freedom, which here is the number of subjects minus 1, i.e. $8 - 1 = 7$.

Turn to Table A2.5 (p. 346). You will see down the left-hand margin a number of df values. Look down the column until you find the df value of 7. To the right of that you will see six critical values of t in the main body of the table:

1.415 1.895 2.365 2.998 3.499 5.405

If your value of t is *equal to* or *larger than* any of the given values, it is significant at the level indicated at the top of the column. For example, 3.499 has an associated p value of 0.005 for a one-tailed test and 0.01 for a two-tailed test. So, if we look at the numbers, we can see that our t value of 2.272 is larger than 1.895 but smaller than 2.365. This means that the probability associated with our t value of 2.272 is somewhere between 0.05 and 0.025 for a one-tailed hypothesis. In other words the p value for $t = 2.272$ must be smaller than 0.05 (or 5%) and larger than 0.025 (or 2.5%).

We would therefore say that for our study and our one-tailed hypothesis, the results are significant at less than 0.05 (or 5%). Because of convention, we would never say that p is greater than 0.025 and so we must focus on the value of 1.895 in the table.

We express this as $p < 0.05$ (< means 'less than'). Had our t value been exactly the same as the critical value of 1.895 in the table, we would have said that $p = 0.05$.

Interpreting the results

Our results have an associated probability of less than 0.05, which means that the chances of random error accounting for the outcome of our experiment are less than 5 in 100. Because the usual cut-off point for claiming that the results are significant is 5%, we can conclude that our results are significant, at less than the 5% level.

However, because we have a one-tailed hypothesis we can only say that our hypothesis has been supported if the results are in the direction predicted. This means that, providing the average amount of time spent with the sports injury patients is greater than the average amount of time spent with the elderly leg fracture patients, we can reject the null hypothesis and accept that our experimental hypothesis has been supported. Since the averages are 57.625 and 50.125 minutes respectively, the results are in the predicted direction and we can conclude that basic-grade physiotherapists spend significantly more time with young sports injury patients than with elderly leg fracture patients. We can state this as follows:

> Using a related t-test on the data ($t = 2.272$, $N = 8$), the results are significant at $p < 0.05$, for a one-tailed test. The experimental hypothesis has been supported, suggesting that young male fracture patients receive significantly more treatment time from basic-grade physiotherapists, than do elderly male fracture patients. The null hypothesis can therefore be rejected.

Remember, had the average time been reversed (i.e. more time spent with the elderly patients), we could not claim that the hypothesis had been supported.

Table 14.3

	Results from experiment		Calculations	
1	2	3	4	5
	Condition 1	Condition 2	d	d^2
Subject pair	'A'-level physics	No 'A'-level physics		
1	64	68		
2	59	60		
3	72	62		
4	68	58		
5	58	49		
6	70	62		
7	65	61		
8	62	50		
9	73	71		
10	45	49		
11	56	54		
12	67	68		

State the t value, the df value, and the p value expressed in a similar format to that above.

Activity 14.1 (Answers on pp. 366–367)

1. To practise looking up t values, look up the following and say whether or not they are significant and at what level.
   (i) df = 11 $t = 2.406$ one-tailed p
   (ii) df = 14 $t = 1.895$ two-tailed p
   (iii) df = 19 $t = 2.739$ one-tailed p
   (iv) df = 7 $t = 3.204$ one-tailed p
   (v) df = 9 $t = 2.973$ two-tailed p
2. Calculate a related t-test on the following data:

   H_1 Student chiropractors with 'A'-level physics do better on their first-year theory exam than students without 'A'-level physics.

Is this hypothesis one- or two-tailed?

Method: Select two groups, each of 12 students, matched on certain key features such as overall 'A'-level points, attendance levels, quality of teaching, etc. Of these, one group has 'A'-level physics and the other does not. Compare the performance of the two groups on their first-year theory exam. The marks are as shown in Table 14.3.

PARAMETRIC TESTS: ONE GROUP OF SUBJECTS AND THREE OR MORE CONDITIONS, OR THREE OR MORE GROUPS OF MATCHED SUBJECTS

ONE-WAY ANALYSIS OF VARIANCE (ANOVA) FOR RELATED- AND MATCHED-SUBJECT DESIGNS

The one-way ANOVA for related- and matched-subject designs is the parametric equivalent of the Friedman test. In other words, it is used for designs which use one subject group in three or more conditions, and the results from these conditions are compared for differences between them. Alternatively, it is used where the experimenter has got three or more groups of matched subjects who do one condition each. The results from each condition are compared for differences (see Designs 1b and 2b, p. 187 and 188).

It is called a 'one-way' ANOVA because it only deals with experiments which manipulate one independent variable. If you ever hypothesised a relationship between two independent variables and a dependent variable (see Ch. 6) you would require a two-way ANOVA, or a relationship between three independent variables and a dependent variable, then you would require a three-way ANOVA. However, these are outside the scope of this book and the reader is referred to Greene & D'Oliveira (2005) and Ferguson and Takane (1989).

Like all parametric tests, the data must be of an interval/ratio level, and the remaining three conditions should be more or less fulfilled.

When calculating an ANOVA you find a value for 'F' which is then looked up in the probability tables for ANOVAs to find out whether this value represents a significant difference between conditions. Like the Friedman test, the ANOVA only tells us whether there are overall differences between conditions, and not the direction of the differences, and so the hypothesis must be two-tailed.

Example

Because the ANOVA is quite complicated to calculate, it may be helpful to explain its purpose beforehand. Let's imagine that you are the manager in charge of patient services for a large unit which employs a range of clinical therapists. You have noticed that your senior clinical therapists seem to show a high degree of clinical skill but they seem less competent in their supervision of trainees and in their interpersonal skills. Obviously, if your observations are correct, you will need to do some staff development on the weaker areas. You therefore decide to make an evaluation of a group of 10 senior clinical

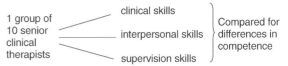

Figure 14.6 Design for comparison of differences in various skills in clinical therapists.

therapists in the three different aspects of their job: clinical skills, interpersonal skills and supervision skills.

Your hypothesis then is:

H_1 Senior clinical therapists show different levels of professional competence in three aspects of their job: clinical, supervisory and interpersonal skills.

To see it there is any difference in the competence shown in these areas you decide to compare the performance of the group on each aspect, giving marks out of 20. As this is an interval/ratio scale of measurement, we can fulfil this requirement of a parametric test.

Therefore we have the design shown in Figure 14.6.

Further suppose that you have collected and set out the results which look as shown in Table 14.4.

You are hypothesising that the performance of the group varies according to the aspect of the job, and therefore you would expect there to be significant differences or *variations* between the *conditions*. This, obviously, is one potential source of variation in the results and is called a between-conditions comparison.

Table 14.4

Subject	Condition 1 Clinical	Condition 2 Interpersonal	Condition 3 Supervisory	Total for Ss (T_s)
1	15	12	11	38
2	12	9	8	29
3	13	10	11	34
4	10	10	12	32
5	17	14	10	41
6	8	12	11	31
7	11	12	9	32
8	14	9	9	32
9	16	8	12	36
10	10	9	8	27
Total T_c	$T_{C1} = 126$	$T_{C2} = 105$	$T_{C3} = 101$	Grand total = 332

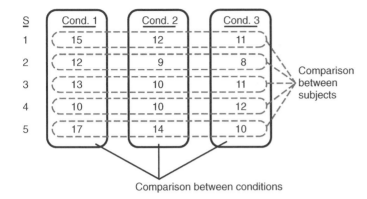

Figure 14.7   Possible sources of variation in the scores, i.e. between subjects and conditions.

However, because each subject is assessed on all three conditions, we can also compare the overall performances of each of the subjects, to see if there is any variation in competence between the clinical therapists, i.e. a comparison of all the T_s totals. This comparison allows us to look at another potential source of variation in the scores: a *between-subjects* comparison. This is illustrated in Figure 14.7 for the example given above using the data from the first five subjects:

The solid lines in Figure 14.7 indicate the comparisons which can be made between conditions, to see if there is any difference in performance on each aspect of the job, as was hypothesised. This comparison concentrates on one source of potential variation in the results: the between-conditions variation.

The dotted lines indicate the comparisons which can be made between subjects, to see if there is any difference in the overall performances among the subjects. This comparison concentrates on a second potential source of variation in the results: the between-subject variation.

There is, of course, a third source of potential variation in scores: that due to random error.

If we consider these sources of variation for a moment, it can be seen that ideally what we would hope to find from our ANOVA is:

a. significant differences between the performance of the job tasks, i.e. a significant *between-conditions* comparison, since this was what was hypothesised, and

b. no significant differences between the subjects, since this would suggest that they were a fairly representative and similar sample, without huge individual differences.

The purpose of the one-way related ANOVA is to find out whether any of these sources of variation are responsible for significant differences in results.

In order to do this, we need a number of values:

the sums of squares (SS)
the degrees of freedom (df)
the mean squares (MS)
the F ratios (F)

for each source of variation. When these have been calculated they are entered into a table the format of which is shown in Table 14.5.

First, do not panic – the calculations are surprisingly easy, if rather laborious! Follow the steps described below (the data are on p. 192)

Calculating the one-way ANOVA

1. We must first calculate the SS values for each source of variation. To do this, you will need several values:

Table 14.5

Source of scores of scores	Sums of squares (SS)	Degrees of freedom (df)	Mean squares (MS)	F variation (F)
Variation between conditions, i.e. aspects of job	SS_{bet}	df_{bet}	MS_{bet}	F_{bet}
Variation between subjects' overall performance	SS_{subj}	df_{subj}	MS_{subj}	F_{subj}
Variation due to random error	SS_{error}	df_{error}	MS_{error}	
Total	SS_{tot}	df_{tot}		

ΣT_C^2 = sum of the squared totals for each condition, i.e. $126^2 + 105^2 + 101^2$

$= 15876 + 11025 + 10201$

$= 37102$

ΣT_S^2 = sum of each subject's performance squared, i.e.

$38^2 + 29^2 + 34^2 + 32^2 + 41^2 + 31^2 + 32^2$
$+ 32^2 + 36^2 + 27^2$

$= 1444 + 841 + 1156 + 1024 + 1681 + 961$
$+ 1024 + 1024 + 1296 + 729$

$= 11180$

n = number of Ss or sets of matched Ss

$= 10$

C = number of conditions

$= 3$

N = total number of scores, i.e. $n \times C$

$= 30$

Σx = grand total (of scores)

$= 332$

$(\Sigma x)^2$ = grand total squared

$= 332^2$

$= 110224$

$\dfrac{(\Sigma x)}{N}$ = a constant to be subtracted from all SS

$= \dfrac{110224}{30}$

$= 3674.133$

x = each individual score

Σx^2 = the sum of each squared individual score

$= 15^2 + 12^2 + 11^2 + 12^2/9^2 + 8^2 + 13^2 + 10^2 +$
$11^2 + 10^2 + 10^2 + 12^2 + 17^2 + 14^2 + 10^2 + 8^2$
$+ 12^2 + 11^2 + 11^2 + 12^2 + 9^2 + 14^2 + 9^2 + 9^2$
$+ 16^2 + 8^2 + 12^2 + 10^2 + 9^2 + 8^2$

$= 3840$

2. To calculate the SS_{bet} the formula is:

$$\frac{\Sigma T_C^2}{n} - \frac{(\Sigma x)^2}{N} = \frac{126^2 + 105^2 + 101^2}{10} - \frac{110224}{30}$$

$$= 3710.2 - 3674.133$$

$$= 36.067$$

3. To calculate the SS_{subj} the formula is:

$$\frac{\Sigma T_S^2}{n} - \frac{(\Sigma x)^2}{N}$$

$$\frac{38^2 + 29^2 + 34^2 + 32^2 + 41^2 + 31^2 + 32^2 + 36^2 + 27^2}{31}$$

$$= \frac{110224}{30}$$

$$= 3726.667 - 3674.133$$

$$= 52.534$$

4. To calculate the SS_{tot} the formula is:

$$\Sigma x^2 - \frac{(\Sigma x)^2}{N}$$

$$= 15^2 + 12^2 + 11^2 + 12^2 + 9^2 + 8^2$$
$$13^2 + 10^2 + 11^2 + 10^2 + 10^2 + 12^2$$
$$+ 17^2 + 14^2 + 10^2 + 8^2 + 12^2 + 11^2$$
$$11^2 + 12^2 + 9^2 + 14^2 + 9^2 + 9^2 + 16^2$$
$$+ 8^2 + 12^2 + 10^2 + 9^2 + 8^2 - \frac{110224}{30}$$

$$= 3840 - 3674.133$$

$$= 165.867$$

5. To calculate the SS_{error} the formula is:

$$SS_{tot} - SS_{bet} - SS_{subj}$$

$$= 165.867 - 36.067 - 52.534$$

$$= 77.266$$

6. To calculate the df values:

$$df_{bet} = \text{number of conditions} - 1$$

$$= 3 - 1$$

$$= 2$$

df_{sub} = number of Ss − 1

(or sets of matched Ss − 1)

= 10 − 1

= 9

df_{tot} = N − 1

= 30 − 1

= 29

$df_{error} = df_{tot} − df_{bet} − df_{subj}$

= 29 − 2 − 9

= 18

7.   To calculate the MS values:

$$MS_{bet} = \frac{SS_{bet}}{df_{bet}}$$

$$= \frac{36.067}{2}$$

$$= 18.034$$

$$MS_{subj} = \frac{SS_{subj}}{df_{subj}}$$

$$= \frac{52.534}{9}$$

$$= 5.837$$

$$MS_{error} = \frac{SS_{error}}{df_{error}}$$

$$= \frac{77.266}{18}$$

$$= 4.293$$

8.   To calculate the F ratios:

F ratio for the between-conditions variation

$$= \frac{MS_{bet}}{MS_{error}}$$

$$= \frac{18.034}{4.293}$$

$$= 4.201$$

F ratio for the between-subjects variation

$$= \frac{MS_{subj}}{MS_{error}}$$

$$= \frac{5.837}{4.293}$$

$$= 1.36$$

Table 14.6

Source of variation in scores	Sums of squares (SS)	Degrees of freedom (df)	Mean squares (MS)	F ratios
Variation in scores between conditions, i.e. aspects of job	36.067	2	18.034	4.201
Variation in scores between subjects	52.534	9	5.837	1.36
Variation in scores due to random error	77.266	18	4.293	
Total	165.867	29		

We can now fill in our table using these values (Table 14.6).

Looking up the values of the F ratios

We need to look up these F ratios to find out whether they represent significant differences between the conditions and/or between the subjects. Turn to Tables A2.6a–d (pp. 347–350), which are the probability tables for the ANOVA.

Table A2.6a shows the critical values of F at $p < 0.05$.

Table A2.6b shows the critical values of F at $p < 0.025$.

Table A2.6c shows the critical values of F at $p < 0.01$.

Table A2.6d shows the critical values of F at $p < 0.001$.

Note again, that as the ANOVA can only tell us whether there are general differences and not whether these differences are in a specific direction, these values are for a two-tailed hypothesis.

On each of these tables you will see that there are values called v_1 across the top and v_2 down the left-hand column. These are df values. To look up the F ratio for the between-conditions comparison, we need the df_{bet} value and the df_{error} value. Taking Table A2.6a first, locate the df_{bet} (i.e. 2) across the top row, and the df_{error} (i.e. 18) down the left-hand column. Where they intersect is the critical value of F for these df values. If our F ratio of 4.21 is equal to or larger than the critical value, it is significant at the p value stated at the top of the table. As 4.021 is larger than 3.55, we can conclude that our results have an associated probability of less than 5%.

But can we do any better? Turn to Table A2.6b and repeat the process. Because our value of 4.201 is smaller than the intersection value of 4.56 our results are not significant at the 0.025 level. Therefore, the probability that our results are due to random error is less than 0.05.

This is expressed, then, as $p < 0.05$.

To find out whether there are differences between the subjects' overall performances (i.e. whether the F ratio of 1.36 is significant), we need the df_{subj} value (in this case 9) and the df_{error} value (in this case 18). Look across the v_1 values in Table A2.6a for 9, and down the left-hand column for 18. You will see that there is no v_1 value of 9, so you must take the next smallest. At the intersection point the critical value is 2.51. As our F ratio is smaller than this, the results can be said to be not significant. In other words, there is no significant difference between subjects in their overall performance.

Interpreting the results

Our results have an associated probability level of less than 5%, which means that the chances of random error accounting for the results are less than 5 in 100. Since the usual cut-off point is 5%, we can say that our results are significant, which means that the clinical therapists perform some parts of their job better than others. However, the between-subjects F ratio is not significant, which suggests that the clinical therapists concerned did not differ from each other in terms of their overall job performance.

If we take these two results together we can conclude that the senior clinical therapists do indeed perform differently on each aspect of their job, and since there is no significant difference in the overall quality of the clinical therapists concerned we may assume that the differences are due to some factor associated with their department, training, attitudes, etc. We can express this in the following way:

Using a one-way ANOVA for related subject samples on the data ($F = 4.201$, $N = 10$) it was found that the results were significant at $p < 0.05$. This suggests that there are significant differences in performance levels on the three aspects

of the clinical therapist's job investigated. These differences cannot be attributed to variations in the subjects since the F ratio for the between-subjects calculations was not significant ($F = 1.36$, $p = NS$). Therefore, the null hypothesis can be rejected.

It must be remembered that the ANOVA tells you that there are significant differences between the conditions and not which condition has better or worse scores. For instance in this example, we know that senior clinical therapists perform differently on three aspects of their job but we do not know whether the difference lies between:

clinical and interpersonal
or
clinical and supervisory
or
interpersonal and supervisory
or
all three.

In order to find out you need to use the Scheffé multiple range test in the next section. However, the Scheffé can only be used if the results from the ANOVA are significant.

Activity 14.2 (Answers on p. 367)

1 To practise looking up F ratios, look up the following and state whether or not they are significant and at what level:

  (i) $F_{bet} = 4.96$ $df_{bet} = 2$ $df_{error} = 10$ p
  (ii) $F_{subj} = 4.22$ $df_{subj} = 7$ $df_{error} = 15$ p
  (iii) $F_{subj} = 2.21$ $df_{subj} = 11$ $df_{error} = 20$ p
  (iv) $F_{bet} = 5.15$ $df_{bet} = 14$ $df_{error} = 8$ p
  (v) $F_{subj} = 3.14$ $df_{subj} = 9$ $df_{error} = 14$ p
  (vi) $F_{bet} = 3.98$ $df_{bet} = 10$ $df_{error} = 12$ p

Remember! Use all the tables to find the smallest p value possible.

2 Calculate a one-way ANOVA for related designs on the following data:

  H_1 There is a relationship between the type of treatment used on hip replacement patients and the distance walked after 1 week of therapy.

Brief method: Select three groups each of six hip replacement patients, matched on age, sex, mobility prior to operation, length of time postoperative, etc.

Each group is treated using one of three different types of therapy. After 1 week, their mobility is measured in terms of yards walked, with the results shown in Table 14.7.

Table 14.7

Subject	Condition A Suspension	Condition B Free exercise	Condition C Hydrotherapy
1	15	16	11
2	12	14	14
3	10	14	12
4	14	15	12
5	22	19	13
6	17	18	15

State your F ratios, df values and p values in the manner suggested above.

SCHEFFÉ MULTIPLE RANGE TEST

The ANOVA only tells you whether there are overall differences between the conditions and not where these differences lie. As a result, it is not possible from this test alone to conclude whether the scores from one condition are significantly better or worse than those from another. If you look back to the example given, the ANOVA only allows us to conclude that clinical therapists perform differently in aspects of their job; it does not permit us to say that their performance on one task is better than their performance on another. However, if you look at the results for each condition (p. 192) it appears that the Clinical scores are better than the Interpersonal scores, with the Supervisory scores being worst. We can find out whether the differences between these sets of results are significant by comparing each pair of mean scores using the Scheffé multiple range test. In other words, we can compare:

1. the mean Clinical score with the mean Interpersonal score
2. the mean Clinical score with the mean Supervisory score
3. the mean Interpersonal score with the mean Supervisory score

to find out if the differences in performance in each area are significant. The Scheffé test should

be carried out after you have calculated the ANOVA because it uses some of the values from the ANOVA table. Remember, too, that it should be carried out only if the results from the ANOVA are significant.

There are a number of other multiple range tests which perform the same function, but the Scheffé has been selected because it is considered to be the best (McNemar 1963) and also because it can be used if there are unequal numbers of subjects in each condition. Obviously this latter point does not apply in same-subject and matched-subject designs (since you will, by definition, have the same number of scores in each condition) but, since the Scheffé can also be used with a one-way ANOVA for unrelated designs and unequal subject numbers, this feature is a useful one.

When calculating the Scheffé, you find two values. First, F is calculated for each comparison of means you wish to make, and, second, a figure called 'F^1' is calculated. Each F is compared with the F^1 value. If it is equal to or larger than the F^1 value, then the result is significant.

Calculating the Scheffé

There are three possible comparisons we can make using the Scheffé on our sample data:

1. Clinical vs Interpersonal scores
2. Clinical vs Supervisory scores
3. Interpersonal vs Supervisory scores.

To make these comparisons, take the following steps:

1. Calculate the mean score for each condition

$$\bar{x} = 12.6; \quad \bar{x}_2 = 10.5; \quad \bar{x}_3 = 10.1$$

2. Find the value of F for the first comparison (i.e. Clinical vs Interpersonal) using the following formula:

$$F = \frac{\left(\bar{x}_1 - \bar{x}_2\right)^2}{\dfrac{MS_{error}}{n_1} + \dfrac{MS_{error}}{n_2}}$$

where

$$\bar{x}_1 = \text{mean for Condition 1}$$
$$= 12.6$$

$\bar{x}_2$ = mean for Condition 2

$= 10.5$

MS_{error} = mean square value for the
random error variation
(from the ANOVA calculations)

$= 4.293$

n_1 = number of subjects in Condition 1

$= 10$

n_2 = number of subjects in Condition 2

$= 10$

If these values are substituted, then

$$F = \frac{(12.6 - 10.5)^2}{\dfrac{4.293}{10} + \dfrac{4.293}{10}}$$

$$= \frac{4.41}{0.858}$$

$$= 5.14$$

3. Repeat the calculations for the other two comparisons, using the appropriate means and n values.

Thus for the comparison of the Clinical and Supervisory scores, the formula is:

$$F = \frac{(\bar{x}_1 - \bar{x}_3)^2}{\dfrac{MS_{error}}{n_1} + \dfrac{MS_{error}}{n_3}}$$

$$= \frac{(12.6 - 10.1)^2}{\dfrac{4.293}{10} + \dfrac{4.293}{10}}$$

$$= 7.284$$

and for the comparison of the Interpersonal and Supervisory scores, the formula is:

$$F = \frac{(\bar{x}_2 - \bar{x}_3)^2}{\dfrac{MS_{error}}{n_2} + \dfrac{MS_{error}}{n_3}}$$

$$= \frac{(10.5 - 10.1)^2}{\dfrac{4.293}{10} + \dfrac{4.293}{10}}$$

$$= 0.187$$

4. Using the df_{bet} and df_{error} values derived from the ANOVA (i.e. 2 and 18 respectively), turn to Table A2.6a and locate the df_{bet} value across the v_1 row, and the df_{error} down the v_2 column. At the

intersection point, you will find the value of 3.55. This is the critical value for F at the <5% or < 0.05 level of significance. The <5% level is selected because of the extreme stringency of the Scheffé test. If a smaller p value were to be selected, you would be far less likely to obtain significant results on the Scheffé. However, should you ever get any results that look as though they are considerably more significant than the 5% level, you can repeat steps 4–6 with Table A2.6b (2.5%), A2.6c (1%) and A2.6d (0.1%).

5. Calculate F^1 using the formula:

$$F^1 = (C - 1)F^0$$

where

C = the number of conditions

$= 3$

F^0 = the figure at the intersection point of the appropriate df values in the table

$= 3.55$

$$F^1 = (3 - 1)3.55$$

$$= 7.1$$

6. Compare the F values derived from the calculations in steps 2 and 3 with the F^1 value above. If the F value is *equal to* or *larger than* the F^1 value it is significant.

Therefore, taking our F values of

5.14

7.284

0.187

we can see that only one is larger than the F^1 value, i.e. the comparison between the Clinical and Supervisory scores.

Interpreting the results

The results from the Scheffé test indicate that there is only one significant difference between pairs of performance scores, that is between the Clinical and Supervisory scores (at $p < 0.05$). This suggests that the main reason for the significant results of the ANOVA is the difference between senior clinical therapists in clinical and supervisory skills.

Activity 14.3 (Answers on pp. 367–368)

Carry out a Scheffé test on the following results:

H_1 There is a difference in the efficacy of four teaching approaches used with student clinical therapists.

Method: A group of six student clinical therapists is given comparable information in four different ways: seminar, tutorial, lecture, and individual reading. They are tested on their understanding and receive marks out of 20. A one-way ANOVA for related designs was computed on the scores and the following relevant results obtained:

$df_{bet} = 3$

$df_{error} = 15$

$MS_{error} = 3.87$

The mean scores for each condition were

Condition 1	Seminar	11.2
Condition 2	Tutorial	13.1
Condition 3	Lecture	10.7
Condition 4	Reading	8.4

Further reading

Cohen L, Halliday M 1996 Practical statistics for students. Paul Chapman Publishing, London

Coolican H 2004 Research methods and statistics in psychology, 4th edition. Hodder and Stoughton, London

Darbyshire P 1986 When the face doesn't fit! Nursing Times 82(39):28–30

Field A, Hole G 2004 How to design and report experiments. Sage, London

Ferguson GA, Takane Y 1989 Statistical Analysis in Psychology and Education, 6th Edition. McGraw Hill, New York

Greene J, D'Oliveira M 2005 Learning to use statistical tests in psychology, 3rd edition. Buckingham, Open University Press

Hicks CM 1993 Effects of psychological prejudices on communication and social interaction. British Journal of Midwifery 1(1):10–16

McNemar Q 1963 Psychological Statistics. Wiley, New York

Polgar S, Thomas S 2007 Introduction to research in the health sciences. Edinburgh, Churchill Livingstone.

Robson C 1994 Experiment, design and statistics in psychology, 3rd edition. Harmondsworth, Penguin

Chapter 15

Non-parametric tests for different- (unrelated-) subject designs

INTRODUCTION

The statistical tests described in this chapter are used when the experimental design involves two or more than two, different unmatched groups of subjects who are compared on a certain task, activity, etc. All the tests covered in this chapter are non-parametric ones, which means that they

- are less sensitive
- are easier to calculate
- can be used on nominal, ordinal or interval/ratio data.

Therefore, if you cannot fulfil the conditions required for parametric tests, you should use its non-parametric equivalent. The designs involved in this chapter, then, are for:

1. **Two different, unmatched subject groups** compared on a certain task, activity, etc. (Figure 15.1).
2. **Three or more different, unmatched subject groups** compared on a certain task, activity, etc. (Figure 15.2).

Results from Design 1 are analysed using the **chi-squared (χ^2) test** if the data are nominal, or the **Mann–Whitney U test** if the data are other than nominal (i.e. ordinal or interval/ratio).

Results from Design 2 are analysed using the **extended chi-squared** test if the data are nominal or the **Kruskal–Wallis** test if the data are other than nominal (i.e. ordinal or interval/ratio).

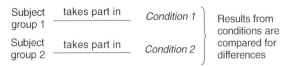

Figure 15.1   Different-subject design: two different unmatched groups of subjects compared on a task.

Figure 15.2   Different-subject design: three or more different, unmatched subject groups compared on a task.

If a trend in the results is predicted, such that subject group 1 is expected to perform better than subject group 2, with subject group 3 performing worst, the **Jonckheere trend test** is used as long as the data are other than nominal (Table 15.1).

NON–PARAMETRIC TEST: TWO DIFFERENT SUBJECT GROUPS AND NOMINAL DATA

CHI-SQUARED (χ^2) TEST

This test is used when you have the sort of experimental design which uses two different, unmatched groups of subjects who are compared on a task, activity, etc. The data for the χ^2 (pronounced 'kie-squared') test must be *nominal*.

To refresh your memory, the nominal level of measurement only allows you to allocate your subjects to named categories (e.g. pass/fail; good/bad; mobile/immobile); it does not allow you to measure your subjects' responses along a dimension, i.e. *how* well they have passed, *how* mobile they are. Check Chapter 4 to make sure you're happy with this concept. As you can see, a subject may only be allocated to one category, since it is impossible to be both mobile and immobile, to pass and to fail. Because of this, the χ^2 can only be used when different subjects are used (an unrelated design) and allocated to different, nominal categories.

With the χ^2 test you may only use two nominal categories and two subject groups. For example,

Table 15.1   Tests for different-subject designs

Design	Non-parametric test
1. Two different groups of subjects, compared on a task	Chi-squared test if data are nominal Mann–Whitney U test (if data are other than nominal, i.e. ordinal or interval/ratio)
2. Three or more different groups of subjects, compared on a task	Extended chi-squared test if data are nominal Kruskal–Wallis (if just a difference in results is predicted and the data are other than nominal, i.e. ordinal or interval/ratio) Jonckheere trend test (if a trend in the results is predicted and the data are other than nominal, i.e. ordinal or interval/ratio)

you may wish to find out whether there is a difference between men and women in terms of which hip (left or right) is more likely to be replaced. You have two groups: 'men' and 'women', and two nominal categories: 'left' and 'right'.

Should you ever wish to allocate two groups to more than two nominal categories you must use the *extended χ^2* (see p. 216).

It should also be noted that when you use the χ^2 test, you should ensure that at least 20 subjects will be in each group. While this may sound off-putting, it rarely takes too much time to collect this amount of data. You do not need to use equal numbers of subjects in each group. When you calculate the χ^2 test, you find a numerical value for χ^2 which you then look up in the probability tables associated with the χ^2 test to see if this value represents a significant difference between the result you observed and those that could be expected by chance.

Example

Let's suppose you were interested in the effects of encouraging early weight bearing after ligamentous ankle sprain. Your hypothesis is:

H_1 Patients who are encouraged to bear full weight after ligamentous ankle sprains are more likely to achieve an early restoration of normal gait pattern.

This is a one-tailed hypothesis, since it predicts a direction to the results.

Method   You select 30 sprained ankle patients and give them full weight-bearing exercise for 15 minutes each day. A further 32 sprained ankle patients are given no exercise. After 3 days, you assess the gait pattern for each group. You count up how many patients have a normal gait pattern and how many do not.

This is a nominal level of measurement because you are using two categories: 'normal gait pattern' and 'abnormal gait pattern' and are simply allocating subjects to one of these groups.

You have a design which looks like Figure 15.3.

In other words you have two groups of subjects who can be allocated to two nominal categories (normal gait pattern or not.)

You end up with the results shown in Figure 15.4.

Calculating the χ^2 test

1. The first step you must always take is to set your data out in a 2×2 table as shown in Figure 15.4. The subject groups should go down the side

and the nominal categories across the top, although it doesn't matter which category is on the left, nor which subject group is at the top. Label your cells A, B, C and D in the same way as above (i.e. from left to right).

2. You must now add up the marginal totals for each row and each column, i.e.

$$A + B = 21 + 9$$
$$= 30$$
$$C + D = 14 + 18$$
$$= 32$$
$$A + C = 21 + 14$$
$$= 35$$
$$B + D = 9 + 18$$
$$= 27$$

3. Calculate the grand total N either by adding up the vertical marginal totals, i.e.

$$30 + 32 = 62$$

or by adding up the horizontal marginal totals, i.e.

$$35 + 27 = 62$$

(The answer will be the same.)

4. Find χ^2 from the formula:

$$\chi^2 = \frac{N\left[(AD - BC) - \frac{N}{2}\right]^2}{(A+B)(C+D)(A+C)(B+D)}$$

where N = the grand total, i.e. 62

$$AD = \text{Cell A} \times \text{Cell D} = 21 \times 18$$
$$= 378$$
$$BC = \text{Cell B} \times \text{Cell C} = 9 \times 14$$
$$= 126$$

The values under the division line are all the marginal totals:

$$A + B = 30$$
$$C + D = 32$$
$$A + C = 35$$
$$B + D = 27$$

Therefore, if we substitute these values in the formula:

Subject group 1 30 sprained ankle patients	takes part in	Condition 1 Full weight-bearing exercises	Assessed as to whether they have normal gait pattern after 3 days. The results are compared.
Subject group 2 32 sprained ankle patients	takes part in	Condition 2 No weight-bearing exercises	

Figure 15.3   Effect of exercises on gait of sprained ankle patients: experimental design.

	Normal gait pattern	Abnormal gait pattern	Marginal total
Subject group 1 Exercises	A 21	B 9	A + B 30
Subject group 2 No exercises	C 14	D 18	C + D 32
Marginal totals	A + C 35	B + D 27	Grand total, N 62

Figure 15.4   Format of data when calculating the χ^2 test.

$$\chi^2 = \frac{62\left[(378-126\,*)-\dfrac{62}{2}\right]^2}{30\times32\times35\times27}$$

(*If you get a minus number from the calculations in the inner brackets, ignore the minus sign.)

$$= \frac{3028142}{907200}$$

$$\chi^2 = 3.338$$

5. Before this χ^2 value can be looked up in the probability tables to see if it represents a significant difference, the df value is required. Use the df formula of:

$$(r-1)(c-1)$$

where

r = the number of rows

c = the number of columns

$$=(2-1)(2-1)$$

$$=1$$

Obviously, in a 2×2 table like this, the df will always equal 1.

Looking up the value of χ^2 for significance

To find out whether the χ^2 value of 3.338 represents a significant difference in gait pattern between patients who have done full weight-bearing exercise and those who have not, it must be looked up in the probability tables associated with the χ^2 test (Table A2.1, p. 341).

Down the left-hand column you will see df values from 1 to 30. Look down this column until you find the df value of 1. To the right of this are five numbers, called critical values of χ^2.

2.71   3.84   5.41   6.64   10.83

Each of these critical values is associated with the probability level at the top of its column, e.g. the critical value of 5.41 is associated with 0.02 for a two-tailed test. You will see that the p values in the table are only associated with two-tailed hypotheses. If you have a one-tailed hypothesis, as we have here, simply look up your χ^2 value as

described, find the two-tailed p value and halve it (see pp. 132–133).

In order for our χ^2 value of 3.338 to be significant at one of these levels, it has to be *equal to* or *larger than* one of these numbers. Our value is larger than 2.71 but smaller than 3.84. Therefore, the probability associated with our obtained χ^2 value must be less than 0.05 (or 5%) but larger than 0.025 (or 2.5%) for a one-tailed hypothesis. (Remember we have had to halve the p values in the table which are for two-tailed hypotheses.) The convention is that we say that p is less than 0.05 (or 5%) rather than greater than 0.025 (or 2.5%). This is expressed as $p < 0.05$.

This means that the probability of our results being due to random error is less than 5%.

Interpreting the results

Our χ^2 value has an associated probability level of less than 0.05 or 5%, which means that the chance of random error being responsible for the results is less than 5%. Because a 5% cut-off point is usually used to claim that the results support the experimental hypothesis, we can say that our results are significant.

However, before we can finally conclude that the hypothesis has been supported, just go back to the 2×2 table and check the results are in the predicted direction, because it is quite possible sometimes to obtain significant results which are opposite to those predicted in the hypothesis and so would not support the hypothesis.

Here we find that more of the exercise group have a normal gait pattern (21 vs 14) and more of the non-exercise group have an abnormal gait pattern (18 vs 9). Therefore the results are as predicted. We can reject the null (no difference) hypothesis on this basis. This can be expressed in the following way:

Using a χ^2 test on the data ($\chi^2 = 3.338$, df = 1) the results were found to be significant at $p < 0.05$, for a one-tailed test. This suggests that the null hypothesis can be rejected and that patients who are encouraged to bear full weight after ligamentous ankle sprain are more likely to achieve an early restoration of normal gait pattern.

Activity 15.1 (Answers on p. 368)

1 In order to practise looking up χ^2 values, look up
   the following and say what the associated p value
   is and whether or not it is significant.
   (i) $\chi^2 = 4.02$ one-tailed   df = 1 p
   (ii) $\chi^2 = 5.91$ two-tailed   df = 1 p
   (iii) $\chi^2 = 3.84$ two-tailed   df = 1 p
   (iv) $\chi^2 = 2.62$ two-tailed   df = 1 p
   (v) $\chi^2 = 6.95$ one-tailed   df = 1 p
2 Calculate a χ^2 test on the following.

H$_1$ Teachers of clinical therapy are more likely to
       study in Open University (OU) degree courses
       than clinical therapist practitioners of
       comparable years of experience since
       qualifying. (Is this a one- or two-tailed
       hypothesis?)

Method: You randomly select 35 teachers of clinical
therapy and 42 clinical therapist practitioners and ask
them whether or not they have ever undertaken an OU
degree course. The results are as shown in Figure 15.5.

	OU course	No OU course
Teachers of clinical therapy	25	10
Clinically-based clinical therapists	15	27

Figure 15.5 Are teachers of clinical therapy more likely
than clinical therapist practitioners to undertake on OU
degree course?

State your χ^2 value, p value, using the sample
format given on p. 204.

NON–PARAMETRIC TEST: TWO DIFFERENT, UNMATCHED SUBJECT GROUPS AND ORDINAL OR INTERVAL/RATIO DATA

MANN–WHITNEY U TEST

This test is used to analyse results from experiments which have compared two different unmatched groups of subjects on a task (see Design 1, pp. 201–202). The Mann–Whitney U test simply compares the results from each group to see if they differ significantly. This test can only be used with ordinal or interval/ratio data. It cannot be used with nominal data.

When calculating this test, you end up with a numerical value, 'U', which you look up in the probability tables associated with the Mann–Whitney test, to see if the U value does, in fact, represent a significant difference between the groups.

Example

Suppose you were interested in testing the hypothesis that there is a difference in the rate of improvement of self-help behaviours among elderly patients with lower limb amputations when treated by two different compensatory techniques.

Your hypothesis would be:

H$_1$ There is a difference in the rate of
       improvement in self-help behaviours
       among elderly lower limb amputation
       patients when treated by two different
       compensatory techniques (techniques 1
       and 2).

This is a two-tailed hypothesis as it does not predict a direction to the results.

In order to do this, you select a group of 28 elderly lower limb amputation patients, all of whom have limited self-help skills. (Assume constant errors have been eliminated, e.g. length of postoperative time.) Randomly allocate 15 patients to technique 1 and 13 to technique 2.

Therefore, we have the design shown in Figure 15.6.

Essentially, you would administer different compensatory treatments to each group and compare the extent of the improvement after a given period of time, e.g. 14 days. Their improvement is recorded along a 9-point ordinal scale. (Note that because we don't have to match the subjects, you can use different numbers in each

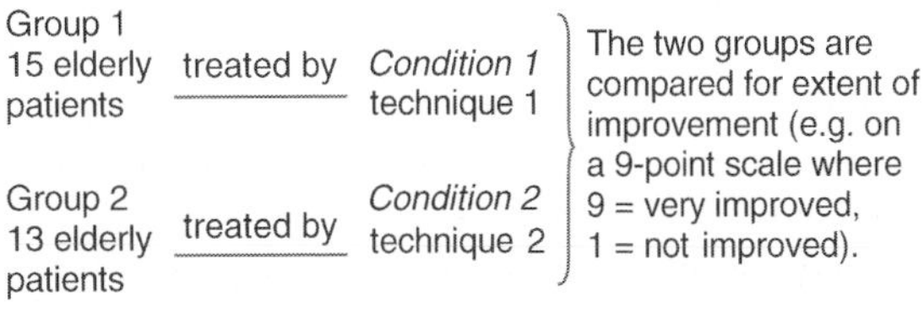

Figure 15.6 Design of experiment to test whether there is a
difference in rates of improvement in self-help behaviours
depending on the compensatory technique used in treatment.

Table 15.2

Subject	Condition 1 Compensatory technique 1	Rank	Subject	Condition 2 Compensatory technique 2	Rank
1	6	18	1	7	22.5
2	5	12.5	2	9	27.5
3	7	22.5	3	6	18
4	3	2.5	4	5	12.5
5	5	12.5	5	6	18
6	4	7	6	7	22.5
7	4	7	7	7	22.5
8	3	2.5	8	8	25.5
9	8	25.5	9	9	27.5
10	6	18	10	6	18
11	5	12.5	11	5	12.5
12	4	7	12	4	7
13	3	2.5	13	5	12.5
14	3	2.5			
15	4	7			
Total	70	159.5		84	246.5
Mean	4.667			6.462	

group.) You might end up with the results shown in Table 15.2.

Calculating the Mann–Whitney U test

To calculate the Mann–Whitney, take the following steps:

1. First calculate the totals (Σ) and means for each condition; i.e.

Condition 1	Total: 70
	Mean: 4.667
Condition 2	Total: 84
	Mean: 6.462

2. *Taking the whole set of scores together* (i.e. all 28 scores) rank them giving the rank of 1 to the lowest, 2 to the next lowest and so on. Where there are two or more scores the same, use the tied rank procedure (see pp. 176–177), i.e. add up the ranks the scores would have obtained had they been different and divide this number by the number of scores that are the same. Thus 3 is the lowest score, but there are four scores of 3. Therefore add up the ranks 1, 2, 3 and 4 (the ranks they would have obtained had they been different) and divide by 4 because there are four scores of 3:

$$\frac{1+2+3+4}{4} = 2.5$$

Assign the rank of 2.5 to all the scores of 3. (See columns labelled 'Rank'.) Remember! Put the scores from both conditions together, as though they were just one set of scores, when you do the ranking. Many students forget to do this.

3. Add the rank totals for each condition separately:

Rank total 1 = 159.5
Rank total 2 = 246.5

4. Select the larger rank total, i.e. 246.5 to use in the formula below.

5. Find U from the formula:

$$U = n_1 n_2 + \frac{n_x(n_x+1)}{2} - T_x$$

where
n_1 = the number of subjects in Condition 1 (i.e. 15)
n_2 = the number of subjects in Condition 2 (i.e. 13)
T_x = the larger rank total (i.e. 246.5)

n_x = the number of Ss in the condition with the larger rank total (i.e. Condition 2 = 13)

Therefore if we substitute these values:

$$U = 15 \times 13 + \frac{13(13+1)}{2} - 246.5$$
$$= 195 + 91 - 246.5$$
$$= 39.5$$

6. Because there are unequal numbers in each condition, it is necessary to repeat the calculations for the smaller rank total (i.e. 159.5) as well.

Here T_x becomes the smaller rank total (159.5), and n_x becomes the number of subjects in the condition with the smaller rank total (i.e. Condition 1 = 15 subjects).

$$U = 15 \times 13 + \frac{15(15+1)}{2} - 159.5$$
$$= 195 + 120 - 159.5$$
$$= 155.5$$

We now have two values of U:

$$U_1 = 39.5$$
$$U_2 = 155.5$$

We need to look up the *smaller* of these two U values in the appropriate table (Tables A2.7a–d, pp. 351–352).

Note: If you use equal numbers of subjects in each condition, you only need to carry out the first calculation of U, using the larger rank total and the appropriate n value. If you use unequal numbers you will have to find both U values and select the smaller one.

Looking up the value of U for significance

In order to find out whether our U value of 39.5 represents a significant difference in healing rates, you have to look up this value in Tables A2.7a–d. There are four probability tables for the Mann–Whitney, each one representing different p values (see headings). Table A2.7a represents the smallest (most significant) p values, while Table A2.7d represents the largest (least significant) p value. To look up your U value you also need the:

n_1 value(15)
n_2 value(13)

Starting with Table A2.7a, look across the top row until you find your n_1 value of 15, and down the left-hand column for your n_2 value of 13. Where these two points intersect is the number 42. In order to be significant at a given level, your U value must be *equal to* or *smaller than* the value at the intersection point. As 39.5 is smaller than 42, our results are significant at either 0.005 for a one-tailed test or 0.01 for a two-tailed test. As we only predicted a general difference in improvement rates in our hypothesis without specifying which compensatory technique would be better, we have a two-tailed hypothesis. Therefore, our results are significant at the 0.01 or 1% probability level.

But, if you notice, our U value of 39.5 is actually smaller than the value of 42 at the intersection point. This means our results are even more significant than the 1% level. This is expressed as:

$$p < 0.01 \, (\text{or} < 1\%)$$

Had our U value been the same as the value at the intersection point, the results would have been significant at exactly the 0.01 or 1% level. This would have been expressed as:

$$p = 0.01 \, (\text{or} \, 1\%)$$

However, our results have a significance level of less than 1% which means that the chance of random error accounting for our results is less than 1%.

Supposing, however, our U value had been 52.5, with our n values the same. Using A2.7a, we would find that the intersection value is 42. Because our U of 52.5 is larger than this value, it would not be significant at the probability levels of 0.005 and 0.01 given in the heading. Therefore, we would move on to Table A2.7b. At this intersection point, for $n_1 = 15$, $n_2 = 13$, the value is 47. Our U value is larger than this and so cannot be classified as significant at this level either. Turn on to Table A2.7c. The intersection value here is 54. Our U value is smaller and so would be significant at the <0.05 level for a two-tailed test.

If you ever find your U value is larger than the relevant intersection values in Table A2.7d, your results would not be significant.

Interpreting the results

Our U value has an associated probability level of less than 1% which means that there is less than a 1% chance of random error causing the results. If you remember, it was said that a good cut-off point for claiming that your results were significant and supported your hypothesis was the 5% level or less. Since our p value is less than 5% we can claim our results are significant; our null (no relationship) hypothesis can therefore be rejected and the experimental hypothesis supported.

Although the hypothesis did not predict which of the two techniques would be better, it is useful to compare the means from each condition to see which method was, in fact, more successful. Here the mean scores are 4.667 and 6.462 for technique 1 and technique 2 respectively, which means that the second technique was more effective. This can be stated in the following way:

Using a Mann–Whitney U test to analyse the data ($U = 39.5$, $n_1 = 15$, $n_2 = 13$), the results were found to be significant at $p < 0.01$ for a two-tailed hypothesis. This means that compensatory techniques 1 and 2 differ significantly in their effectiveness in improving self-help skills in elderly lower limb amputation patients. Further inspection of the results suggests that compensatory technique 2 produces better results.

Method   Randomly select 28 patients all of whom are within 1 week post removal of plaster following forearm fracture. Randomly allocate 14 to paraffin wax treatment and the other 14 to a hot soak. Rate the ease of movement of the wrist joint, following 30 minutes of mobilising exercises, on a 7-point scale (7 = extremely easy to move, 1 = very difficult to move).

The results might be as shown in Table 15.3

Table 15.3

	Condition 1			Condition	
Subject	Paraffin wax	Rank	Subject	2 Hot soak	Rank
1	5		1	3	
2	4		2	3	
3	5		3	5	
4	6		4	4	
5	3		5	2	
6	3		6	1	
7	4		7	3	
8	5		8	4	
9	6		9	5	
10	5		10	5	
11	6		11	3	
12	6		12	3	
13	4		13	4	
14	3		14	2	

State the U value and the p value in a format similar to that suggested earlier.

Activity 15.2 (Answers on p. 368)

1. To practise looking up U values, look up the following and state whether or not they're significant and at what level.
   (i) $n_1 = 12$ $n_2 = 12$ $U = 33.5$ two-tailed p
   (ii) $n_1 = 10$ $n_2 = 10$ $U = 27$ one-tailed p
   (iii) $n_1 = 14$ $n_2 = 12$ $U = 37.5$ one-tailed p
   (iv) $n_1 = 20$ $n_2 = 18$ $U = 87.5$ one-tailed p
   (v) $n_1 = 15$ $n_2 = 15$ $U = 70.5$ one-tailed p
   (vi) $n_1 = 18$ $n_2 = 15$ $U = 92.5$ two-tailed p
2. Calculate a Mann–Whitney U test on the following:

   H_1 Paraffin wax is more effective than a hot soak as a preparation for mobilising exercise for post-fracture patients.

   Is this a one- or two-tailed hypothesis?

NON–PARAMETRIC TESTS: THREE OR MORE DIFFERENT, UNMATCHED SUBJECT GROUPS AND ORDINAL OR INTERVAL/RATIO DATA

KRUSKAL–WALLIS TEST

This test is simply an extension of the Mann–Whitney test, in that it is used:

- when different subject groups are involved
- when the data are ordinal, or interval/ratio
- when the conditions for its parametric equivalent cannot be fulfilled.

However, while the Mann–Whitney can only be used to analyse the results from designs with two different groups of subjects, the Kruskal–

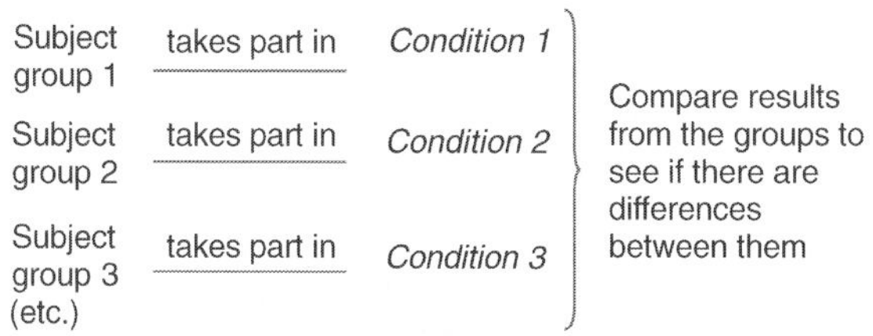

Figure 15.7 A different-subject design with three or more groups of subjects. The Kruskal–Wallis test is used to analyse the results.

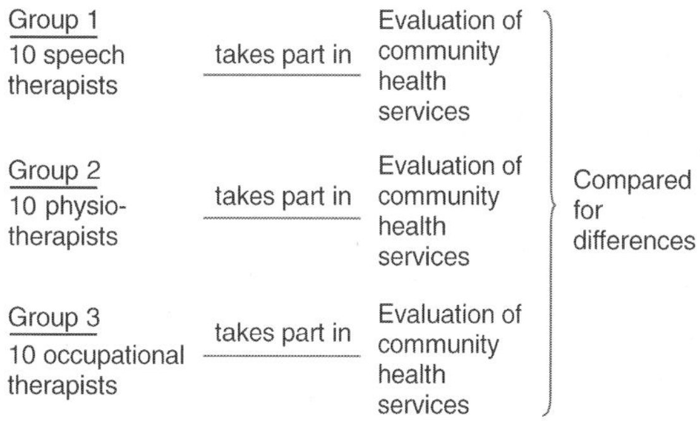

Figure 15.8 Design of experiment to test whether there is a difference between speech therapists, occupational therapists and physiotherapists in their evaluations of community health services for non-comatose stroke patients.

Wallis is used with designs employing three or more different groups of subjects (Figure 15.7).

The Kruskal–Wallis test, however, only tells you whether there are differences between these groups and not which results are better or worse than the others. Therefore, the associated hypothesis must be two-tailed (i.e. just predicting differences in the results with no specific direction to them). Should you ever predict a trend in your results (e.g. that Group 1 will perform better than Group 2, which in turn will perform better than Group 3, etc.) with this sort of unrelated design, you would use a **Jonckheere trend test** to analyse your results.

However, with the Kruskal–Wallis test, you calculate a value H, which you then look up in the probability tables associated with the Kruskal–Wallis test, to find out whether the H value represents significant differences between the groups.

Example

Let's suppose you are conducting an audit of clinical practitioners' satisfaction with the quality of community health services for non-comatose stroke patients. You are interested to find out whether the main service providers (physiotherapy, speech therapy and occupational therapy) have different perceptions of the quality of the clinical service they provide.

Your hypothesis, then, is:

H_1 There is a difference in the perceptions of three main service providers (physiotherapy, speech therapy and occupational therapy) of the quality of clinical services provided for non-comatose stroke patients.

In order to test this out, you select 10 community speech therapists, 10 community physiotherapists and 10 community occupational therapists and ask them to evaluate the overall quality of their cognate service provision for non-comatose stroke patients, using a 5-point scale (1 = very poor, 5 = very good).

Your design looks like Figure 15.8, and your results look like Table 15.4.

Calculating the Kruskal–Wallis test

1. Calculate the totals and mean scores for each condition:

Condition 1   Total = 24 $\bar{x} = 2.4$
Condition 2   Total = 39 $\bar{x} = 3.9$
Condition 3   Total = 25 $\bar{x} = 2.5$.

2. Taking *all* the scores together, as though they were a single set of 30 scores, rank the scores, giving a rank of 1 to the lowest score, a rank of 2 to the next lowest, etc. Where two or more scores are the same, apply the average ranks procedure (see pp. 176–177); i.e. add up the ranks the scores would have obtained had they been different and divide this number by the total number of scores that are the same. Thus, in the example, 1 is the lowest score, but there are four scores of 1. Had these been different, they would have been ranked 1, 2, 3 and 4. So add these ranks up (10) and divide by 4 because there were four scores of 1, giving 2.5. Give the rank of 2.5 to all the scores of 1. Remember that you have now used up ranks 1–4, so you must start with 5 next.

Remember! Rank all the scores together, as though they were just one set of 30 scores.

Table 15.4

Subject*	Condition 1 Speech therapists	Rank	Subject	Condition 2 Physiotherapists	Rank	Subject	Condition 3 Occupational therapists	Rank
1	3	16	1	4	24	1	2	8
2	4	24	2	5	29	2	3	16
3	2	8	3	5	29	3	3	16
4	2	8	4	4	24	4	4	24
5	1	2.5	5	4	24	5	1	2.5
6	3	16	6	3	16	6	3	16
7	4	24	7	2	8	7	2	8
8	1	2.5	8	3	16	8	1	2.5
9	2	8	9	5	29	9	3	16
10	2	8	10	4	24	10	3	16
Total	24	117.0		39	223		25	125.0
Mean	2.4			3.9			2.5	

*Because this is a different-, unmatched-subject design, you do not have to have equal numbers of subjects in each group, although it is easier if you do.

3. Add the rank total for each condition separately to give T:

$$T_{C1} = 117.0$$
$$T_{C2} = 223$$
$$T_{C3} = 125.0$$

4. Find the value of H from the following formula:

$$H = \left[\frac{12}{N(N+1)} \left(\sum \frac{T_c^2}{n_c} \right) \right] - 3(N+1)$$

where

N = total number of subjects (i.e. 30)

n_C = number of subjects in each group (i.e. $n_1 = 10$; $n_2 = 10$; $n_3 = 10$)

T_C = rank totals for each condition (i.e. $T_{C1} = 117$; $T_{C2} = 223$; $T_{C3} = 125$)

T_C^2 = rank total for each condition squared (i.e. 117^2; 223^2; 125^2)

Σ = total of any calculations following the sign

$\sum \dfrac{T_c^2}{n}$ = each rank total squared and divided by the number of subjects in that condition i.e. $\dfrac{117^2}{10} + \dfrac{223^2}{10} + \dfrac{125^2}{10}$

Substituting these values:

$$H = \left[\frac{12}{30(30+1)} \times \left(\frac{117^2}{10} + \frac{223^2}{10} + \frac{125^2}{10} \right) \right]$$

$$- 3 \times 31$$

$$= \left[\frac{12}{930} \times (1368.9 + 4972.9 + 1562.5) \right] - 93$$

$$= (0.013 \times 7904.3) - 93$$

$$= 102.756 - 93$$

$$= 9.756$$

Looking up the H value for significance

To find out whether $H = 9.756$ represents significant differences between the results from each group, you will also need the df value. This is the number of conditions minus 1, i.e. $3 - 1 = 2$. Turn to Tables A2.1 and A2.8 (pp. 341 and 353–354). Table A2.8 covers the probability levels for experiments using three groups of subjects, with 1–5 subjects in each group, while Table A2.1 covers the probability levels for experiments with more subjects and more conditions. (This is also the chi-squared table.)

Because we have 10 subjects in each condition we use Table A2.1. Down the left-hand column you will see various df values. Look down the column until you find our df of 2. To the right of this are five numbers:

$$4.60 \quad 5.99 \quad 7.82 \quad 9.21 \quad 13.82$$

These are called critical values and each one is associated with the probability level indicated at the top of the column, e.g. 7.82 has a p value of 0.02. To be significant at a given level, our H value has to be *equal to* or *larger than* one of these numbers. So, with our H of 9.756, we can see that it is larger than 9.21, but smaller than 13.82. This means that for our two-tailed hypothesis, the probability associated with the obtained H value of 9.756 must be somewhat less than 0.01 (or 1%) but somewhat greater than 0.001 (or 0.1%). To comply with convention, we would say that p is less than 0.01 (or 1%). (Remember with the Kruskal–Wallis, we can only predict general differences in our results, therefore any hypothesis must be two-tailed.) This is expressed as $p < 0.01$ or <1%. This means that there is less than a 1% chance that our results are due to random error. (Had our H value been equal to the critical value, p would have been 0.01 exactly. This would have been expressed as $p = 0.01$ or 1%.)

Interpreting the results

Our H value of 9.756 has a probability of <0.01 (or <1%) which means that the probability of random error accounting for the results is less than 1%. As you will remember, it was noted earlier that the usual cut-off point for assuming support for the experimental hypothesis is the 5% level or less. As our p value is less than 1%, it is smaller than the cut-off point of 5% and therefore we can say that our results are significant. This means we can reject the null hypothesis and accept the experimental hypothesis. This can be expressed in the following way:

Using a Kruskal–Wallis test on the data ($H = 9.756$, $N = 30$) the results were found to be significant at $p < 0.01$. This suggests that there is a significant difference between speech therapists', occupational therapists' and physiotherapists' evaluations of community health services for non-comatose stroke patients. This means that the experimental hypothesis has been supported.

Remember that the Kruskal–Wallis will only tell you that there are differences between your conditions and not which particular group of practitioners had the most positive perceptions of the services. If you had hypothesised a trend in the results, e.g. that physiotherapists would evaluate their community services more positively than would occupational therapists, who in turn would evaluate them higher than would speech therapists and had used the same unmatched design, you would have used a Jonckheere trend test to analyse your results (see p. 212).

Because we used more than five Ss in our experiment, we had to use Table A2.1 to look up our H value. Suppose, however, that we had used instead, 5 Ss in condition 1 (i.e. 5 speech therapists), 4 physiotherapists (Condition 2) and 3 occupational therapists (Condition 3), and had obtained an H value of 5.438. We would now need to use Table A2.8. You will see that there is a heading 'Size of groups', under which there is every permutation of n values. Your n values are $n_1 = 5$, $n_2 = 4$ and $n_3 = 3$. Therefore you need to find these n values (in any order) in the columns and to the right of these you will see six values of H:

$$7.4449$$
$$7.3949$$
$$5.6564$$
$$5.6308$$
$$4.5487$$
$$4.5231$$

and to their right, the relevant p values. (You do not need the df value here.)

To be significant at a given level, our H value must be *equal to* or *larger than* the critical values here. Our H value of 5.438 is larger than 4.5487 but smaller than 5.6308. These values are associated with probabilities of 0.050 and 0.099, and so our obtained H value must have a probability of less than 0.099 but greater than 0.050. Because of convention, we would say that our H of 5.438 has a probability of less than 0.099. Because our cut-off point is 0.05, we must accept the null (no relationship) hypothesis, i.e. our results would not be significant.

Activity 15.3 (Answers on p. 368)

1. To practise looking up H values, look up the following and state whether or not they are significant and at what level.
   (i) $n_1 = 3$ $n_2 = 4$ $n_3 = 3$ $H = 5.801$ p
   (ii) $n_1 = 5$ $n_2 = 5$ $n_3 = 4$ $H = 5.893$ p
   (iii) $n_1 = 12$ $n_2 = 10$ $n_3 = 10$ $N_4 = 10$
        $df = 3$ $H = 8.5$ p
   (iv) $n_1 = 3$ $n_2 = 3$ $n_3 = 5$ $H = 7.0234$ p
   (v) $n_1 = 10$ $n_2 = 12$ $n_3 = 14$ $N_4 = 14$
       $n_5 = 14$ $df = 4$ $H = 15.23$ p
   (vi) $n_1 = 10$ $n_2 = 10$ $n_3 = 8$ $N_4 = 10$
        $df = 3$ $H = 6.86$ p

2. Calculate a Kruskal–Wallis on the following data:

   H_1 Compliance with lumbar mobility exercise instructions varies according to whether the instructions are (a) oral, (b) written by the clinical therapist, or (c) written by the patient her/himself.

   Method: Select 15 patients with restricted lumbar mobility, and randomly allocate 5 to oral instruction, 5 to clinical therapist-written instructions and 5 to self-written instructions. After 1 week compare their self-reported compliance (on a 5-point scale where 5 = did every exercise daily, 1 = did no exercises at all). The results are as shown in Table 15.5.

Table 15.5 Self-reported compliance score on a 5-point scale

	Condition 1 Oral			Condition 2 Therapist-written			Condition 3 Self-written		
Subject	Score	Rank	Subject	Score	Rank	Subject	Score	Rank
1	3		1	3		1	4	
2	2		2	3		2	3	
3	2		3	3		3	4	
4	3		4	2		4	3	
5	1		5	3		5	5	

State the H and p values in the format recommended earlier.

JONCKHEERE TREND TEST

This test is used with the same experimental designs as the Kruskal–Wallis, i.e.

- three or more different- (unmatched-) subject groups are being compared
- the data is ordinal or interval/ratio
- the conditions required for a parametric test cannot be fulfilled (see p. 202 for the design).

However, the one major difference which determines whether you use a Kruskal–Wallis or Jonckheere trend test relates to your hypothesis. If you simply predict that there will be differences between the groups, without specifying which group will perform best or worst then you use the Kruskal–Wallis. However, if you predict a trend in your results, for example, Group A will do better than Group B who in turn will do better than Group C, then you are predicting a definite direction to your results and you should use the Jonckheere to analyse them. Therefore any hypothesis associated with the Jonckheere must be one-tailed.

When calculating the Jonckheere, you end up with a numerical value called 'S', which you look up in the probability tables associated with the Jonckheere test, to see whether this value represents a significant trend in the results.

It should be stressed here that you must have the same numbers of subjects in each group for the Jonckheere. This is not necessary for the Kruskal–Wallis, but it is essential here.

Example

If we look back at the example given on p. 209 i.e. that there will be a difference in the physiotherapists', speech therapists' and occupational therapists' evaluations of the quality of community health provision for non-comatose stroke patients, we can see that because we only predicted a difference in compliance levels without specifying which service provider would report greatest satisfaction, we used a Kruskal–Wallis test. However, that hypothesis can be restated to predict a specific direction to the results:

H_1 There is a difference in the evaluation of the quality of community health service provision for non-comatose stroke patients, with physiotherapists reporting higher evaluations than occupational therapists, who in turn report higher evaluations than speech therapists.

In which case, we are predicting a specific directional trend to the results which would require the Jonckheere trend test to analyse them. We would therefore have the design shown in Figure 15.9.

If we use the previous data, we can see whether or not there was a definite trend in results. These results are as in Table 15.6.

Calculating the Jonckheere trend test

So, taking the data from the previous example, we first have to set out the conditions such that the condition expected to obtain the lowest scores is on the left, and the condition expected to obtain the highest scores is on the right, the remaining condition in the middle. In other words, the conditions must be ordered from lowest on the left, to highest on the right, with any intermediary conditions ordered accordingly.

Therefore, because we have predicted that the speech therapists will provide the lowest evaluations, followed by the occupational therapists, and with the physiotherapists recording the highest evaluations, we must re-order the above data to put the speech therapists on the left, the occupational therapists in the middle and physiotherapists on the right as in Table 15.7.

To calculate the Jonckheere:

1. First calculate the mean score for each condition (Condition 1 = 2.4, Condition 2 = 2.5 and Condition 3 = 3.9).
2. Starting with the extreme left-hand condition and the first score (i.e. 3) count up all the scores to the right of Condition 1 (i.e. in Conditions 2 and 3) which are larger than this score. Do not count any scores which are the same.

Therefore, in Condition 2, only Subject 4 with a score of 4 achieved a higher score, while in

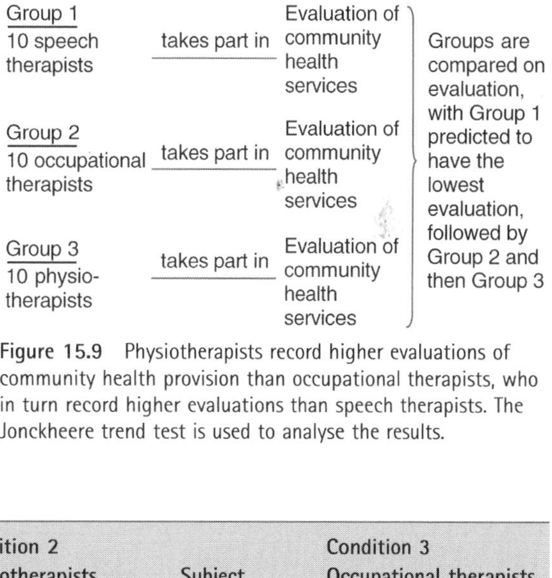

Figure 15.9   Physiotherapists record higher evaluations of community health provision than occupational therapists, who in turn record higher evaluations than speech therapists. The Jonckheere trend test is used to analyse the results.

Table 15.6

Subject	Condition 1 Speech therapists	Subject	Condition 2 Physiotherapists	Subject	Condition 3 Occupational therapists
1	3	1	4	1	2
2	4	2	5	2	3
3	2	3	5	3	3
4	2	4	4	4	4
5	1	5	4	5	1
6	3	6	3	6	3
7	4	7	2	7	2
8	1	8	3	8	1
9	2	9	5	9	3
10	2	10	4	10	3

Table 15.7

Subject	Condition 1 Speech therapists	Subject	Condition 2 Occupational therapists	Subject	Condition 3 Physiotherapists
1	3 (8)	1	2 (9)	1	4
2	4 (3)	2	3 (7)	2	5
3	2 (15)	3	3 (7)	3	5
4	2 (15)	4	4 (3)	4	4
5	1 (18)	5	1 (10)	5	4
6	3 (8)	6	3 (7)	6	3
7	4 (3)	7	2 (9)	7	2
8	1 (18)	8	1 (10)	8	3
9	2 (15)	9	3 (7)	9	5
10	2 (15)	10	3 (7)	10	4
$\bar{x}$	2.4		2.5		3.9

Condition 3, Ss 1, 2, 3, 4, 5, 9 and 10 all obtained higher scores. This means that in total, 8 scores in Conditions 2 and 3 are higher than the score of 3. This number is put in brackets by the Subject 1, Condition 1 score.

Do exactly the same for the second score (4) in Condition 1. There are no scores in Condition 2 which are larger and 3 scores in Condition 3 which are larger. Thus the total of 3 is put in brackets by Subject 2, Condition 1. Continue in this way for the rest of the scores in Condition 1.

Do the same for each score in Condition 2, although, of course, you will only be comparing these with Condition 3 since it is only these scores which are to the right of Condition 2.

Because Condition 3 has no scores to the right, the procedure terminates with the last subject in Condition 2.

3. Before we can calculate S, we need two more values: A and B. To find A: add up *all* scores in brackets to give the value A, i.e.

$$A = 8+3+15+15+18+8+3+18+15+15$$
$$+9+7+7+3+10+7+9+10+7+7$$
$$= 194$$

In order to find out B, which is the maximum value A could have been, had all the scores in Conditions 2 and 3 been bigger than those in Condition 1 and all the scores in Condition 3 been bigger than those in Condition 2, we use the formula:

$$B = \frac{C(C-1)}{2} \times n^2$$

where
   n = number of Ss in each condition
   C = number of conditions
Therefore $n = 10$
   $C = 3$

$$B = \frac{3(3-1)}{2} \times 10^2$$
$$= 300$$

4. Calculate S using the following formula:

$$S = (2 \times A) - B$$
$$= (2 \times 194) - 300$$
$$= 88$$

Looking up the value of S for significance

To look up $S = 88$, turn to Table A2.9 (p. 355) where you will see two tables: the top one is for significance levels of <5% and the lower one for levels of <1%. Both are for one-tailed hypotheses because a specific direction to the results must be predicted in order to use the Jonckheere test.

Start with the top table first. In order to look up your S value, you need the number of conditions and the number of subjects in each condition (i.e. 3 and 10 respectively). Look across the top row for the appropriate value of n and down the left-hand column for the appropriate value of C. At the intersection point you will find the figure 88. If our S value is *equal to* or *larger than* this figure, then the results are significant at the level stated in the heading of the table. As our S value is exactly 88, our results are significant at the <0.05 or <5% level. This means that there is less than a 5% probability that our results are due to random error.

Had our S value been larger than the intersection figure of 88 (say 131), we would move down to the second table which is associated with a probability level of <0.01 and repeat the process. The intersection figure is 124, which means the result is larger than this value and the probability of our results being due to random error is less than 0.01 or 1%.

Interpreting the results

Because our usual cut-off point is 5% and our results have a probability level of <5%, the results can be classified as significant and we can reject the null (no relationship) hypothesis. There is

less than a 5% chance that random error is responsible for our results. This means that there is a significant trend in our results with physiotherapists recording the highest evaluations of the community health services, followed by occupational therapists, who in turn report greater satisfaction than the speech therapists. This can be expressed thus:

> Using a Jonckheere trend test on the data ($S = 88$, $n = 10$), the results were found to be significant at <5% level. This means that there is a significant trend in the evaluations of community health provision for non-comatose stroke patients, with physiotherapists reporting most satisfaction with the quality of service, followed by occupational therapists, and with speech therapists recording the lowest satisfaction scores. The null hypothesis can be rejected.

Activity 15.4 (Answers on p. 368)

1. To practise looking up S values, look up the following and state whether or not they are significant and at what level.

   (i) $C = 3$ $n = 6$ $S = 61$ p
   (ii) $C = 5$ $n = 5$ $S = 68$ p
   (iii) $C = 5$ $n = 8$ $S = 151$ p
   (iv) $C = 3$ $n = 10$ $S = 124$ p
   (v) $C = 3$ $n = 7$ $S = 55$ p
   (vi) $C = 4$ $n = 5$ $S = 48$ p

2. Calculate a Jonckheere trend test on the following data:

   H_1 There is a difference in the number of appointments kept at an outpatients' clinic according to the social class to which the patients belong, with social class 3 being better than social class 2, who in turn are better than social class 4.

   Method: Randomly select 8 patients belonging to each of the social classes and calculate the percentage of kept appointments. The data are as shown in Table 15.8.

Table 15.8

Subject	Condition 1 Social class 3	Subject	Condition 2 Social class 2	Subject	Condition 3 Social class 4
1	100	1	100	1	75
2	90	2	100	2	70
3	100	3	80	3	50
4	75	4	75	4	30
5	75	5	60	5	60
6	80	6	80	6	80
7	90	7	50	7	70
8	70	8	50	8	75

Remember! You must arrange your data such that the condition expected to have the lowest results is on the left, while the condition expected to have the highest results is on the right.

State the values of A, B, S and p; express the results in the format given earlier in the section.

NON-PARAMETRIC TEST: THREE OR MORE DIFFERENT SUBJECT GROUPS AND NOMINAL DATA

EXTENDED CHI-SQUARED (χ^2) TEST

As the name implies this test is an extension of the χ^2 test described earlier in the chapter. Like the earlier test it is used:

- with different subject groups
- with nominal data (re-read Chapter 4 if you need to refresh your memory on levels of measurement)
- when the remaining conditions required for a parametric test cannot be fulfilled.

However, there is an important point which relates to the extended χ^2 test. The ordinary χ^2 test only allows you to use two groups of subjects which you can allocate to two nominal categories. This means you arrange your data in a 2×2 table as in Figure 15.10.

However, the extended χ^2 allows you to use one of the following:

- Two groups of subjects and three (or more) nominal categories. This means you arrange your data in a 2×3 table as in Figure 15.11.
- Three (or more) groups of subjects and two nominal categories. This means you arrange your data in a 3×2 table, as in Figure 15.12.
- Three (or more) groups of subject and three (or more) nominal categories. This means you arrange your data in a 3×3 table as in Figure 15.13.

So you may wish to ask the opinions of senior clinical therapists and newly qualified clinical therapists (two groups) on the issue of reviewing clinical skill mix: 'Approve', 'Disapprove' and 'Don't know' (three nominal categories). This would be a 2×3 table. You would need to use the extended χ^2 test to analyse the results.

(By the way, I recognise that the heading of this subsection may be confusing, in that it implies the extended χ^2 can only be used with three or more subject groups, whereas it can be used with two groups as long as they are being allocated to more than two nominal categories. I apologise for this, but as you can see, a clear, succinct title was difficult to achieve.)

The extended χ^2 test only tells you whether there are overall differences between the groups and not where these differences lie. As a result any hypothesis associated with the extended χ^2 must be two-tailed, in that it cannot predict a specific direction to the results.

The data you obtained in your experiment are called the 'observed' data. The main point of the χ^2 test is to compare your observed data with the data you would have expected had your results been due to totally random distributions. In other words you are comparing the results obtained from your experimental hypothesis (observed data) with those predicted by your null (no relationship) hypothesis (expected data). Obviously, the greater the discrepancies between the

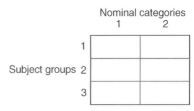

Figure 15.12 A 3×2 table for calculating the extended χ^2 test, with three subject groups and two nominal categories.

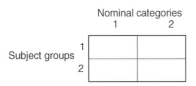

Figure 15.10 A 2×2 table for calculating the χ^2 test.

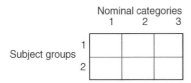

Figure 15.11 A 2×3 table for calculating the extended χ^2 test, with two subject groups and three nominal categories.

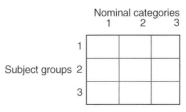

Figure 15.13 A 3×3 table for calculating the extended χ^2 test with three subject groups and three nominal categories.

observed and the expected data, the more likely your results are to be significant. Always ensure that you have tested sufficient subjects to obtain expected frequencies of more than 5. The easiest way to do this is by using at least 20 subjects in each group. You do not need to use equal numbers of subjects in each group.

When calculating the extended χ^2, the value of χ^2 is found and this is then looked up in the probability tables associated with the test to find out whether this value represents significant differences between the observed and expected frequencies.

Example

Suppose in the course of your work you had to treat a very large number of patients presenting with back pain. Over the years, a pattern seems to emerge, which makes you wonder whether the stress levels associated with some jobs predispose people to generalised rather than localised back pain. You decide to find out whether your hunch is correct, by selecting three groups representing different occupational stress levels and assessing whether they had specific low back pain or general back pain. Your hypothesis is:

H$_1$ Occupations associated with different levels of stress vary with respect to the type of back pain they experience (specific low back pain vs general back pain).

You might then go into two or three back clinics and select three groups of patients (with at least 20 subjects in each group) representing the occupational groups: 'High stress', 'Medium stress' and 'Low stress'. You might then simply count up how many patients in each group had been referred either for low back pain or for other forms of back pain (two nominal categories). Thus you would have:

Subject group 1
High stress jobs   ⎫
⎪
Subject group 2   ⎪   Compared for differ-
Medium stress jobs ⎬   ences in type of back
⎪   pain (specific/general)
Subject group 3   ⎪
Low stress jobs   ⎭

There are, then, three unrelated groups of subjects. Each subject's response is allocated to one of two categories (specific back pain/other back pain) and the relative numbers in each category are compared using the extended χ^2.

Imagine that you have carried out some research to test the hypothesis just quoted and you have obtained the following data:

High stress jobs	low back pain	9
	other back pain	21
Medium stress jobs	low back pain	22
	other back pain	13
Low stress jobs	low back pain	25
	other back pain	28

These data are then set out as in Figure 15.14.

You should ensure that the cells are numbered as shown in Figure 15.14, i.e. from left to right. Make sure your subject groups are down the left-hand side, and the nominal categories across the top, although the order in each case is irrelevant.

Calculating the extended χ^2 test

So, to calculate the χ^2 test, take the following steps:

1. Add up the numbers in each row to give the marginal total for

High stress jobs	i.e. $9 + 21 = 30$
Medium stress jobs	i.e. $22 + 13 = 35$
Low stress jobs	i.e. $25 + 28 = 53$.

	Low back pain	Other back pain	Marginal totals of patients
Group 1 High stress	Cell 1 9 $E = 14.237$	Cell 2 21 $E = 15.763$	30
Group 2 Medium stress	Cell 3 22 $E = 16.61$	Cell 4 13 $E = 18.39$	35
Group 3 Low stress	Cell 5 25 $E = 25.153$	Cell 6 28 $E = 27.848$	53
Marginal totals of types of pain	56	62	Grand total (N) 118

Figure 15.14   An example of data for the extended χ^2 test, with three subject groups and two nominal categories.

2. Add up the numbers in each column to give the marginal totals for

low back pain   i.e. 9 + 22 + 25 = 56
other back pain   i.e. 21 + 13 + 28 = 62

3. Add up either the marginal totals for patients, i.e.

$$30 + 35 + 53 = 118$$

or the marginal totals for types of pain, i.e.

$$56 + 62 = 118$$

to give the grand total (N):

$$N = 118$$

4. Calculate the expected frequency (E) for each cell by multiplying the two relevant marginal totals together and dividing by N.

$$\text{Cell 1 } E = \frac{30 \times 56}{118}$$
$$= 14.237$$

$$\text{Cell 2 } E = \frac{30 \times 62}{118}$$
$$= 15.763$$

$$\text{Cell 3 } E = \frac{35 \times 56}{118}$$
$$= 16.61$$

$$\text{Cell 4 } E = \frac{35 \times 62}{118}$$
$$= 18.39$$

$$\text{Cell 5 } E = \frac{53 \times 56}{118}$$
$$= 25.153$$

$$\text{Cell 6 } E = \frac{53 \times 62}{118}$$
$$= 27.848$$

Enter each expected frequency in the lower left-hand corner of the appropriate cell.

5. Calculate the following formula for χ^2

$$\chi^2 = \sum \frac{(O-E)^2}{E}$$

where
O = observed frequencies for each cell (i.e. your actual data)
E = expected frequencies for each cell
Σ = sum or total of all calculations to the right of the sign.

$$\text{Cell 1} = \frac{(9-14.237)^2}{14.237}$$
$$= 1.926$$

$$\text{Cell 2} = \frac{(21-15.763)^2}{15.763}$$
$$= 1.74$$

$$\text{Cell 3} = \frac{(22-16.61)^2}{16.61}$$
$$= 1.75$$

$$\text{Cell 4} = \frac{(13-18.39)^2}{18.39}$$
$$= 1.58$$

$$\text{Cell 5} = \frac{(25-25.153)^2}{25.153}$$
$$= 0$$

$$\text{Cell 6} = \frac{(28-27.848)^2}{27.848}$$
$$= 0$$

6. All these values are added together to give χ^2:

$$\chi^2 = \sum \frac{(O-E)^2}{E}$$

i.e.

$$\chi^2 = 1.926 + 1.74 + 1.75 + 1.58 + 0 + 0$$
$$= 6.996$$

7. To look up the value $\chi^2 = 6.996$, you will also need the degrees of freedom (df) value, i.e.

$$(r-1) \times (c-1)$$

where
r = number of rows (3)
c = number of columns (2)
Therefore:

$$df = (3-1) \times (2-1) = 2$$

Looking up the value of χ^2 for significance

Turn to Table A2.1 (p. 341). You will see down the left-hand column, different df values. Find our df = 2 value. To the right of this are 5 numbers, called critical values of χ^2:

$$4.60 \quad 5.99 \quad 7.82 \quad 9.21 \quad 13.82$$

Each critical value is associated with the p value at the top of its column, e.g. 9.21 has a p value of 0.01. To be significant at a particular level, our χ^2 values must be equal to or larger than one of these critical values. (Remember that the extended χ^2 can only determine whether there are overall differences in the results, so the associated hypothesis must be two-tailed.)

Our χ^2 value of 6.996 is larger than 5.99 but smaller than 7.82. This means that our results are not good enough to be significant at 0.02, but they are slightly better than the 0.05 level. Therefore, by convention we express this as $p < 0.05$ (less than 0.05). Had our χ^2 value been 5.99 exactly we would have expressed this as $p = 0.05$. This means that our χ^2 value is significant at the <0.05 level or <5% level. In other words, the chances of our results being due to random error are less than 5%.

Interpreting the results

Our χ^2 value has an associated probability value of <0.05. This means that there is less than a 5% chance that our results could be accounted for by random error. As the usual cut-off point of 5% or less is used to claim support for the experimental hypothesis and our results have a probability of less than 5%, we can say they are significant. The null hypothesis can be rejected and the experimental hypothesis accepted. This means that there is a significant relationship between job stress and type of back pain.

This can be expressed in the following way:

Using the extended χ^2 on the data ($\chi^2 = 6.996$, df = 2) the results were found to be significant at $p < 0.05$ for a two-tailed test. This suggests that occupational stress levels (Low, Medium and High) are significantly associated with type of back pain (low back pain or general back pain).

Activity 15.5 (Answers on pp. 368–369)

1 To practise looking up χ^2 values, look up the following and state whether or not they are significant.

    (i) $\chi^2 = 3.45$ df = 2 p
    (ii) $\chi^2 = 8.91$ df = 3 p
    (iii) $\chi^2 = 6.77$ df = 2 p
    (iv) $\chi^2 = 9.42$ df = 4 p
    (v) $\chi^2 = 7.95$ df = 2 p

2 Calculate an extended χ^2 on the following data. You are concerned about the missed appointments at the outpatients' clinic and think it may be to do with the ease of getting to the clinic by public transport. Your hypothesis, then, is:

H_1 Keeping an outpatient appointment is related to the ease of access to the hospital, when using public transport.

So you select 25 patients who have a single bus journey with no changes, 30 who have to make one change of bus and 29 who have to make more than one change of bus. You simply note whether or not they missed their next appointment. You obtain the data in Figure 15.15.

		Attended	Missed
	1 No change of bus	20	5
Subject group	2 One change of bus	17	13
	3 More than one change of bus	15	14

Figure 15.15   Is keeping outpatient appointments related to the ease of getting to the clinic? What are the χ^2 and p values for these data?

Calculate an extended χ^2 on these data, and state what the χ^2 value is and the p value. Present your results in the format suggested earlier.

FURTHER READING

Cohen L, Halliday M 1996 Practical statistics for students. Paul Chapman Publishing, London

Coolican H 2004 Research methods and statistics in psychology, 4th edition. Hodder and Stoughton, London

Field A, Hole G 2004 How to design and report experiments. Sage, London

Greene J, D'Oliveira M 2005 Learning to use statistical tests in psychology, 3rd edition. Open University Press, Buckingham

Pett M 1997 Non-parametric statistics in health care research. Sage, London

Polgar S, Thomas S 2007 Introduction to research in the health sciences. Edinburgh, Churchill Livingstone.

Robson C 1994 Experiment, design and statistics in psychology, 3rd edition. Penguin, Harmondsworth

Siegel S 1956 Non-parametric statistics for the behavioural sciences. McGraw-Hill Kogakusha, Tokyo

Chapter 16

Parametric tests for different- (unrelated-) subject designs

INTRODUCTION

The statistical tests described in the previous chapter are used to analyse results from unrelated designs, i.e. any design which uses two or more than two groups of different, unmatched subjects. They are also used when the conditions necessary for a parametric test (see Chapter 9) cannot be fulfilled. The tests covered in this chapter are the parametric equivalent to those in the previous chapter, in other words they are used when:

- Two or more than two different (unmatched) groups of subjects are used in the research and the results from each are compared for differences.
- The conditions essential for a parametric test can be fulfilled (especially the interval/ratio level of measurement).

Therefore, the sorts of designs involved are:

1. **Two different, unmatched subject groups,** compared on a task (Figure 16.1).
2. **Three or more different, unmatched subject groups,** compared on a task (Figure 16.2).

Results from experiments using Design 1 (two unmatched groups) are analysed by the unrelated *t*-test, while results derived from experiments using Design 2 (three or more unmatched groups) are analysed by the one-way analysis of variance (ANOVA) for unrelated designs. In addition, the Scheffé multiple range test can be used

Subject group 1 — takes part in — *Condition 1*
Subject group 2 — takes part in — *Condition 2*
} Results compared for differences

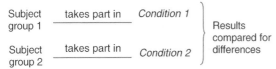

Figure 16.1 Different-subject design: two groups of different, unmatched subjects each taking part in one condition.

Subject group 1 — takes part in — *Condition 1*
Subject group 2 — takes part in — *Condition 2*
Subject group 3 etc. — takes part in — *Condition 3* etc.
} Results compared for differences

Figure 16.2 Different-subject design: three or more groups of different, unmatched subjects each taking part in one condition.

Table 16.1 Parametric tests for different- (unrelated-) subject designs

Design	Parametric test
1. Two groups of different, unmatched, subjects, each taking part in one condition. Results from conditions compared for differences.	Unrelated *t*-test
2. Three or more groups of different, unmatched subjects, each taking part in one condition. Results from conditions compared for differences.	One-way analysis of variance (ANOVA) for unrelated designs, and Scheffé multiple range test

in conjunction with the ANOVA for further analysis of the results. This will be explained later in the chapter (Table 16.1).

Remember that a parametric test is much more powerful than the non-parametric equivalent, in that if there are differences in the results from the different subject groups, the parametric test is more likely to pick them up. This said, there are, however, a number of points you should remember:

1. The parametric test and its non-parametric equivalent do essentially the same job in that they compare results from the subject groups to find out whether any differences between them are significant.
2. In order to use a parametric test you must ensure that you fulfil the necessary conditions. (see pp. 124–125).
3. If you are in any doubt as to whether a parametric test should be used, always use the non-parametric equivalent.
4. Parametric tests, although more sensitive, are more difficult to calculate.

Group 1: 10 meniscectomy patients, within 48 hours postoperative — *Condition 1* Audiobiofeedback
Group 2: 10 meniscectomy patients, within 48 hours postoperative — *Condition 2* Muscle stimulation
} Compare percentage range of movement for each group to see if there are any differences

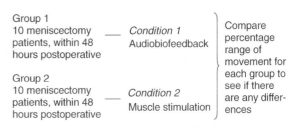

Figure 16.3 Is audiobiofeedback more effective than muscle stimulation for rehabilitation for meniscectomy patients?

PARAMETRIC TEST: TWO GROUPS OF DIFFERENT SUBJECTS

UNRELATED *t*-TEST

This test is used when the experimental design compares two separate or different unmatched groups of subjects participating in different conditions (see Design 1, this page). It is the parametric equivalent of the Mann–Whitney *U* test. The fact that it is parametric means, principally, that you must have *interval/ratio data*. Do note that you do not need to have equal numbers in each group.

When calculating the unrelated *t*-test, you find the value called 't', which you then look up in the probability tables associated with the *t*-test to find out whether the *t* value represents a significant difference between the results from your two groups.

Example

In order to rehabilitate meniscectomy patients more efficiently, you wish to compare two treatments commonly in use in your department: audiobiofeedback and muscle stimulation, to see

Table 16.2

| | Group 1*, audiobiofeedback | | | Group 2, muscle stimulation | |
Subject	Scores (X_1)	X_1^2	Subject	Scores (X_2)	X_2^2
1	40	1600	1	20	400
2	30	900	2	25	625
3	35	1225	3	30	900
4	25	625	4	25	625
5	30	900	5	15	225
6	40	1600	6	40	1600
7	45	2025	7	35	1225
8	35	1225	8	40	1600
9	25	625	9	25	625
10	40	1600	10	30	900
$\Sigma X_1=$	345	$\Sigma X_1^2 = 12325$	$\Sigma X_2=$	285	$\Sigma X_2^1 = 8725$
$\bar{x}_1=$	34.5		$\bar{x}_2=$	28.5	

*It does not matter whether audiobiofeedback is Condition 1 or 2.

which one produces greater movement in the knee joint. Your hypothesis, then, is:

H_1 Meniscectomy patients who have lost some movement improve more quickly when treated by audiobiofeedback than by muscle stimulation.

This is a one-tailed hypothesis because it is predicting a specific direction to the results.

You might select 20 meniscectomy patients, all within 48 postoperative hours, and randomly allocate 10 patients to audiobiofeedback and 10 to muscle stimulation. After, five treatment sessions, you might compare percentage range of movement for each group. Therefore, you would have the design shown in Figure 16.3.

In other words you are comparing the results of two different groups of subjects; a design and type of measurement which requires an unrelated t-test.

You obtain the results shown in Table 16.2.

Calculating the unrelated t-test

In order to calculate t, you should take the following steps (the unrelated t-test formula looks very formidable, but please don't panic! As long as you work through the following stages systematically, you shouldn't have too much difficulty).

1. Find the total (Σ) of the scores for each condition:

Condition 1 = 345
Condition 2 = 285

2. Find the average score ($\bar{x}$) for each condition:

Condition 1 = 34.5
Condition 2 = 28.5

3. Square every individual score and enter the results in the columns headed X_1^2 and X_2^2, e.g. Subject 1, Group 1, scored 40, which when squared becomes 1600.

4. Add up the squared scores for each condition separately to give ΣX^2, i.e.

$$\sum X_1^2 = 12325$$
$$\sum X_2^2 = 8725$$

5. Take the total for each condition separately, and square it, to give $(\Sigma X)^2$, i.e.

$$\left(\sum X_1\right)^2 = 345^2$$
$$= 119025$$
$$\left(\sum X_2\right)^2 = 285^2$$
$$= 81225$$

Do make a note of the difference between the symbol 'ΣX^2', which means 'square each individual score, and then add up all the squared, scores', and $(\Sigma X)^2$, which means 'add up all the individual scores for the condition and then square the result'.

6. Now (take a deep breath!) calculate t from the formula:

$$t = \frac{\bar{x}_1 - \bar{x}_2}{\left[\sqrt{\dfrac{\left(\Sigma X_1^2 - \dfrac{(\Sigma X_1)^2}{n_1}\right) + \left(\Sigma X_2^2 - \dfrac{(\Sigma X_2)^2}{n_2}\right)}{(n_1 - 1) + (n_2 - 1)}} \times \sqrt{\left(\dfrac{1}{n_1} + \dfrac{1}{n_2}\right)}\right]}$$

where

$\bar{x}_1$ = mean of scores from Condition 1
   = 34.5

$\bar{x}_2$ = mean of scores from Condition 2
   = 28.5

ΣX_1^2 = the square of each individual score from Condition 1 totalled
   = 12325

ΣX_2^2 = the square of each individual score from Condition 2 totalled
   = 8725

$(\Sigma X_1)^2$ = the total of the individual scores from Condition 1 squared
   = 345$_2$
   = 119025

$(\Sigma X_2)^2$ = the total of the individual scores from Condition 2 squared
   = 285^2
   = 81225

n_1 = number of Ss in Condition 1
   = 10

n_2 = number of Ss in Condition 2
   = 10

If we substitute these values in the formula:

$$t = \frac{34.5 - 28.5}{\left[\sqrt{\dfrac{\left(12325 - \dfrac{119025}{10}\right) + \left(8725 - \dfrac{81225}{10}\right)}{(10 - 1) + (10 - 1)}} \times \sqrt{\left(\dfrac{1}{10} + \dfrac{1}{10}\right)}\right]}$$

$$= \frac{6}{\sqrt{\dfrac{422.5 + 602.5}{18} \times \dfrac{1}{5}}}$$

$$= \frac{6}{\sqrt{56.944 \times 0.2}}$$

$$= \frac{6}{3.375}$$

$$= 1.778$$

(Note: it does not matter if your t value is + or −, because you ignore the sign anyway.)

7. Calculate the degrees of freedom (df) from the formula:

$$df = (n_1 - 1) + (n_2 - 1)$$
$$= (10 - 1) + (10 - 1)$$
$$= 18$$

Looking up the value of t for significance

To look up the value $t = 1.778$, with df = 18, turn to Table A2.5 (p. 346). Down the left-hand column, you will find values of df. Look down the column until you find df = 18. To the right of this, you will see six numbers, called critical values of t:

1.330 1.734 2.101 2.552 2.878 3.922

Each critical value represents a different level of probability as indicated by the bold type at the top of the table. Therefore, 2.552, for example, is associated with a probability of 0.01 for a one-tailed test and 0.02 for a two-tailed test. To be significant at one of these levels, our t value must be *equal to* or *larger than* the associated critical t value in the table.

Our t value is larger than 1.734, but smaller than 2.101. This means that for our one-tailed hypothesis, the probability associated with our t value of 1.778 comes somewhere between 0.05

(5%) and 0.025 (2.5%). In other words the probability for $t = 1.778$ is less than 5%, but greater than 2.5%. According to convention, we always say that p is less than a given level, and so here the p value for $t = 1.778$ is less than 5% (or 0.05). This is expressed as:

$$p < 0.05 (\text{or } 5\%)$$

as < means 'less than'.

This means that the chances of random error accounting for our results are less than 5%.

Had our t value been 1.734 exactly, the associated probability level would have equalled 0.05. This would be expressed as $p = 0.05$.

Interpreting the results

Our t value of 1.778 has an associated probability level of less than 5%, which means that the possibility of random error being responsible for the outcome of our experiment is less than 5 in 100. As the usual cut-off point for claiming support for the experimental hypothesis is 5% we can say that our results are significant. However, because we predicted a specific direction to the results (i.e. a one-tailed hypothesis), we must check that the results are in the predicted direction (i.e. audiobiofeedback being more effective than muscle stimulation); sometimes significant results are obtained which are in the opposite direction to the hypothesis and therefore do not support it.

Here, if we look at the mean scores for each condition, we can see that the average score for the audiobiofeedback condition is larger (34.5 as opposed to 28.5). Therefore, the experimental hypothesis has been supported. This can be stated in the following way:

Using an unrelated t-test on the data ($t = 1.778$, df = 18) the results were found to be significant ($p < 0.05$ for a one-tailed hypothesis). The null hypothesis can therefore be rejected. This means that audiobiofeedback is more effective than muscle stimulation for developing movement in meniscectomy patients.

Activity 16.1 (Answers on p. 369)

1 To practise looking up t values, look up the following and state whether or not they are significant and at what level:

(i) $t = 2.149$	df = 10	one-tailed	p
(ii) $t = 2.596$	df = 16	two-tailed	p
(iii) $t = 3.055$	df = 12	two-tailed	p
(iv) $t = 1.499$	df = 15	one-tailed	p
(v) $t = 3.204$	df = 18	two-tailed	p

2 Calculate an unrelated t-test on the following data

H$_1$ Absenteeism is greater among basic-grade clinical therapists than among senior clinical therapists.

Method: Randomly select 15 basic grade clinical therapists and 12 senior clinical therapists, and count up the number of days each subject was absent during the previous 12 months. The results are as shown in Table 16.3.

Table 16.3

Condition 1, basic grade		Condition 2, senior	
Subject	Score	Subject	Score
1	18	1	17
2	22	2	12
3	10	3	15
4	14	4	10
5	25	5	19
6	19	6	8
7	17	7	5
8	28	8	14
9	18	9	18
10	14	10	21
11	15	11	20
12	22	12	16
13	23		
14	19		
15	24		

State the t, df and p values, using the format outlined earlier.

PARAMETRIC TEST: THREE OR MORE GROUPS OF DIFFERENT SUBJECTS

ONE-WAY ANALYSIS OF VARIANCE (ANOVA) FOR UNRELATED- (DIFFERENT-) SUBJECT DESIGNS

The one-way ANOVA for unrelated designs is the parametric equivalent of the Kruskal–Wallis test, i.e. it is used to compare results from three or more conditions, with different, unmatched subject groups in each condition, as shown in Figure 16.2 (p. 222).

It is used when the prerequisite conditions for a parametric test can be fulfilled, the most important of which is that the data are of an interval/ratio level.

The one-way ANOVA is so-called because it analyses results from experiments where only one independent variable (IV) is manipulated. (All the statistical tests and designs covered in this book relate solely to the manipulation of one IV.) More complex designs which manipulate two IVs simultaneously are analysed using a two-way ANOVA; those which manipulate three IVs simultaneously require a three-way ANOVA. (Refresh your memory by rereading Chapter 6.) All this is outside the domain of this book, but the reader is referred to Ferguson and Takane (1989) and Cohen and Holliday (1996) for more information on this topic.

The ANOVA only tells you whether there are general, non-specified differences in the results from the different conditions; it does not tell you which group is better than the others. (To find this out, once you have calculated your ANOVA, you will need to use the Scheffé test, but more of that later.) Because of this, any hypothesis associated with the ANOVA must, of necessity, be two-tailed.

Essentially, what the one-way unrelated ANOVA does is to tell you whether the differences in scores from each condition are sufficiently large to be classified as significant. But if you look back to the outline design on p. 222 you will see that different subject groups are doing different conditions. Therefore, any variation between the scores from the conditions must also reflect the variations between the subject groups.

This source of variation is called *between-conditions variance*. However, because different subjects are involved in each condition, it is conceivable that any outcome in the results is due not to differences between conditions, but to individual differences amongst the subjects, of inherent variations in personality, ability, reactions to the study, etc., i.e. the result of random error. Thus, this is another source of potential variation in the results and is known as *error variance*.

Obviously, you would wish your results to be the outcome of the different conditions and not random error. Thus, the degree of between-condition variance should be much larger than the error variance. What the one-way unrelated ANOVA does is to tell you whether your results are due to real differences between the experimental conditions or alternatively to random error in the form of individual differences.

Example

An actual example might clarify all this. If we go back to the hypothesis quoted for the unrelated *t*-test, i.e. meniscectomy patients who have lost some movement improve more quickly when treated by audiobiofeedback than by muscle stimulation. Suppose we add a further treatment group of ice-packs to this, such that our hypothesis becomes:

H₁ There is a difference in the degree of movement of the knee joint among meniscectomy patients according to whether they have been treated with audiobiofeedback, muscle stimulation or ice-packs.

(Note the inevitable change to a two-tailed hypothesis in this example.)

Obviously, what you are predicting here are differences in percentage range of movement between the groups as a result of different treatments. Therefore, you are anticipating a significant degree of between-group variation. However, suppose you picked your subjects badly, such that all the most motivated were accidentally put in the audiobiofeedback group. Almost inevitably, this type of treatment would produce the best results, not because of the nature of the treatment, but because of the idiosyncrasies of the subjects. In other words random error would account for your results. Obviously, the sort of situation which has all the most moti-vated subjects inadvertently allocated to one group is very unlikely to occur, particularly if you randomly allocate your subjects to condi-tions, but the point is this: your results could be due to genuine differences in terms of treatment, or to some quirks of your subjects. Obviously, you want your results to be due to the former and what the one-way unrelated ANOVA does is to tell you how probable it is that your results are due to the IV and not to random error.

Thus, when you calculate the one-way unre-lated ANOVA, you have to find out the degree of variation in the scores due to the differences between experimental conditions (between-con-ditions variance) and that due to random error (error variance). This will give you an 'F ratio' which you then look up in the probability tables associated with the ANOVA to see if it represents a significant result. Please note, however, that the following formula is only appropriate for designs with *equal numbers of subjects* in each group.

Let's suppose, then, that we added this third treatment group to our earlier experiment, such that we were now comparing the degrees of movement in three groups of meniscectomy patients following different kinds of treatment: audiobiofeedback, muscle stimulation and ice-packs. Thus we have the sort of design shown in Figure 16.4.

When we calculate the one-way unrelated ANOVA we need to set out a table for the sources of variance in scores, like Table 16.4.

So, using the scores from the unrelated *t*-test, together with some new data for the ice-pack group, we have the scores shown in Table 16.5.

Calculating the one-way ANOVA for unrelated designs

To calculate the sums of squares (SS) for each source of variation, take the following steps:

1. Calculate the value ΣT_c^2, which is the sum of the squared total for each condition, i.e.

$$T_1^2 = 345^2$$
$$= 119\,025$$
$$T_2^2 = 285^2$$
$$= 81\,225$$
$$T_3^2 = 300^2$$
$$= 90\,000$$

Therefore:

$$\sum T_c^2 = 119\,025 + 81\,225 + 90\,000$$
$$= 290\,050$$

2. Find the value of n, which is the number of subjects in each condition

$$n = 10$$

3. Calculate the value of N, which is the total number of scores, i.e.

$$N = 10 + 10 + 10$$
$$= 30$$

4. Calculate $(\Sigma x)^2$ which is the grand total of all the scores, squared, i.e.

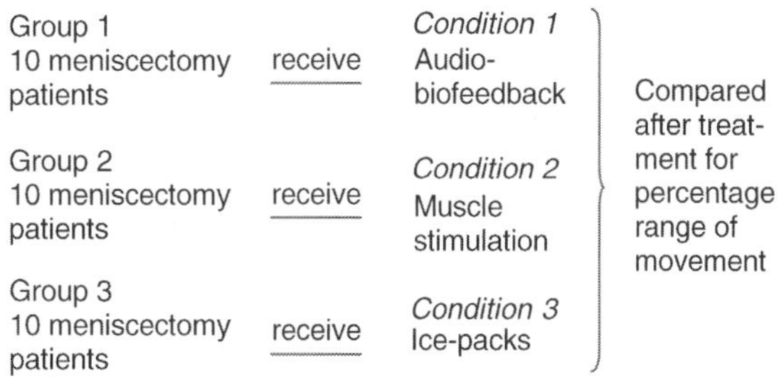

Group 1 10 meniscectomy patients	receive	*Condition 1* Audio- biofeedback	⎫ ⎪ Compared ⎪ after treat-
Group 2 10 meniscectomy patients	receive	*Condition 2* Muscle stimulation	⎬ ment for ⎪ percentage ⎪ range of ⎪ movement
Group 3 10 meniscectomy patients	receive	*Condition 3* Ice-packs	⎭

Figure 16.4   Comparison of three different rehabilitation procedures for meniscectomy patients.

Table 16.4

Source of variance	Sums of squares (SS)	Degrees of freedom (df)	Mean squares (MS)	F ratio
Variation in results due to treatment (between conditions)	SS_{bet}	df_{bet}	MS_{bet}	F_{bet}
Variation in results due to random error	SS_{error}	df_{error}	MS_{error}	
Total	SS_{tot}	df_{tot}		

Table 16.5

	Condition 1 Audiobiofeedback		Condition 2 Muscle stimulation		Condition 3 Ice-packs
Subject	Score	Subject	Score	Subject	Score
1	40	1	20	1	25
2	30	2	25	2	30
3	35	3	30	3	40
4	25	4	25	4	35
5	30	5	15	5	25
6	40	6	40	6	25
7	45	7	35	7	20
8	35	8	40	8	30
9	25	9	25	9	35
10	40	10	30	10	35
	$\Sigma T_1 = 345$		$\Sigma T_2 = 285$		$\Sigma T_3 = 300$

Table 16.6

Source of variance	SS	df	MS	F ratio
Variation due to treatment, i.e. between-conditions	195	2	97.5	1.915
Variation due to random error	1375	27	50.926	
Total	1570	29		

$$\left(\sum x\right)^2 = (345 + 285 + 300)^2$$
$$= 930^2$$
$$864\,900$$

5. Calculate the value of $\frac{\left(\sum x\right)^2}{N}$ (this value is subtracted from all calculations), i.e.

$$\frac{\left(\sum x\right)^2}{N} = \frac{(930)^2}{30}$$
$$= \frac{864900}{30}$$
$$= 28830$$

6. Thus to calculate the SS_{bet} use the formula:

$$\frac{\sum T_c^2}{n} - \frac{\left(\sum x\right)^2}{N} = \frac{345^2 + 285^2 + 300^2}{10} - \frac{864900}{30}$$
$$= \frac{119025 + 81225 + 9000}{10} - 28830$$
$$= 195$$

7. Calculate SS_{tot} from the following formula:

$$\sum x^2 - \frac{\left(\sum x\right)^2}{N}$$

where Σx^2 = the square of each individual score, all added together:

$$\sum x^2 = 40^2 + 30^2 + 35^2 + 25^2 + 30^2 + 40^2 + 45^2$$
$$+ 35^2 + 25^2 + 40^2 + 20^2 + 25^2 + 30^2 + 25^2$$
$$+ 15^2 + 40^2 + 35^2 + 40^2 + 25^2 + 30^2 + 25^2$$
$$+ 30^2 + 40^2 + 35^2 + 25^2 + 25^2 + 20^2 + 30^2$$
$$+ 35^2 + 35^2$$
$$= 30\,400$$

Therefore

$$SS_{tot} = 30\,400 - 28\,830$$
$$= 1570$$

8. Calculate SS_{error} from the formula $SS_{tot} - SS_{bet}$

$$SS_{error} = 1570 - 195$$
$$= 1375$$

9. Calculate the df values:

$$df_{bet} = \text{number of conditions} - 1$$
$$= 3 - 1$$
$$= 2$$

$$df_{tot} = N - 1$$
$$= 30 - 1$$
$$= 29$$

$$df_{error} = df_{tot} - df_{bet}$$
$$= 29 - 2$$
$$= 27$$

10. Divide each SS value by its own df value to obtain the MS value, i.e.:

$$MS_{bet} = \frac{SS_{bet}}{df_{bet}}$$
$$= \frac{195}{2}$$
$$= 97.5$$

$$MS_{error} = \frac{SS_{error}}{df_{error}}$$
$$= \frac{1375}{27}$$
$$= 50.926$$

11. Calculate the F ratio by using

$$\frac{MS_{bet}}{MS_{error}}$$
$$= \frac{97.5}{50.926}$$
$$= 1.915$$

Insert all these values into the appropriate slots in your ANOVA table (see p. 228), as in Table 16.6.

To look the F ratio up in Tables A2.6a–d, you also need the df values for each source of variation, i.e. 2 and 27. If you turn to Tables A2.6a–d (pp. 347–350) you will see that they each deal with critical values of F for different significance levels:

Table A2.6a: $p < 0.05$
Table A2.6b: $p < 0.025$
Table A2.6c: $p < 0.01$
Table A2.6d: $p < 0.001$

Starting with Table A2.6a which represents the largest and therefore least significant probabilities ($p < 0.05$) you will see various numbers associated with v_1, which are the df_{bet} values across the top, and v_2 values down the left-hand side which are the df_{error} values. Therefore, locate your df_{bet} of 2 along the top and the df_{error} of 27 down the left-hand column. Where these two lines intersect you will see the number 3.35. To be significant at the $p < 0.05$ level, our F value has to be *equal to* or *larger than* the given value of 3.35. Since $F = 1.915$ is smaller, we must conclude our results are not significant.

Interpreting the results

Because our F value of 1.915 is smaller than the number observed at the appropriate intersection point on Table A2.6a, we have to conclude that our results are not significant at <0.05, and that the probability of our results being due to random error is greater than 5%. Since the normal cut-off level for claiming support for the experimental hypothesis is 5% or less, we have to accept the null (no relationship) hypothesis. This means that there is no relationship between type of treatment for meniscectomy patients (audiobiofeedback, muscle stimulation or ice-packs) and percentage movement of the knee joint. This can be expressed as:

Using a one-way ANOVA for unrelated designs ($F = 1.915$, $df_{bet} = 2$, $df_{error} = 27$) the results were not significant (p is greater than 5% for a two-tailed hypothesis). Therefore the null hypothesis must be accepted. This indicates that there is no relationship between type of treatment given to meniscectomy patients (audiobiofeedback, muscle stimulation and ice-packs) and subsequent degree of movement of the knee joint.

Had our F value been larger, say 5.234, it would obviously have been significant on Table A2.6a's probabilities. But could we do any better? Turn to Table A2.6b ($p < 0.025$) and repeat the process. The value at the intersection point using df values of 2 and 27 is 4.24. Our F value of 5.234 is larger than this and so is significant at the <0.025 level. Repeat the process with Table A2.6c ($p < 0.01$). The value at the intersection point is 5.49. Our F ratio is smaller and so is not significant at this level. Therefore, in this case we would conclude that the F value of 5.234 is significant at the $p < 0.025$ level.

Remember that, because an ANOVA only tells us whether there are differences and not in which direction these differences lie, the p values are for a two-tailed hypothesis. Had you obtained significant results and you wanted to find out which group did significantly better than the others, you would need to use the Scheffé if you obtained significant results from your ANOVA.

Activity 16.2 (Answers on p. 369)

1. To practise looking up F ratios, look up the following and state whether or not they are significant and at what level.
   (i) df = 3   df = 12 $F = 6.103$ p
   (ii) df = 2   df = 10 $F = 15.76$ p
   (iii) df = 3   df = 15 $F = 4.01$ p
   (iv) df = 3   df = 12 $F = 5.95$ p
2. Calculate a one-way unrelated ANOVA on the following data:

   H_1 Traumatic brain injury patients make differential progress according to whether they receive computer-assisted cognitive rehabilitation, speech therapy or occupational therapy.

Method: Select 21 traumatic brain injury patients and randomly assign 7 to computer-assisted cognitive rehabilitation (CACR), 7 to speech therapy and 7 to occupational therapy. Take a measure of their neuropsychological ability before the start of treatment and again 1 month later. Results are in percentages, which are compared between the three groups. Results are shown in Table 16.7.

Table 16.7

Subject	CACR	Speech therapy	Occupational therapy
1	25	15	10
2	35	30	20
3	30	20	20
4	20	15	25
5	20	25	15
6	25	30	10
7	15	15	20

State your F ratio and p value in a format similar to that suggested. Also, present your values in an ANOVA table.

SCHEFFÉ MULTIPLE RANGE TEST FOR USE WITH ONE-WAY ANOVAS FOR UNRELATED DESIGNS

The analysis of variance only tells us whether there are significant differences between the results from each condition. It does not tell us which group(s) did better or worse than the others. For example, let's take the hypothetical case given in Activity 16.2 that various therapies are differentially effective in aiding the progress of traumatic brain injured patients. Further, let's imagine that the results were significant. These results only tell us that the therapies have differential impacts on neuropsychological progress; they do not tell us which therapy is significantly better than the others. In other words, we can't tell from the results of the ANOVA alone whether there are significant differences between:

computer-assisted cognitive rehabilitation
    (CACR) and speech therapy
and/or
CACR and occupational therapy
and/or
speech therapy and occupational therapy.

If we want to find this out, we must use a Scheffé multiple range test. There are three important points which relate to the use of the Scheffé:

- The Scheffé can only be used if the results from the ANOVA are significant.
- The formula for the Scheffé has already been presented in conjunction with the one-way ANOVA for related samples. The formula for the Scheffé for use with the ANOVA for unrelated samples is the same, but is presented again here for ease and clarity.
- The Scheffé can only be carried out after an ANOVA has been performed. It cannot be used independently.

Essentially what the Scheffé does is to compare the mean scores from each condition to see if the difference between them is significant.

When calculating the Scheffé you have to find two values: F is computed first for each comparison of means you wish to make. This is then

Table 16.8

Subject	Condition 1 CACR	Condition 2 Speech therapy	Condition 3 Occupational therapy
1	35	20	10
2	30	25	15
3	33	30	15
4	30	20	20
5	25	25	20
6	25	15	10
Σ	178	135	90
$\bar{x}$	29.667	22.5	15.0

Table 16.9

Source of variance	SS	df	MS	F ratio
Variation due to treatment, i.e. between-conditions	645.445	2	322.723	15.088
Variation due to random error	320.833	15	21.389	
Total	966.278	17		

compared with a second value: F_1. If any F is equal to or larger than F_1 then the difference between the two relevant means is significant.

Example

Let's take the example given in Activity 16.2, i.e. that there is a relationship between the type of therapy used with traumatic brain injury patients and the neuropsychological progress made. Suppose you repeated the experiment, with six subjects in each group this time and you obtained the data shown in Table 16.8.

You can perform a one-way ANOVA for unrelated designs on the data. The outcome looks like Table 16.9.

$$F = 15.088 \text{ is significant at } p < 0.001$$

This means that there are significant differences in before/after neuropsychological levels between the three treatment groups. However, in order to find out which therapy group does significantly better than the others we need to compare

1. CACR and speech therapy
2. CACR and occupational therapy
3. Speech therapy and occupational therapy

using the Scheffé multiple range test.

Calculating the Scheffé multiple range test

1. Calculate the mean score for each group, i.e.

Condition 1 CACR = 29.667 ($\bar{x}_1$)
Condition 2 Speech therapy = 22.5 ($\bar{x}_2$)
Condition 3 Occupational therapy = 15.0 ($\bar{x}_3$)

2. Find the value of F for the first comparison you wish to make, i.e. CACR vs speech therapy, using the following formula:

$$F = \frac{(\bar{x}_1 - \bar{x}_2)^2}{\dfrac{MS_{error}}{n_1} + \dfrac{MS_{error}}{n_2}}$$

where

$\bar{x}_1$ = mean for Condition 1
$= 29.667$

$\bar{x}_2$ = mean for Condition 2
$= 22.5$

MS_{error} = the MS_{error} value from the ANOVA table
$= 21.389$

n_1 = the number of subjects in Condition 1
$= 6$

n_2 = the number of subjects in Condition 2
$= 6$

Substituting these values:

$$F = \frac{(29.667 - 22.5)^2}{\dfrac{21.389}{6} + \dfrac{21.389}{6}}$$

$$= \frac{(7.167)^2}{3.565 + 3.565}$$

$$= \frac{51.366}{7.13}$$

$$= 7.204$$

3. Repeat the calculations for the second comparison, i.e. CACR vs occupational therapy. Substitute the appropriate means and n values:

$$F = \frac{\left(\bar{x}_1 - \bar{x}_3\right)^2}{\dfrac{MS_{error}}{n_1} + \dfrac{MS_{error}}{n_3}}$$

$$= \frac{\left(29.667 - 15\right)^2}{\dfrac{21.389}{6} + \dfrac{21.389}{6}}$$

$$= 30.171$$

4. Repeat the calculations for the third comparison, i.e. speech therapy and occupational therapy.

Substitute the appropriate means and n values:

$$F = \frac{\left(\bar{x}_2 - \bar{x}_3\right)^2}{\dfrac{MS_{error}}{n_2} + \dfrac{MS_{error}}{n_3}}$$

$$= \frac{\left(22.5 - 15\right)^2}{\dfrac{21.389}{6} + \dfrac{21.389}{6}}$$

$$= 7.889$$

5. To calculate F_1, use the df_{bet} and the df_{error} values derived from the ANOVA table (i.e. 2 and 15 respectively). Turn to Table A2.6a: critical values of F at $p < 0.05$. Locate df_{bet} (2) across the top row and df_{error} (15) down the left-hand column. At their intersection point, you will see the figure 3.68 (F^0).

Find the F^1 from the formula:

$$F_1 = (C - 1)F^\circ$$

where
F^0 is the figure at the intersection point = 3.68
C is the number of conditions = 3

Therefore:

$$F^1 = (3 - 1)3.68$$

$$= 7.36$$

6. Compare each F value derived from the comparison of pairs of means with the F^1 value above. If the F value is equal to or larger than F^1, then the result is significant at $p < 0.05$ (because we used the $p < 0.05$ table to calculate F^1).

If we take our F values:

1. 7.204
2. 30.171
3. 7.889

we can see that only Comparison 1 is not significant (CACR vs speech therapy).

This means that the differences between CACR and occupational therapy, and speech therapy and occupational therapy are significant and that there is less than a 5% probability that the results are due to random error.

It is important to point out that to derive F^1 we used the $p < 0.05$ table. The reason for this relates to the extreme stringency of the Scheffé; if we were to derive F^1 from the smaller p value tables, we would rarely get significant results using this test.

However, should you ever obtain results from the Scheffé which look as though they might be significant at a lower p value, just recalculate F^1 using Tables A2.6a–d. Here, the F value of 30.171 (Comparison 2) above seems to be significant at a smaller probability level. If we recalculate F^1 using Table A2.6d ($p < 0.001$) we get

$$F^1 = (3 - 1)11.34$$

$$= 22.68$$

The F value of 30.171 is larger than this and so this comparison (CACR vs occupational therapy) is significant at $p < 0.001$.

Interpreting the results

We have obtained the following results:

1. The comparison between CACR and speech therapy was not significant. This means that any differences between these two groups could be explained by random error. Therefore there is no significant difference in neuropsychological improvement between these two treatment groups.

2. The comparison between the CACR group and the occupational therapy group is significant at $p < 0.001$. This means that there is less than a 0.1% chance that the differences between these groups are attributable to random error. Therefore, we can conclude that CACR is significantly more effective than occupational therapy in improving neuropsychological performance (mean scores 29.667 and 15.0 respectively).

3. The comparison between the speech therapy group and the occupational therapy group is significant at $p < 0.05$. Therefore, there is less than a 5% probability that random error could account for the differences between these groups. Speech therapy is significantly more effective than occupational therapy in improving the neuropsychological performance of traumatic brain injured patients.

These results might be expressed in the following way:

Having calculated a one-way ANOVA for unrelated designs on the data and obtained significant results ($F = 15.088$, $p < 0.001$), comparisons of means were performed using the Scheffé multiple range test. The results indicated that: (a) there was no significant difference between the CACR group and the speech therapy group ($F = 7.204$); (b) the comparison between the CACR group and the occupational therapy group was significant at $p < 0.001$ ($F = 30.171$) with the CACR group benefiting more from treatment; (c) the comparison between the speech therapy and occupational therapy groups was significant at $p < 0.05$ ($F = 7.889$) with the speech therapy group benefiting more from treatment.

Activity 16.3 (Answers on p. 369)

Carry out a Scheffé on the following results:

H_1 There is a difference in the 'A'-level standards of students accepted at a school of chiropractic over the last decade.

Method   Randomly select 10 students who were accepted for training in 1992, 10 who were accepted in 1997 and 10 who were accepted in 2002. For each student, count up their total 'A'-level points (Grade A = 5 marks, Grade E = 1). Perform a one-way ANOVA for unrelated subject designs on the data. You obtain the following figures:

$F = 6.01$; $p < 0.01$
$df_{bet} = 2$
$df_{error} = 27$
$MS_{error} = 2.11$
$\bar{x}_1$ (1992 'A'-level results) $= 6.3$
$\bar{x}_2$ (1997 'A'-level results) $= 7.75$
$\bar{x}_3$ (2002 'A'-level results) $= 10.15$

FURTHER READING

Cohen L, Halliday M 1996 Practical statistics for students. Paul Chapman Publishing, London

Coolican H 2004 Research methods and statistics in psychology, 4th edition. Hodder and Stoughton, London

Ferguson GA, Takane Y 1989 Statistical analysis in psychology and Education. 6th Edition. McGraw Hill, New York

Field A, Hole G 2004 How to design and report experiments. Sage, London

Greene J, D'Oliveira M 2005 Learning to use statistical tests in psychology, 3rd edition. Open University Press, Buckingham

Polgar S, Thomas S 2007 Introduction to research in the health sciences. Churchill Livingstone, Edinburgh

Robson C 1994 Experiment, design and statistics in psychology, 3rd edition. Penguin, Harmondsworth

Chapter 17

Non-parametric and parametric tests for correlational designs

INTRODUCTION

All the tests described in this chapter are for use with correlational designs rather than experimental designs. Let's recap on the characteristics of correlational designs.

First, while the experimental design is concerned with finding differences between sets of scores, the correlational design looks for the degree of association between them. Furthermore, with a correlational design neither of the two variables in the hypothesis is manipulated. Therefore, there is no independent variable (IV) or dependent variable (DV). As a result, a correlational design cannot ascertain which variable is having an effect on the other and thus, no cause and effect can be determined. All that can be concluded is whether or not there is any association in the scores for the two variables. Although this failure to ascribe cause and effect in correlational designs means that the researcher ends up with less precise information than would be obtained from experimental designs, it should also be pointed out that correlational designs are more acceptable if any ethical considerations are involved, because the researcher is not manipulating anything. Therefore, correlational designs are frequently used as a first stage in medical and paramedical research.

The way in which this association between sets of scores is assessed involves using the appropriate statistical test, which calculates a correlation coefficient between the sets of scores.

This will result in a figure somewhere between −1 and +1. The closer the figure is to −1, the stronger the negative correlation between the scores. This means that large scores on one variable are associated with small scores on the other. The closer the figure is to +1, the stronger the positive correlation between the scores. In other words, high scores on one variable are associated with high scores on the other (and by definition, low scores on one variable are associated with low scores on the other). The closer the correlation coefficient is to 0, the weaker the relationship is between the scores. It should be noted that if large samples are used for correlational studies, then statistically significant results can be obtained for correlations that are actually very small (ie close to 0). Therefore, while a correlation of, say, 0.31 may be statistically significant, it may have little clinical relevance. Therefore, I would recommend that you take into account the actual correlation coefficient when interpreting your results, using the following guidelines suggested by Cohen (1988):

Correlation coefficients of +0.10 to +0.29 and −0.10 to −0.29 are considered to be small

Correlation coefficients of +0.30 to +0.49 and −0.30 to −0.49 are considered to be medium

Correlation coefficients of +0.50 to +1.0 and −0.50 to −1.0 are considered to be large

To carry out a correlational design, you might decide to look at the number of hospital admissions for hypothermia over a 3 month period, to see whether there is a correlation between temperature and the number of patients admitted. Or alternatively, you might select one group of subjects who represent a whole range of scores on one of the variables in the hypothesis and then assess them on the other variable of interest to see if there is a correlation between these two data sets. The implication of this is that in order to cover a range of numbers, the data must be ordinal or interval/ratio. It is possible to carry out a correlational study with non-dimensional nominal data, and this will be covered in Chapter 24 (Cohen's Kappa).

For instance, if we take the example that the greater the number of cigarettes smoked, the greater the incidence of bronchitis, we could select a group of subjects who vary in terms of the number of cigarettes they smoked, i.e. repre-

Table 17.1

Subject	No. of cigarettes
1	0
2	15
3	10
4	20
5	30
6	0
7	5
8	25
9	40
10	20

Table 17.2

Subject	Cigarettes	Bronchitis
1	0	0
2	15	2
3	10	2
4	20	4
5	30	5
6	0	0
7	5	1
8	25	4
9	40	6
10	20	4

sented a whole range of scores on the smoking variables as in Table 17.1.

We would then collect information on their incidence of bronchitis over the last few years. We would expect that the subject who smoked fewest cigarettes would have the lowest incidence of bronchitis, while the one who smoked most would have the highest incidence, with the other subjects ranging in between accordingly (see Table 17.2).

By computing the appropriate statistical test, we could find out whether there is a correlation between the scores shown in Table 17.2. Such a design differs from an experimental design in that, although the experimental design would also predict a relationship between smoking and lung disease, it would have to manipulate the smoking variable in order to assess its effects on bronchitis. This would be done by selecting two groups of subjects, smokers and non-smokers, measuring the incidence of bronchitis for each and comparing the results to see if there are differences between the groups.

Obviously, whether you use an experimental or a correlational design depends on what you are predicting and the sort of research area you are involved in. If you're still unsure about the differences in assumptions and approach between experimental and correlational designs, re-read Chapter 6. When you have done this, plan out a correlational and an experimental design for the hypothesis in Activity 17.1.

Activity 17.1 (Answers on pp. 369–370)

H_1 There is a relationship between age of patient and vital capacity.

STATISTICAL TESTS FOR CORRELATIONAL DESIGNS

The tests that are covered in this chapter are appropriate for two sorts of correlational design:

1. Those that compare two sets of scores to see if there is a correlation between them. In addition, a further test will be provided in this section, which allows you to predict scores on one variable, if you know the scores on the other.
2. Those that compare three or more sets of scores to see if there is a correlation between them.

Therefore, the tests shown in Table 17.3 are included in this chapter. These are both non-parametric and parametric. Each will be outlined separately. (The test for nominal data—Cohen's Kappa—will be covered in Chapter 24.)

STATISTICAL TESTS THAT COMPARE TWO SETS OF SCORES

Within this section, we shall look at two statistical tests, each of which can be used to assess the correlation between two sets of scores. In other words, you would typically take a group of subjects who represented a whole range of scores on one variable, and you would compare these with just one set of scores on the other variable, to see if they were associated in some way. Like the statistical tests for experimental designs, you can use either a non-parametric test to analyse your results, or, as long as you can fulfil the necessary conditions (see pp. 124–125), a parametric test. The most important of these conditions is the sort of data you have. In order to use a parametric test, you must have interval/ratio data.

The tests are:

1. *Non-parametric*: Spearman rank order correlation coefficient if the data are at least ordinal or interval/ratio.
2. *Parametric*: Pearson product moment correlation coefficient if the data are interval/ratio.

NON-PARAMETRIC TEST: CORRELATIONAL DESIGNS THAT COMPARE TWO SETS OF SCORES

SPEARMAN RANK ORDER CORRELATION COEFFICIENT TEST

Example

Let's suppose you were interested in the hypothesis:

Table 17.3

Design	Non-parametric test	Parametric test
One group of subjects; two sets of scores compared for the degree of association between them	Spearman rank order correlation coefficient	Pearson product moment correlation coefficient
	If you wish to predict scores on one variable from your knowledge of scores on the other, use a linear regression equation	If you wish to predict scores on one variable from your knowledge of scores on the other, use a linear regression equation
One group of subjects; three or more sets of scores compared for the degree of association between them	Kendall's coefficient of concordance	

H$_1$ There is a correlation between the length of rest in support splints and the degree of pain experienced by rheumatoid arthritis patients, such that the longer the time in splints, the lower the degree of pain (i.e. a negative correlation). (This is a one-tailed hypothesis as it is predicting the type of correlation anticipated, i.e. negative.)

You would select a number of patients who had been in support splints for varying periods and assess the intensity of the pain experienced (say on a 7-point scale: 7 = intense, 1 = none). You anticipate that, if your hypothesis is correct, the patients who had been in splints the longest would have least pain, while the patients who had been in splints the shortest time would have the most pain.

Your results might look like Table 17.4.

Because one set of scores (the pain measure) is only ordinal, we cannot fulfil the conditions necessary for a parametric test and so the Spearman must be used. It should be remembered that it does not matter at all that one variable is of an interval/ratio type (number of days in splints) and that the other is of an ordinal type, since all this correlational test does is to tell you whether the highest scores on one variable are associated with the highest or lowest scores on the other, irrespective of the nature of the scores. Therefore, as long as your data are not nominal, you can compare anything using the Spearman: weight with height, percentage range of movement with pain, etc.

When calculating the Spearman you will find a correlation coefficient called 'r_s' or 'rho', which you then look up in the probability tables associated with the Spearman test to see whether this value represents a significant correlation between the two variables.

Calculating the Spearman test

To calculate the Spearman test, take the following steps:

1. Rank order the scores on Variable A, giving the rank of 1 to the smallest score, the rank of 2 to the next smallest and so on. Enter these ranks in the column 'Rank A'. Repeat the procedure for the scores in Variable B and enter the ranks in the column 'Rank B'.

If some scores are the same, follow the procedure for tied ranks (see pp. 176–177). In other words add up the ranks these scores would have had if they had been different and divide this total by the number of scores that are the same. For example, in Variable B, the lowest score is 1, but subjects 3, 6 and 7 all had this score. Thus, had these scores been different they would have had the ranks 1, 2 and 3. Therefore, add these ranks up, and divide by 3 (because there are three scores of 1), i.e.

$$\frac{1+2+3}{3} = 2$$

Table 17.4

	Results from the experiment		Calculations from the statistical test			
	Variable A*	Variable B			d	d^2
Subject	No. of days in splints	Pain felt on a 7–point scale	Rank A	Rank B	$(A - B)$	$(A - B)^2$
1	4	5	2	7.5	−5.5	30.25
2	10	3	5	4.5	+0.5	0.25
3	15	1	8	2	+6	36
4	7	3	3	4.5	−1.5	2.25
5	2	6	1	9	−8	64
6	21	1	9	2	+7	49
7	14	1	7	2	+5	25
8	12	4	6	6	0	0
9	8	5	4	7.5	−3.5	12.25
						$\Sigma d^2 = 219$

*It does not matter which is Variable A and which is B.

Assign the average rank of 2 to each score of 1.

2. For each subject take the Rank B score from the Rank A score to give d.

Enter these differences in the column entitled 'd (A – B)', i.e.

Subject 1, Rank A – Rank B = 2 – 7.5 = –5.5

3. Square each d to give d^2, and enter this in the appropriate column, entitled 'd^2', i.e.

$$-5.5^2 = 30.25$$

4. Add up all the d^2 figures to give Σd^2 (Σ means 'sum or total of').

$$\Sigma d^2 = 219$$

5. Find r_s from the following formula:

$$r_s = 1 - \frac{6\sum d^2}{N(N^2-1)}$$

where

Σd^2 = the total of all the d^2 values

= 219

N = the number of subjects or pairs of scores

= 9

If we substitute these values then

$$r_s = 1 - \frac{6 \times 219}{9(81-1)}$$

$$= 1 - \frac{1314}{720}$$

$$= 1 - 1.825$$

$$= -0.825$$

(Do not forget to put in the + or – sign in front of the r_s figure, since this indicates a positive or negative correlation, respectively.)

Looking up the value of r_s

Turn to Table A2.10 (p. 355). Down the left-hand column you will find values of N, while across the top you will see levels of significance for a one-tailed test and for a two-tailed test. First, find your value of N down the left-hand column. To the right you will see four numbers, called critical values of r_s:

0.600 0.683 0.783 0.833

Each of these values is associated with the level of significance indicated at the top of the column, e.g. 0.600 is associated with 0.05 for a one-tailed test and 0.10 for a two-tailed test.

If your r_s value is *equal to* or *larger than* one of these four critical values, then your results are associated with the probability level indicated at the top of the appropriate column.

Our r_s value of –0.825 (ignore the minus sign for the time being) is larger than 0.783, but smaller than 0.833. This means that for our one-tailed hypothesis, the probability associated with our r_s value of 0.825 must be less than 0.01 (or 1%) but greater than 0.005 (or 0.5%). Convention dictates that we say that our p value is less than 0.01 (rather than saying it is greater than 0.005). In other words the probability of our results being due to random error is even less than 0.01 or 1%. This is expressed as:

$$p < 0.01 \,(\text{or} < 1\%)(< \text{means 'less than'})$$

Had our r_s value been equal to the critical value of 0.783 the associated probability level would be exactly 0.01. This would be expressed as:

$$p = 0.01 \,(\text{or } 1\%).$$

Interpreting the results

Our r_s value of –0.825 is associated with a probability level of less than 1%. This means that the chance of random error accounting for our results is less than 1 in 100. Now, given that the usual cut-off point for claiming results as significant is 5% or less, we can say that the results obtained in this experiment are significant. Furthermore, using the guidelines outlined on p. 236, this correlation coefficient of –0.825 would be considered to be large.

As we had a one-tailed hypothesis we must check that the results are in the predicted direction before claiming that our hypothesis has been supported. We have an r_s value of *minus* 0.825. This means that the two variables are negatively correlated; in other words, the longer the time in support splints, the less the pain. This is exactly what was predicted and so we can safely reject the null hypothesis and accept the experimental hypothesis. This can be expressed in the following way:

Using a Spearman test on the data ($r_s = -0.825$, $N = 9$) the results were found to be significant ($p < 0.01$ for a one-tailed test). This means that there is a large negative correlation between the variables, such that the longer the time spent in support splints, the less the degree of pain experienced. The null hypothesis can therefore be rejected.

Activity 17.2 (Answers on p. 370)

1 To practise looking up r_s values, look up the following and state whether or not they are significant and at what level.

   (i) $r = 0.784$ $N = 10$ one-tailed p
   (ii) $r = 0.812$ $N = 6$ two-tailed p
   (iii) $r = 0.601$ $N = 16$ two-tailed p
   (iv) $r = 0.506$ $N = 12$ two-tailed p
   (v) $r = 0.631$ $N = 18$ one-tailed p

2 Calculate a Spearman on the following data:

   H_1 There is a relationship between the length of lunch-break taken (in minutes) by newly qualified clinical therapists and their degree of clinical competence (on a 7-point scale, 7 = excellent, 1 = very poor).

Method: You select a group of 10 newly qualified clinical therapists who take varying lunch-break times and assess their clinical competence. The data are as shown in Table 17.5.

Table 17.5

Subject	Condition A Lunch–break time	Condition B Clinical competence
1	45	4
2	65	3
3	50	5
4	30	5
5	75	2
6	40	6
7	55	5
8	80	2
9	35	6
10	70	3

State your r_s and p values in a format similar to the one outlined earlier.

PARAMETRIC TEST: CORRELATIONAL DESIGNS THAT COMPARE TWO SETS OF SCORES

PEARSON PRODUCT MOMENT CORRELATION COEFFICIENT

As was noted earlier, the Pearson is the parametric equivalent of the Spearman test, in that it is used for correlational designs that compare two sets of data for their degree of association. It may be used when the prerequisite conditions for a parametric test can be fulfilled, in particular interval/ratio data (see pp. 124–125).

As long as the data are of an interval/ratio level, it does not matter if one variable is measured in yards, feet, etc. and the other in kilos, percentages, minutes. The Pearson formula can accommodate different sorts of measurement as long as they are of an interval/ratio level.

Example

Let's suppose you were interested in finding out whether there is a correlation between body weight and range of movement in the hip among osteoarthritis patients. Your hypothesis is:

H_1 There is a negative correlation between body weight and range of movement of the hip in osteoarthritis patients (i.e. high body weights are associated with low ranges of movement).

This is a one-tailed hypothesis as it is predicting the type of correlation expected, i.e. negative.

In order to test your hypothesis, you select 10 40–50-year-old female osteoarthritis patients who represent a range of body weights, and each of whom has suffered from the condition for between 36 and 42 months. You measure the percentage range of movement in their hip joints, and take the average of these scores. The results are as shown in Table 17.6.

Calculating the Pearson test

The Pearson formula involves some rather large numbers, as you will see. These may look very off-putting initially, but you should be all right as long as you have a calculator.

Table 17.6

| | Results from the experiment | | Calculations | | |
Subject	Variable A Weight (lbs)	Variable B Range of movement	$A \times B$	A^2	B^2
1	140	40	5600	19600	1600
2	128	45	5760	16384	2025
3	170	25	4250	28900	625
4	132	40	5280	17424	1600
5	154	30	4620	23716	900
6	135	35	4725	18225	1225
7	143	45	6435	20449	2025
8	149	50	7450	22201	2500
9	158	30	4740	24964	900
10	162	25	4050	26244	625
Σ	$\Sigma A = 1471$	$\Sigma B = 365$	$\Sigma(A \times B) = 52\,910$	$\Sigma A^2 = 218\,107$	$\Sigma B^2 = 14\,025$

1. Add up all the scores on Variable A to give ΣA, i.e.

$$\Sigma A = 1471$$

2. Add up all the scores on Variable B to give ΣB, i.e.

$$\Sigma B = 365$$

3. Multiply each subject's Variable A score by their Variable B score, e.g.

$$\text{Subject } 1 = 140 \times 40$$
$$= 5600$$

$$\text{Subject } 2 = 128 \times 45$$
$$= 5760$$

Enter each result in Column '$A \times B$'
4. Add up all the scores in Column $A \times B$ to give $\Sigma(A \times B)$, i.e.

$$\Sigma(A \times B) = 52\,910$$

5. Square each subject's Variable A score and enter the result in column 'A^2', e.g.

$$\text{for Subject } 1, A^2 = 140^2$$
$$= 19\,600$$

6. Square each subject's Variable B score and enter the result in Column 'B^2', e.g.

$$\text{for Subject } 1, B^2 = 40^2$$
$$= 1600$$

7. Add up all the scores in Column A^2 to give ΣA^2, i.e.

$$\Sigma A^2 = 218\,107$$

8. Add up all the scores in Column B^2 to give ΣB^2, i.e.

$$\Sigma B^2 = 14\,025$$

9. Find the value of r from the following formula:

$$r = \frac{N\sum(A \times B) - \left(\sum A \times \sum B\right)}{\sqrt{\left[N\sum A^2 - \left(\sum A\right)^2\right]\left[N\sum B^2 - \left(\sum B\right)^2\right]}}$$

where

$$N = \text{number of subjects}$$
$$= 10$$

$\sum(A \times B) = $ the total of the scores in the $A \times B$ column
$$= 52\,910$$

$\sum A = $ the total of the scores in the Variable A column
$$= 1471$$

$\sum B = $ the total of the scores in the Variable B column
$$= 365$$

ΣA^2 = the total of the scores in the A^2 column

$= 218\,107$

ΣB^2 = the total of the scores in the B^2 column

$= 14\,025$

$(\Sigma A)^2$ = the total of the scores in the Variable A column, squared

$= 1471^2$

$= 2\,163\,841$

$(\Sigma B)^2$ = the total of the scores in the Variable B column, squared

$= 365^2$

$= 133\,225$

Therefore, if we substitute these values in the formula:

$$r = \frac{(10 \times 52910) - (1471 \times 365)}{\sqrt{[(10 \times 218107 - 2163841)][(10 \times 14025) - 133225]}}$$

$$= \frac{529100 - 536915}{\sqrt{[2181070 - 2163841][140250 - 133225]}}$$

$$= \frac{-7815}{\sqrt{11001.533}}$$

$$= -0.710$$

Looking up the value of r

To find out whether r is significant, you also need a df value, which here is the number of subjects minus 2, i.e.

$$df = N - 2$$

$$= 10 - 2$$

$$= 8$$

Turn to Table A2.11 (p. 356). Down the left-hand column you will see a number of df values. Find our df = 8. You will see five numbers, called critical values of r to the right of df = 8.

0.5494 0.6319 0.7155 0.7646 0.8721

Each of these is associated with the level of significance indicated at the top of its column, e.g. 0.5494 is associated with a level of significance, for a one-tailed test of 0.05 and for a two-tailed test of 0.10.

To be significant at one of these levels, our r value has to be *equal to* or *larger than* the corresponding critical value. Ignoring the minus sign in front of our r value for the time being, we can see that our r of 0.71 is larger than 0.6319 but smaller than 0.7155. Since we have a one-tailed test, our r value has an associated probability which is less than 0.025 (or 2.5%) but greater than 0.01 (1%). According to convention we must say that our r has a p value of less than 0.025, (rather than saying it is greater than 0.01).

This is expressed as:

$$p < 0.025$$

This means that there is less than a 2.5% chance that our results are due to random error. Had our r value been the same as the critical value of 0.6319 the associated probability value would have been exactly 0.025. This is expressed as:

$$p = 0.025$$

Interpreting the results

Our r value has an associated probability value of <0.025, which means that the chance of random error being responsible for the results is less than 2.5 in 100. In addition, if we look at the guidelines for interpreting the size of correlation coefficients (p. 236), our r value would be considered to be large.

Because the standard cut-off point for claiming results to be significant is 5% we can conclude that the results here are significant. But before we can definitely state that they support the experimental hypothesis, we must check that the direction of the results was the one predicted. In other words, did we obtain the negative correlation between the two variables that we anticipated? Our r value was minus 0.71, which means that the results do, in fact, confirm the hypothesis and that there is a large negative correlation between body weight and range of movement in the hip joint of osteoarthritis patients. We can therefore reject the null hypothesis and accept the experimental hypothesis. This can be expressed in the following way:

Using a Pearson product moment correlation test on the data ($r = -0.71$, df = 8), the results were significant ($p < 0.025$ for a one-tailed test). This means that there is a large negative correlation in osteoarthritis patients, between weight and range of movement (the higher the weight, the lower the range of movement). The null hypothesis can therefore be rejected.

Activity 17.3 (Answers on p. 370)

1 To practise looking up *r* values, look up the following and state whether or not they are significant and at what level.
   (i) $r = 0.632$ $df = 6$ one–tailed p
   (ii) $r = 0.567$ $df = 10$ two–tailed p
   (iii) $r = 0.779$ $df = 8$ one–tailed p
   (iv) $r = 0.612$ $df = 12$ two–tailed p
   (v) $r = 0.784$ $df = 13$ two–tailed p
2 Calculate a Pearson on the following data:

H$_1$ There is a positive correlation between students' marks on their first-year examination and their averaged continuous assessment mark throughout the year.

Method: Randomly select eight first-year students to represent a range of examination marks. Average their continuous assessment marks for the year's assignments.
The results are as shown in Table 17.7.

Table 17.7

Subject	Variable A Examination	Variable B Continuous assessment
1	70	66
2	60	64
3	49	54
4	54	50
5	66	70
6	72	68
7	40	49
8	62	65

State your *r* and *p* values in the suggested format.

NON–PARAMETRIC TEST THAT COMPARES THREE OR MORE SETS OF SCORES

Both the Spearman and the Pearson tests are used for correlational designs that look for the degree of association between only two sets of scores, for instance, comparing the theory and

practice exam marks for a group of students to see if they correlate.

However, there will be many occasions when you may want to see if three or more sets of scores are associated in some way.

For example, you may be involved in chairing an interview panel of four people which is concerned with appointing a new senior clinical therapist in the department. There are six candidates for the post. You decide to ask each member of the panel to rank order these candidates in terms of their suitability for the job. Obviously, if there were consensus in terms of choice the decision would be easy, but you know that is unlikely to be the case. So, you will have to analyse the rankings in order to see whether there is *overall* agreement. In other words, you have *one* group of six candidates, each of whom is ranked by four people. You need to assess the four sets of rankings given to each candidate to see how far the opinions of the panel agree.

Therefore, in this case, rather than having two sets of scores to analyse for correlations, you have four sets. Such a design requires a test called the **Kendall coefficient of concordance**.

KENDALL COEFFICIENT OF CONCORDANCE 1

This is a non-parametric test which can only be used when the data are ordinal, i.e. when you have three or more sets of rank orderings. This does not, of course, mean that you cannot use this test when you have interval/ratio data; all you would do here is to rank order your data and use the rank orderings in the test.

A further point to remember is that this particular formula of the Kendall coefficient of concordance can only be used if the number of people or objects being ranked is seven or less. So, for instance, you might ask four clinical therapists to rank order six patients in terms of how compliant they are. Thus there are four judges (or sets of rankings) and six objects or people being ranked. If you want to design an experiment where more than seven objects or people are being ranked, you will need the formula given in the next section, entitled 'Kendall coefficient of concordance 2'.

One other point to note about this test: both the Spearman and Pearson tests produce a correlation coefficient which may be somewhere between −1 (negative correlation) through 0 (no correlation) to +1 (positive correlation), whereas the Kendall coefficient of concordance only gives us a value from 0 to 1, i.e. an indication of whether there is no correlation at all between the sets of scores (0) or a positive correlation (+1). It does not give a negative correlation. If we think about this a bit more, the reason for this becomes clear. Where three or more sets of rankings are being compared, they cannot all disagree completely. So in the previous example, Interviewer A may produce a set of rankings which are absolutely the reverse of Interviewer B's. If we only had two interviewers, we could analyse this with a Spearman and we would end up with a negative correlation between the scores. But here, if Interviewers A and B disagree so completely from each other, what about Interviewers C and D? If C also disagrees with A, it means by definition they must agree with B and hence there is some measure of agreement among the rankings. If D disagrees with C, it means these rankings must agree with those of A, because C disagrees with A. Therefore, all we may conclude from the Kendall coefficient of concordance is whether there is a positive correlation between the scores or whether there is no relationship. Because the Kendall coefficient of concordance only tells us whether or not there is a positive correlation between our results our hypothesis must be one-tailed.

When calculating the Kendall coefficient of concordance, a value called 's' is found. This is then looked up in the probability table associated with the Kendall coefficient of concordance, to see whether the value of s represents a significant agreement among the rankings. Remember that because the Kendall only deals with positive correlations, any hypothesis associated with it must be one-tailed.

Example

Let's imagine that the practice placement assessments of your student clinical therapists appear to be inconsistent, with some students achieving very high marks in some clinical areas but very poor grades in others. Having spoken to the clinical assessors involved in student supervision you realise that the students' performance seems to

be less a function of the clinical area in which they have their placement, but more to do with wide differences of opinion among the clinical assessors as to which clinical skills are deemed most important. In other words, the variation in marks is the result of the assessor rather than the student. Clearly, if the clinical assessors have different views regarding the most salient competencies, then it is hardly surprising that the marks awarded differ so widely from one placement to the next. So, you decide to ask the three senior clinical therapists who have most supervisory responsibility for student therapists to rank order six core competencies in order of importance. If some agreement emerges, this can be used in a future training programme for clinical educators, as one means by which performance criteria can be standardised. Therefore, you have three judges and six core competencies being ranked. Your hypothesis therefore, is

H_1 There is significant agreement between the three clinical therapists' judgements of the most important core competencies for student clinical therapists.

You ask the clinical therapists to rank all six competencies, giving a rank of 1 to the most important. The results you obtain are shown in Table 17.8. (When calculating the Kendall coefficient of concordance, always set the results out such that the rank orderings from each judge go across the page.)

Table 17.8

	Competency					
	1	2	3	4	5	6
Clinical therapist						
1	6	4	2	1	3	5
2	6	2	3	4	1	5
3	6	5	3	1	2	4
Total of ranks for each student	18	11	8	6	6	14

Calculating the Kendall coefficient of concordance

1. For each competency add up the total of the ranks assigned, i.e.

$$1 = 18$$
$$2 = 11$$

$3 = 8$
$4 = 6$
$5 = 6$
$6 = 14$

Obviously, if all three clinical therapists had been in perfect agreement, the most important core competency would have been assigned three ranks of 1 (total 3), the next most important core competency, three ranks of 2 (total 6), etc. right up to the least important core competency which would have had three ranks of 6 (18). On the other hand, had there been no agreement whatever, every competency would have ended up with an identical rank total, because the ranks would have been randomly assigned by the sample. In other words, they would not reflect any common understanding of the importance of the competencies.

What the formula aims to do is to assess how far the actual rankings accord with the rankings for no agreement whatever between the judges.

2. Add up all the rank totals to give ΣR, i.e.

$$\Sigma R = 18 + 11 + 8 + 6 + 6 + 14$$

$$= 63$$

3. Divide ΣR by the number of competencies being ranked to obtain the average of the rank totals, $\bar{x}_R$, i.e.

$$\bar{x}_R = 63 \div 6$$

$$= 10.5$$

4. Take each rank total away from the average rank total and square the result, i.e.

1. $(10.5 - 18)^2 = 56.25$
2. $(10.5 - 11)^2 = 0.25$
3. $(10.5 - 8)^2 = 6.25$
4. $(10.5 - 6)^2 = 20.25$
5. $(10.5 - 6)^2 = 20.25$
6. $(10.5 - 14)^2 = 12.25$

5. Add up all these squared differences to give s, i.e. 115.5.

6. Find W from the formula:

$$W = \frac{s}{\frac{1}{12}n^2(N^3 - N)}$$

where

s = the total of all the squared differences between each individual rank total and the average rank total

$= 115.5$

n = the number of judges or sets of rankings

$= 3$

N = the number of people or objects being ranked

$= 6$

Substituting these values:

$$W = \frac{115.5}{\frac{1}{12}3^2(6^3 - 6)}$$

$$= \frac{115.5}{\frac{1}{12}9 \times 210}$$

$$= \frac{115.5}{157.5}$$

$$= 0.733$$

Looking up the value of s for significance

To find out whether these results are significant you need the s value (the total of squared differences between each individual rank total and the average rank total), the n value (the number of judges or sets of rankings) and N (the number of objects or people ranked):

$$s = 115.5$$
$$n = 3$$
$$N = 6$$

Turn to Table A2.12 (p. 357). This gives critical values of s associated with particular values of p. You will see that two tables are presented, one for p values of 0.05 and one for p values of 0.01. (Note again that because this test only tells you whether or not there is a positive correlation between the scores, these values are associated with one-tailed hypotheses only.)

Down the left-hand column you will see values of n, while across the top there are values of N. Taking the $p = 0.05$ table first, locate your n and N values and identify the number at the intersection point, i.e. 103.9. To be significant at the 0.05

level, our s value must be *equal to* or *larger than* 103.9. Our s value is larger (115.5) which means that our results are associated with a probability value of 0.05.

But are they significant at the 0.01 level? Repeat the process. You will find the figure at the intersection point is 122.8. Our s value is smaller than this, so the results are not significant at the 0.01 level. So, we must go back to the first table.

Now, because our s value is larger than the value at the intersection point, it means that the associated probability comes between the 0.05 probability of the first table and the 0.01 probability of the second. In other words, for our s of 115.5, the associated probability is less than 5% (or 0.05) but greater than 1% (or 0.01). To comply with convention we have to say that our probability is less than 0.05 or 5%. This is expressed as:

$$p < 0.05$$

This means that the probability of random error being responsible for the results is less than 5%. Had our s value been exactly the same as the number at the intersection point, our results would have been associated with a probability value which equalled 0.05. This is stated as:

$$p = 0.05$$

Interpreting the results

Our results have an associated probability value of <0.05, which means that there is less than a 5% chance that random error could account for the outcome of the experiment. If we use the usual cut-off point of 5% to claim significance, we can state that the results here are, in fact, significant, and that we can reject the null hypothesis and accept the experimental hypothesis. This can be stated thus:

Using a Kendall's coefficient of concordance on the data ($s = 115.5$, $W = 0.733$, $n = 3$, $N = 6$) the results were found to be significant ($p < 0.05$ for a one-tailed test). This means that there is significant agreement among the senior clinical therapists as to which core competencies are most important in student therapist training. The null hypothesis can therefore be rejected.

Should you ever have a situation where there are a number of tied ranks, i.e. where, for instance, a judge has ranked three objects or people equally, this will have the effect of reducing the signifi-

cance of your results. Try, then, to ensure that your data do not contain too many tied ranks.

One final point. Many students ask why W is calculated, since it is not used to look up the significance of the results. The answer is that W is the correlation coefficient, and the researcher often finds it useful to know this value in order to assess, in absolute terms, the extent of the correlation between results. In other words, the correlation coefficient is often as meaningful as the actual probability to the experimenter (see section on clinical vs statistical significance of research findings).

Activity 17.4 (Answers on page 370)

1 To practise looking up s values, look up the following s values and state whether or not they are significant and at what level.

(i) $s = 96.1$ $n = 4$ $N = 5$ p
(ii) $s = 117.5$ $n = 5$ $N = 6$ p
(iii) $s = 124.5$ $n = 3$ $N = 6$ p
(iv) $s = 103.7$ $n = 6$ $N = 4$ p
(v) $s = 619.2$ $n = 10$ $N = 7$ p

2 Calculate a Kendall coefficient of concordance on the following data. You are concerned about the variability in measurements of lumbar mobility using the double inclinometer method. You decide to put this to the test.

H_1 There is a significant agreement between chiropractors' measurements of lumbar movement using the double inclinometer method.

Method: Five chiropractors each measure the degrees of lumbar movement of four patients using the double inclinometer method. The range of movement recorded is noted.

The results are as shown in Table 17.9.

Table 17.9

	Patient			
	1	2	3	4
Chiropractor				
1	45	30	50	65
2	45	40	55	70
3	25	30	65	55
4	50	55	30	60
5	60	50	65	80

(Remember the data must be rank ordered!) State your s, W and p values in the format outlined earlier.

KENDALL COEFFICIENT OF CONCORDANCE 2

Sometimes more than seven objects, skills people or whatever have to be ranked, and in these cases, you will need an extension of the previous Kendall formula, which uses the χ^2 probability tables.

Let's imagine that instead of ranking six core competencies, the three senior clinical therapists were instead asked to rank 10 of them. To find out whether there is any agreement between the rankings of these ten core competencies, we proceed as follows:

1. Calculate steps 1–6 as in the earlier Kendall in order to obtain a value of W. Rather than repeating all these computations, let's just suppose that we obtained a W value for this of 0.677.

2. We now need to use this W value in a further formula, which is used in situations where more than seven objects are being ranked. This formula is:

$$\chi^2 = n(N-1)W$$

where

n = the number of judges or sets of rankings
N = the number of people or objects being ranked
W = the correlation coefficient obtained from calculating steps 1–6 above.

3. If we substitute our data, we get:

$$\chi^2 = 3(10-1)0.677$$
$$= 27 \times 0.677$$
$$= 18.279$$

We now need to look this up in the probability tables associated with the χ^2, and to do this we need the df value, which is obtained from the formula:

$$df = N-1$$
$$= 10-1$$
$$= 9$$

Looking this up in Table A2.1, we find that for a df of 9 and a χ^2 value of 18.279, the results are significant at $p < 0.025$ for a one-tailed hypothesis. This means that there is a significant level of agreement between the three senior clinical therapists about the relative importance of the 10 core competencies.

LINEAR REGRESSION: PREDICTING SCORES ON ONE VARIABLE FROM SCORES ON THE OTHER

We have already seen that correlational designs are used when we want to find out whether two variables are associated with each other; that is, whether high scores on one variable are related to high scores on the other, or alternatively, whether high scores on one variable are related to low scores on the other. This is a particularly valuable sort of approach in medical and paramedical research because ethical issues are rarely involved.

Correlational designs can tell us whether, for example, blood pressure and reaction to a particular drug are related, or whether traction weights and degree of improvement in back pain are associated, or which treatment is more effective for hallux valgus, although they cannot say which of the two variables causes an effect on the other; all they tell us is whether or not two variables co-vary together in a related way.

Now, there will be occasions when you might be quite happy to leave your research at this point, having found out whether or not the variables are correlated. For example, in the earlier illustration, you may be content with the knowledge that blood pressure and reaction to Drug A are positively correlated, i.e. that the higher the blood pressure, the more adverse the reaction to the drug. This reaction, let's say, induces drowsiness.

However, let's suppose that having completed this research, you are faced with a new patient with a blood pressure reading of, say, 170/90. Now, from the results of your correlational design, you will know that this person's reaction to Drug A is likely to be adverse, since they have high blood pressure. However, let's further suppose that this person drives a public transport vehicle. It is obviously essential to establish whether the degree of drowsiness induced is likely to be a danger to him or his passengers. In other words, it would be extremely useful to you to be able to predict this man's reaction more precisely from your knowledge of his blood pressure. In other words, what you want to be able to do is to predict with some degree of accuracy the scores on one variable from your knowledge of the scores on the other. What you need, therefore, is a formula whereby you can calculate the unknown score. This formula is known as a regression formula or equation and is of enormous use in medical research. For example, as long as you know that the two variables are correlated, it can tell you:

- the vital capacity of a man who smokes 55 cigarettes a day
- the heart rate of someone who regularly jogs 2 miles a day
- the theory exam performance of a student who achieved 32% in the practical exam.

So, providing you know that two variables are related, you can make predictions about one variable from your knowledge of scores on the other, using a regression formula. The linear regression technique can be used in conjunction with either the Pearson or the Spearman test, but the data should be of a type which assumes equal intervals. In other words it should be interval/ratio or a point scale which implies comparable distances between the points (see Chapter 4).

The convention when using regression formulae is to call the variable whose score you are trying to predict, 'Y', and the variable whose scores you already know, 'X'. Therefore, in the above example, we are trying to predict the patient's reaction to Drug A (Y) from our knowledge of his blood pressure (X).

Now, it is important to reiterate that you can only use a regression equation if the two variables you are interested in have been shown to be correlated. If you look back to pp. 80–86, you will see that there are two types of correlation: a positive correlation whereby high scores on one variable are associated with high scores on the other; and a negative correlation whereby high scores on one variable are associated with low scores on the other. If scattergrams are plotted for both of these, we find that a positive correlation is represented by an uphill slope, while a negative correlation is represented by a downhill one. Furthermore, it was pointed out that a perfect one-to-one correlation would produce an absolutely smooth, straight line. However, there are very few things in this world which produce a perfect correlation, but supposing we found that the amount of time a clinical therapist spent with a patient produced a one-to-one correlation with

the patient's reported satisfaction with the treatment (on a 9-point scale) such that the longer time spent, the greater the satisfaction. If we plotted the data from this we might end up with the scattergram shown in Figure 17.1. For the sake of the example, we shall treat this 9-point scale as though it were interval data and assume that the distances between each point are equal (see pp. 41–43).

We can draw a perfectly straight line through all the dots and it is this line which is used in your future predictions. For example, you would know from this scattergram that if you were to treat a patient for 17 minutes, the degree of reported satisfaction would be 3.6, because all you would have to do would be to locate the appropriate time along the bottom axis, and trace it vertically up to the sloping line and then move horizontally across to the satisfaction scores (see dotted line on Figure 17.1).

You could also predict that if you treated someone for 3 minutes, their satisfaction would be 0.6; again you simply take the 3-minute time along the bottom axis, trace this up to the slope and then move left from the slope to the satisfaction scores. In other words, from your existing knowledge that these two variables are related, should you ever treat someone for a period of time which has not been incorporated in your previous calculations, you can predict how satisfied they will be.

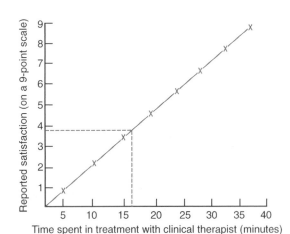

Figure 17.1   Scattergram showing relationship between patient satisfaction and time spent with clinical therapist, supposing the correlation were perfect.

Table 17.10

Patient	Reported satisfaction	Time spent in treatment (min)
1	7	29
2	4	10
3	6	18
4	8	17
5	2	8
6	3	5
7	5	15
8	6	16
9	5	16
10	1	5

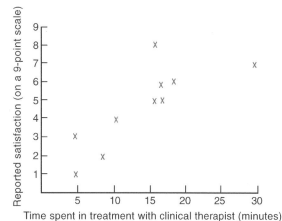

Figure 17.2   A more likely scattergram showing the relationship between patient satisfaction and time spent with clinical therapist.

You can see that this sloping line is obviously extremely important if you need to make this sort of prediction and therefore it has to be drawn in. However, while it is easy to draw it in when the correlation is perfect, because all the dots are lined up, it is not as easy when the correlation is imperfect and the dots are more randomly scattered.

However, as has already been pointed out very little in life conforms to a perfect correlation. It would be far more likely in the previous example that the data obtained were as shown in Table 17.10.

Statistical analysis using the Pearson test (see earlier section of this chapter) shows that the data are correlated ($r = 0.836$, $p < 0.005$).

If these data were plotted on a scattergram, we would find the pattern shown in Figure 17.2. There is still a general upward slope but it is far from smooth. In this case, if you had to draw a straight line through the dots, so that you could perform the same sort of prediction as before, where would you draw it? You obviously cannot connect all the dots as you would with the perfect correlation and still obtain a straight line so you need to make a decision about where to put the line so that it achieves the 'best fit'. The line of best fit is the straight sloping line which when drawn in, means that every dot is as close as possible to the line, and consequently produces fewest errors when predicting the value of variable Y from knowledge of variable X.

Now, if you look at the scattergram (Figure 17.2), you can see that it is almost impossible to

draw in the line of best fit by eye, and if you cannot draw in this line, then how can you make predictions? For instance, if you treated someone for 12 minutes, what would the level of satisfaction be? If you only have the scattergram and no line of best fit; you can't answer this question.

What you need, then, is a regression formula such that this line of best fit can be calculated and the prediction made. This equation is:

$$Y = bX + a$$

where

   Y is the variable to be predicted

   X is the known score

   a and b are constants which have to be calculated.

(Note that the regression we are dealing with is called linear regression, because it is concerned with simple linear relationships; see the scattergram.)

Calculating the linear regression equation

In order to calculate these constants, take the following steps:

1. Calculate the Spearman or Pearson test (whichever is appropriate) on your data to establish whether or not there is a significant correlation. If there isn't a significant correlation, don't proceed any further, since you cannot make any predictions from variables that don't correlate.

Table 17.11

Subject	Variable Y Satisfaction	Variable X Treatment time	X × Y	X²
1	7	29	203	841
2	4	10	40	100
3	6	18	108	324
4	8	17	136	289
5	2	8	16	64
6	3	5	15	25
7	5	15	75	225
8	6	16	96	256
9	5	16	80	256
10	1	5	5	25
Σ	$\Sigma Y = 47$	$\Sigma X = 139X$	$\Sigma(X \times Y) = 774$	$\Sigma X^2 = 2405$

2. Having established that the data are correlated, make a note of whether the correlation is positive or negative. If you wish, you can plot a scattergram of the data, but it isn't essential.

3. Set out your data in the format shown in Table 17.11, remembering that Y is the variable to be predicted and X is the variable from which the prediction will be made. Here, we will take the sample data already provided for the last scattergram. So, the $X \times$ column is ariable score X multiplied by variable score Y, i.e.

$$\text{for Subject } 1, 7 \times 29 = 203$$

The X^2 column is simply the squared variable X score. Therefore:

$$\text{for Subject } 1, 29 \times 29 = 841$$

4. Add each column up to give the totals (Σ)

$\Sigma Y = 47$
$\Sigma X = 139$
$\Sigma(X \times Y) = 774$
$\Sigma X^2 = 2405$

5. To calculate the constants a and b, first find b from the formula:

$$b = \frac{N\sum(X \times Y) - \left(\sum X\right)\left(\sum Y\right)}{N\sum X^2 - \left(\sum X\right)^2}$$

where

N = the total number of Ss
$= 10$

$\Sigma(X \times Y)$ = the total of the X × Y column
$= 774$

ΣX = the total of the Variable X column
$= 139$

ΣY = the total of the Variable Y column
$= 47$

ΣX^2 = the total of the X^2 column
$= 2405$

$\left(\Sigma X\right)^2$ = the total of the Variable X column squared
$= 139^2$
$= 19\,321$

If we substitute our values:

$$b = \frac{(10 \times 774) - (139 \times 47)}{(10 \times 2405) - 19321}$$

$$= \frac{7740 - 6533}{24050 - 19321}$$

$$= \frac{1207}{4729}$$

$$= 0.255$$

6. Find a from the formula:

$$a = \frac{\sum Y}{N} - b\frac{\sum X}{N}$$

where

N = the total number of Ss
$= 10$

ΣY = the total of the Variable Y column

$= 47$

ΣX = the total of the Variable X column

$= 139$

b = the result of the earlier calculation in step 5.

$= 0.255$.

Substituting the values:

$$a = \frac{47}{10} - 0.255 \times \frac{139}{10}$$
$$= 4.7 - (0.255 \times 13.9)$$
$$= 4.7 - 3.545$$
$$= 1.155$$

7. We can now substitute the values of a and b into the regression formula

$$Y = bX + a$$

to find any value of Y we require from the known value of X. Therefore:

$$Y = 0.255X + 1.155$$

Interpreting the results

Suppose, then, a patient was treated for 22 minutes (Variable X); we can predict his level of satisfaction (Variable Y) using the calculated values for the regression equation.

$$Y = (0.255 \times 22) + 1.155$$
$$= 5.61 + 1.155$$
$$= 6.765$$

Therefore, this patient's predicted level of satisfaction would be 6.765. So it is possible to calculate from any treatment time the associated degree of satisfaction.

Activity 17.5 (Answers on p. 370)

Imagine that the data in Table 17.12 were obtained from a correlational study which looked at the relationship between the amount of weight gained during pregnancy and length of labour.

Table 17.12

Subject	Weight gain (lbs)	Length of labour (hours)
1	17	8.3
2	35	16.2
3	28	12.8
4	21	9.9
5	20	10.0
6	30	15.8
7	24	14.0
8	32	17.5
9	20	11.6
10	26	12.2

The two variables correlate significantly ($p < 0.005$).

Three women come in for the last antenatal visit. Their weight gains are: (i) 23 lbs, (ii) 16 lbs, (iii) 29 lbs.

What is the estimated length of labour for each woman?

FURTHER READING

Cohen J 1988 Statistical power analysis for the behavioural sciences, 2nd edition. Lawrence Erlbaum Associates, Hillsdale, NJ

Cohen L, Halliday M 1996 Practical statistics for students. Paul Chapman Publishing, London

Coolican H 2004 Research methods and statistics in psychology, 4th edition. Hodder and Stoughton, London

Field A, Hole G 2004 How to design and report experiments. Sage, London

Greene J, D'Oliveira M 2005 Learning to use statistical tests in psychology, 3rd edition. Open University Press, Buckingham

Pett M 1997 Non-parametric statistics in health care research. Sage, London

Polgar S, Thomas S 2007 Introduction to research in the health sciences. Edinburgh, Churchill Livingstone

Robson C 1994 Experiment, design and statistics in psychology, 3rd edition. Penguin, Harmondsworth

Siegel S 1956 Non-parametric statistics for the behavioural sciences. McGraw-Hill Kogakusha, Tokyo

Chapter 18

Estimation

INTRODUCTION

Estimation is a particularly useful statistical technique for any clinical therapist who is involved in resource management or planning. It can be thought of as a sort of statistical 'best guessing' system which, like other methods of inferential statistics, allows us to make predictions about certain characteristics of a population based on our knowledge of a small sample of that population.

However, unlike the statistical tests which we have looked at so far in this book, estimation does not involve testing a hypothesis. Instead, we collect data on the characteristics we are interested in from a sample of people, equipment or whatever, and then, using a statistical formula, we can make predictions or estimates about how far the population also possesses these characteristics. (If you are unclear about the terms it might be worth refreshing your memory by re-reading pp. 32–33.) The characteristics we are interested in estimating are called **parameters**.

These concepts may be best illustrated by using an example. Let's imagine you are the head of a school of clinical therapy and each year you have places for 40 new students to start their training. However, over the last 3 years you have had at least five to eight students drop out before the start of the course, which leaves you under the establishment figure. Clearly, if you could make an accurate estimate of potential drop-out for the forthcoming year, you could offer that number of extra places over and above the 40 students you normally take in. This means that when the new course starts, you will have the correct number of students and no resources will be wasted. However, the success of this strategy depends heavily on the accuracy of your estimates. From this example, it can be seen that formal, statistical techniques of estimation are particularly important to any planning activities, whether it be for training places, financial predictions, service delivery or whatever.

However, in order to make good and accurate estimates, the following conditions must be fulfilled:

1. You must define your area of interest clearly, avoiding vague concepts such as 'service delivery', 'patients', etc. If you mean by service delivery the treatment of frozen shoulder patients by megapulse, then you must say so. In the same way, you must also be precise about the parameters you wish to estimate. For example, if you are managing a budget for the coming year and need to consider how much must be allocated for staff development and top-up training courses, you must specify what type of course you are budgeting for. Are they local 1-day events? Are they residential? Over 1-week/1-month/1-term duration? The characteristics must be properly defined if estimates made about them are to have any value and precision. Therefore, the first rule of estimation is:

Define your terms and focus of interest precisely.

2. The next stage involves the selection of a **random sample,** so that the estimates are based on a reasonably representative subgroup of the population in which you are interested. Random sampling was covered in Chapter 3 but essentially involves ensuring that every member of the relevant population has an equal chance of being selected. This can be achieved using random number tables, pulling names out of hats, etc. (see pp. 30–31).

The sample should also be of an adequate number in relation to the population size. The concept of adequacy is difficult to define because it depends on the population being studied and the topic under investigation (see pp. 110–118). However a good rule-of-thumb is to select as many subjects as time and budget will afford. Thus the second rule of estimation is:

Select your subjects randomly and try to ensure that the sample is of an adequate size.

3. The third stage in the estimation process is the data collection phase. Like all other forms of research, it is essential that the data collected are a valid measure of the characteristic you are interested in. Let us imagine you are interested in estimating stress levels among senior clinical therapists. If you simply monitored blood pressure it would not be an adequate measure, since there may be: (a) many reasons for elevated blood pressure readings, and (b) other additional symptoms such as subjective reports of stress, all of which may be a valuable contribution to your stress indices.

Therefore, the third rule of estimation is:

Ensure the data collected are a suitable and valid measure of the characteristics being studied.

4. The last stage in the estimation process is the application of the appropriate estimation formula. There are different formulae available, and their use is determined by what it is the researcher wishes to find out. These formulae and their functions are described below. The last rule of estimation is therefore:

Apply the appropriate statistical formula for what it is you wish to estimate.

TECHNIQUES OF ESTIMATION

The two main types of estimation procedures are 'point estimations' and 'interval estimations'.

POINT ESTIMATES

These are simply a single figure (usually a percentage or an average), which is derived from your sample and which is used as an estimate for the relevant population. For example, you might be interested in planning patient treatment sessions for your lumbar back-pain patients over the coming year. In order to do this, you select a sample of lumbar back-pain patients from those who have attended for treatment over the previous year, and calculate the average number of treatments required before discharge. Let's imagine that the average comes out at seven 30-minute treatments per patient (210 minutes in total). On this basis you could estimate the amount of therapy time required for new lumbar back-pain patients as being 210 minutes. This figure is therefore a point estimate of the average treatment time for lumbar back-pain patients within your clinic.

What you have done here is to select a sample of patients (i.e. a selection from those who attended during the previous year) and you have calculated the average figure for the parameter in which you are interested (i.e. treatment time). From this you have made an estimate for that parameter for the population of lumbar back-pain patients who are likely to require treatment during the coming year.

However, this may not provide you with all the essential information you might need for accurate planning of resources. What you might also need to know is the proportion or percentage of the total patient numbers attending the clinic that lumbar back-pain patients constitute. By knowing this, you could fine-tune your provision a bit more. Consequently, then, you need to obtain a percentage point estimate of lumbar back-pain patients relative to the whole population of patients in your clinic. You might find that these patients constituted 12% of the total patients for the previous 12 months and therefore you could estimate a similar percentage for the forthcoming year. This percentage point estimate of 12% coupled with the average point estimate for treatment (210 minutes per patient) would give you useful information when planning resources and finances in your unit.

I feel sure you are not too impressed by estimation thus far, since it is something that many of us do all the time at a routine and informal level, whether it be estimating our time on domestic tasks so that we know how much can be fitted into a 2-hour slot, or calculating next month's financial outgoings in order to work out whether we can afford new curtains or whatever. However, the accuracy, and thus the value, of estimation depends very largely on the quality of the random sample selected for study; in other words, how representative was the particular sample bank-balance you used when predicting next month's expenditure? A truly representative sample is almost impossible to achieve, but even if we managed it, it is still quite possible for any estimates based on the sample to be wrong, if only minutely. Where patient wellbeing or limited budgets are at stake, even minor inaccuracies in estimates could prove to be disastrous and consequently, it might be useful, in these circumstances, to know what degree of confidence you can place on your estimate.

INTERVAL ESTIMATION

The last point leads us into another variant of estimation, **interval estimation,** which involves the calculation of two figures (rather than a single one), between which we can be confident our estimate falls. So, in the example above concerning our lumbar back-pain patients, instead of saying that the estimate for average treatment time is 210 minutes, we would calculate a lower and upper limit of treatment time, for example 150 minutes to 240 minutes, and we could then estimate with a reasonable degree of confidence that the treatments for other lumbar back-pain patients would fall within this interval.

This procedure clearly allows a bit more leeway in our predictions but it also gives the researcher some confidence about the estimates. This concept of confidence is a crucial one in interval estimation and distinguishes interval estimates from point estimates. The amount of confidence a researcher has in his or her estimate is expressed as a percentage, and the higher the percentage, the more confident they are. Therefore an estimate made with 99% confidence should be more reliable than one made with 95%.

To illustrate this distinction between the point and interval estimates, suppose a researcher asks the question:

How much treatment on average are future lumbar back-pain patients going to need?

A point estimate would answer:

I don't know precisely, but my guess is an average of 210-minute sessions.

Whereas the interval estimate would reply:

I don't know precisely but I am 95% confident that average treatment needs will be between 150 minutes and 240 minutes in total.

The higher figure in this last answer (i.e. 240 minutes) is called the **upper confidence limit,** while the lower figure (i.e. 150 minutes) is called the **lower confidence limit.** The difference between these two numbers is known as the **confidence interval.** How much confidence that can be expressed in any given interval estimate depends on the formula used to calculate the estimate. These formulae are given later in the chapter.

THE THEORY BEHIND INTERVAL ESTIMATES

In order to understand the theoretical basis underpinning interval estimates, it is important that you have read the sections on the normal distribution (pp. 65–67) and on the standard deviation (pp. 59–60).

Just to refresh your memory on the key points, a normal distribution is a frequency distribution graph, which is bell-shaped as in Figure 18.1.

This curve has a number of important properties which are essential to statistics.

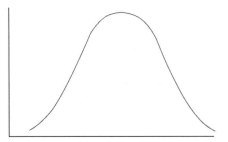

Figure 18.1 The normal distribution curve.

The standard deviation is a number which represents how much a set of data varies, on average, from the mean of those data (see pp. 59–60).

It is the relationship between the normal distribution and the standard deviation that is important to estimation. In any set of normally distributed data, a fixed percentage of that data lies within given areas on either side of the average score.

These 'given areas' are related to the standard deviations of that set of data and are as follows:

- 68% of the scores fall within one standard deviation either side of the mean.
- 95% of the scores fall within two standard deviations either side of the mean.
- 99.73% of the scores fall within three standard deviations either side of the mean.

These figures may be more clearly illustrated by looking back to Figure 5.16 (p. 66).

If you reread the example regarding heart rate given on pp. 66–67, then the implications all this has for estimation can be explored further.

On the hypothetical basis that the average heart rate is 72 beats per minute, and the standard deviation is 5, you would know that 68% of the population have heart rates of between 67 and 77 beats per minute, 95% have heart rates between 62 and 82 beats per minute, and 99.73% have heart rates between 57 and 87 beats per minute.

These (fictitious) figures would have been calculated on a *sample* of people. If, for example, you wanted to make an interval estimate on the average heart rate for the *whole population* with 95% confidence in that estimate, then you need to use the mean score and add two standard deviations to it to get the upper confidence limit (i.e. 82 beats). You then take two standard deviations away from the mean to get the lower confidence limit (i.e. 62 beats). This would give us the confidence interval of 62–82 beats per minute. Because 95% of any normally distributed data lie within two standard deviations either side of the mean, you could say with 95% confidence that the heart rates of the whole population lie within that interval. This 95% figure is called the **level of confidence** and is a statement of belief that the average heart rate of the population will fall within the upper and lower confidence limits stated.

In the same way, you could make estimates with 68% confidence by using one standard deviation either side of the mean, or with 99.73% confidence by using three standard deviations either side of the mean. However, it is more common to use confidence levels of 90% and 99% in addition to 95% and these clearly have no direct correspondence with the standard deviations. Therefore, we need to use the appropriate estimation formulae. These are provided in the next section. These formulae also allow the researcher to make estimates from large samples (over 30) about characteristics which are not normally distributed throughout the population.

CALCULATING INTERVAL ESTIMATES

There are several different formulae for calculating interval estimates and which one you use will depend on the following points:

1. Whether your sample size is greater than, equal to or less than 30.
2. Do you want to estimate the population *average* for the parameter in question (such as the average number of visits the community clinical therapist makes to elderly Parkinson's disease patients), or do you require *proportions* or *percentages* (for example, the proportion of the secretarial population who sustain repetitive strain injury)?
3. The confidence level you need in your estimate. The usual level is 95%, but you may need to have more confidence (i.e. 99%) or less (90%) depending on what it is you are estimating. The more disastrous the effects of an inaccurate estimate, the more confidence you will need.

SAMPLES LARGER THAN 30

ESTIMATING CONFIDENCE LIMITS FOR THE POPULATION AVERAGE

If you wish to estimate population averages from data derived from samples larger than 30 the formulae contained in this section are appropriate. The first formula provided is for the most commonly used 95% confidence level. The other formulae are for the 99% and 90% levels respectively.

Supposing you were interested in the average absenteeism rate for senior clinical therapists across your region. To calculate your estimate for this population, you might select a random sample of 75 senior clinical therapists and work out their average absence rate over the previous 12 months. Let's say this works out at 19.0 units per annum with a standard deviation of 4.5.

What you have here is:

- a sample larger than 30
- an average or mean score for the parameter in which you are interested (i.e. absenteeism).

The 95% confidence level

If you need the usual 95% confidence level in your estimate, the formula is:

$$1.96 \times \frac{SD}{\sqrt{n}}$$

where
  1.96 = a constant for the 95% confidence level
  SD = the standard deviation of the population
  n = the sample size
  $\sqrt{}$ = is the square root of the sample size.

It is important to note that very often the standard deviation of the population is not known. In such cases you can use the standard deviation of the sample instead.

If we now translate these figures, from the example about senior clinical therapists' absenteeism rates, into the formula, we get:

$$1.96 \times \frac{4.5}{\sqrt{75}}$$
$$= 1.96 \times \frac{4.5}{8.66}$$
$$= 1.96 \times 0.52$$
$$= 1.02$$

This figure of 1.02 is then added to the average absenteeism rate of 19.0 units to give the upper confidence limit, i.e.

$$19.0 + 1.02 = 20.02$$

It is then subtracted from the average to give the lower confidence limit, i.e.

$$19.0 - 1.02 = 17.98$$

This gives us the confidence interval of 17.98–20.02. We can therefore say with 95% confidence that average absenteeism rates among the senior clinical therapist population in the region will fall within these figures.

The 99% confidence level

Should you want to make your estimates with more confidence, the formula becomes

$$2.58 \times \frac{SD}{\sqrt{n}}$$

So, using the above example, and substituting the relevant figures we get

$$2.58 \times \frac{4.5}{\sqrt{75}}$$
$$= 2.58 \times \frac{4.5}{8.66}$$
$$= 2.58 \times 0.52$$
$$= 1.34$$

The upper confidence limit is then:

$$19.0 + 1.34 = 20.34$$

and the lower confidence limit is:

$$19.0 - 1.34 = 17.66$$

So we can now say with 99% confidence that the average absenteeism will fall between 17.66 and 20.34 units.

The 90% confidence level

If we don't need such a high level of confidence in our estimate, we can use the less stringent 90% formula:

$$1.64 \times \frac{SD}{\sqrt{n}}$$

Therefore, using the same data we get

$$1.64 \times \frac{4.5}{\sqrt{75}}$$
$$= 1.64 \times \frac{4.5}{8.66}$$
$$= 1.64 \times 0.52$$
$$= 0.85$$

The confidence interval is therefore:

$$18.15 - 19.85$$

We can estimate with 90% confidence that the average absenteeism rate for the population of senior clinical therapists will be between 18.15 and 19.85 units per annum.

ESTIMATING CONFIDENCE LIMITS FOR PROPORTIONS OF THE POPULATION

If, rather than estimating confidence limits for population averages, you wish to calculate population proportions or percentages, you will need the following formulae instead. Three formulae are provided, the first for the 95% confidence limits, the second for the 99% limits and the third for the 90% limits.

Let's imagine you are interested in the topic of carpal tunnel syndrome in pregnancy. You wish to estimate what proportion of the pregnant women population are likely to suffer this problem. You select a sample of 90 pregnant women of 35+ weeks' gestation and find that 27 of them have carpal tunnel syndrome. You therefore have a sample larger than 30 and are concerned with proportion and percentage estimates of the population.

The following formulae are therefore appropriate for this purpose.

The 95% confidence limit

The formula for this calculation is:

$$1.96 \times \sqrt{\frac{pq}{n}}$$

where
  1.96 = a constant to be used for the 95% confidence limits
  p = the proportion of the sample which possesses the characteristic
  q = the proportion of the sample which does not possess the characteristic
  n = the sample size
  $\sqrt{}$ = the square root of the calculations under this sign.

The proportion of a sample is calculated by dividing the actual number of people possessing the characteristic by the total number of people in the sample. For example, here the proportion of women with carpal tunnel syndrome would be:

$$\frac{27}{90} = 0.3$$

while the proportion of women without the syndrome is

$$\frac{63}{90} = 0.7$$

Therefore substituting these figures in the formula we get:

$$1.96 \times \sqrt{\frac{0.3 \times 0.7}{90}}$$

$$= 1.96 \times \sqrt{\frac{0.21}{90}}$$

$$= 1.96 \times \sqrt{0.0023}$$

$$= 1.96 \times 0.05$$

$$= 0.1$$

This figure of 0.1 is now added to the proportion of the sample who have carpal tunnel syndrome to get the upper confidence limit, i.e.

$$0.1 + 0.3 = 0.4$$

It is then subtracted from the proportion of the sample who have carpal tunnel syndrome to get the lower confidence limit, i.e.

$$0.3 - 0.1 = 0.2$$

This gives us the confidence interval of 0.2–0.4, which means that we can now estimate with 95% confidence that the proportion of the population of pregnant women who suffer carpal tunnel syndrome will lie between 0.2 and 0.4.

The 99% confidence limit

Should you need to have greater confidence in your estimate then the following formula should be used:

$$2.58 \times \sqrt{\frac{pq}{n}}$$

If we use the example and figures above then we get

$$2.58 \times \sqrt{\frac{0.3 \times 0.7}{90}}$$

$$= 2.58 \times \sqrt{\frac{0.21}{90}}$$

$$= 2.58 \times \sqrt{0.0023}$$

$$= 2.58 \times 0.05$$

$$= 0.13$$

This number is then added to the proportion of the sample who have carpal tunnel syndrome to get the upper confidence limit, i.e.

$$0.3 + 0.13 = 0.43$$

It is then subtracted from the proportion of the sample with carpal tunnel syndrome to get the lower confidence limit, i.e.

$$0.3 - 0.13 = 0.17$$

Therefore, the 99% confidence interval for the proportion of the population of pregnant women with carpal tunnel syndrome is 0.17 to 0.43.

The 90% confidence limit

If you don't need such a high level of confidence in your estimate, you can use the 90% confidence limit formula instead:

$$= 1.64 \times \sqrt{\frac{pq}{n}}$$

$$1.64 \times \sqrt{\frac{0.3 \times 0.7}{90}}$$

$$= 1.64 \times \sqrt{\frac{0.21}{90}}$$

$$= 1.64 \times \sqrt{0.0023}$$

$$= 1.64 \times 0.05$$

$$= 0.08$$

This number is now added to the proportion of the sample with carpal tunnel syndrome to give the upper confidence limit, i.e.

$$0.3 + 0.08 = 0.38$$

It is then subtracted from the proportion of the sample with carpal tunnel syndrome to give the lower confidence limit, i.e.

$$0.3 - 0.08 = 0.22$$

Therefore, it can be predicted with 90% confidence that the proportion of the pregnant woman population who have carpal tunnel syndrome falls somewhere between 0.22 and 0.38.

SAMPLES OF 30 SUBJECTS OR FEWER

Before proceeding with estimates for samples of 30 or fewer it is important to emphasise two points. First, these particular calculations should only be performed if the parent population is known to be normally distributed on the characteristic in question. The second important point to note is that proportions of a population are not usually calculated from samples of 30 or fewer, because the estimates are likely to be unreliable. Consequently, only the formulae associated with estimating means will be provided.

Let's suppose you are interested in the promotion prospects of newly qualified clinical therapists. You select a random sample of 15 and follow them up over a 10-year period. You find that the average length of time taken to achieve promotion is 4.7 years. From this sample mean you wish to calculate the population mean. Therefore, your interest is in averages and you have a sample of 30 or fewer. The following formulae are therefore appropriate.

The formula for the 99%, 95% and 90% confidence limits requires that you first calculate the standard deviation from the sample data, thus

$$SD = \sqrt{\frac{\sum (x - \bar{x})^2}{N-1}}$$

where
Σ = the total
x = the individual score
$\bar{x}$ = the average score
N = the total number of scores in the sample
$\sqrt{}$ = the square root of all the calculations under this sign.

To refresh your memory on how to do this calculation, turn back to pp. 59–60. Imagine for the purpose of this example that the standard deviation is 2.1 years.

The estimation calculations for the confidence limits of 99%, 95% and 90% all start off in the same way:

1. Calculate $N - 1$ where N is the number in your sample, i.e.

$$15 - 1 = 14$$

2. Turn to the probability tables associated with the t test (Table A2.5, p. 346), where you can see that down the left-hand column are df values from 1 to 120. Look down this column until you find our $N - 1$ value of 14. To the right of this are the numbers

1.345 1.761 2.145 2.624 2.977 4.140

The procedures for calculating the different levels of confidence limits now change slightly, and each will be dealt with separately.

Calculating the 95% confidence limits

We are only interested in the figure under the heading '0.05 level of significance for a two-tailed test' (see top of the table). This terminology is explained in Chapter 9 but is of no relevance to us here. The figure at the intersection point of this column with $N - 1 = 14$, is 2.145 and is used to provide us with the 95% confidence limit, thus:

$$t \times \frac{SD}{\sqrt{N}}$$

where

t = the figure derived from the probability table for t

= 2.145

SD = the standard deviation of the sample's score

= 2.1 years

N = the number of subjects in the sample

= 15

$\sqrt{}$ = the square root
Therefore, substituting these figures we get:

$$2.145 \times \frac{2.1}{\sqrt{15}}$$

$$= 2.145 \times \frac{2.1}{3.87}$$

$$= 2.145 \times 0.54$$

$$= 1.16$$

This figure is added to the average sample score to give the upper confidence limit, i.e.

$$4.7 + 1.16 = 5.86$$

It is then subtracted from the average sample score to give the lower confidence limit, i.e.

$$4.7 - 1.16 = 3.54$$

Therefore we can estimate with 95% confidence that, for the whole population of newly qualified clinical therapists the average time for achieving promotion is between 3.54 and 5.86 years after qualifying.

The 99% confidence limits

To calculate this value we need to look under the '0.01 level of significance for a two-tailed test' heading in Table A2.5 for $N - 1$. Our $N - 1$ value is 14 and the relevant figure at the intersection point is 2.977.

Using the formula

$$t \times \frac{SD}{\sqrt{N}}$$

and substituting our values we get

$$2.997 \times \frac{2.1}{\sqrt{15}}$$

$$= 2.997 \times \frac{2.1}{3.87}$$

$$= 2.997 \times 0.54$$

$$= 1.61$$

We now add 1.61 to the sample mean of 4.7 to get the upper confidence limit, i.e.

$$4.7 + 1.61 = 6.31$$

We then subtract 1.61 from the sample mean of 4.7 to get the lower confidence limit, i.e.

$$4.7 - 1.61 = 3.09$$

Therefore the 99% confidence limits are 3.09–6.31 years.

The 90% confidence limits

To obtain the 90% confidence limits we need to select the number under the heading '0.10 level of significance for a two-tailed test' (in Table A2.5), to the right of $N - 1$.

Here for our $N - 1$ value of 14, the relevant figure is 1.762.

Using the formula

$$t \times \frac{SD}{\sqrt{N}}$$

and substituting our values we get

$$1.761 \times \frac{2.1}{\sqrt{15}}$$

$$= 1.761 \times \frac{2.1}{3.87}$$

$$= 1.761 \times 0.54$$

$$= 0.95$$

This figure is now added to the sample mean of 4.7 to give the upper confidence limit, i.e.

$$4.7 + 0.95 = 5.65$$

It is then subtracted from the sample mean of 4.7 to give the lower confidence limit, i.e.

$$4.7 - 0.95 = 3.75$$

The 90% confidence limits for this example are therefore 3.75–5.65 years.

Key Concepts

- Estimation is a technique of making scientific 'best guesses' about events.
- It is particularly useful to anyone who is involved in service planning (e.g. budgets, service delivery, etc.).
- The technique of estimation involves making predictions about a particular population characteristic known as a **parameter** from knowledge about a small sample of that population.
- There are two types of estimation: **point estimates** and **interval estimates.**
- Point estimates make a prediction of a single figure about the population parameter, whereas interval estimates make a prediction that the population parameter will fall between two figures.
- These two figures are called **confidence limits** and the gap between them is called the **confidence interval.**

- When using interval estimates, the predictions about the population can be made with different levels of confidence.
- The degree of confidence is dictated by the nature of the research and the formula used to calculate the estimates.

Activity 18.1 (Answers on p. 370)

1 You are in charge of an outpatients' clinic. The non-attendance levels are becoming increasingly worrying because of resource wastage and length of waiting lists. If you could make an accurate estimate of non-attendance over the next 6 months, you could double-book appointments in order to reduce wastage.

   You find that the number of non-attenders of a sample of 150 patients was 57. Estimate the confidence limits for the proportion of non-attenders in the outpatient population, using the 95% confidence level.

2 You are trying to plan care activities in a new respite centre for learning disabled children. As many of these children have physical handicaps which impair their mobility and self-care activities you will need to estimate how much clinical therapy time on average, will be required per child, per day.

   You select a sample of 25 learning disabled children and find that the average amount of clinical therapy time needed is 3.2 hours, with a SD of 1.7 hours. Estimate the average amount of time that will be required by the children in this new centre, using the 99% confidence level.

3 You are responsible for the equipment budget in your district health authority. One activity involves you in estimating the mean life expectancy of your ultrasound machines over the next financial year. You look at the lifespan of a sample of 40 of these machines and find that the mean length of service is 4.3 years, with a standard deviation of 0.9 years. Using the 90% confidence level, estimate the average life expectancy of the ultrasound machines in your area, so that you can get some idea of how many replacements will be needed.

FURTHER READING

Cohen L, Holliday M 1996 Practical statistics for students. Paul Chapman Publishing, London

Crichton N 2005 Principles of statistical analysis in nursing and health care research. http://www.nursing-standard.co.uk/nurseresearcher/resources/archive/GetArticleById.asp?ArticleId=6171

Ferguson GA, Takane Y 1989 Statistical analysis in psychology and education. 6th Edition. McGraw-Hill, New York

http://davidmlane.com/hyperstat/B12386.html

http://nurseresearcher.rcnpublishing.co.uk/resources/archive/GetArticleById.asp?ArticleId=6171

SECTION 3

Research applications

This section is intended to illustrate the application of some of the statistical processes described earlier, using seven different examples. The first example relates to the development of valid and reliable attitude scales which can be customised for use in any area of health research. The second example describes a useful technique known as repertory grid analysis, which has a range of uses, for example, to establish which aspects of health care delivery provide work satisfaction and dissatisfaction for the health care professionals involved. The third application is called Receiver Operating Characteristics, which is especially valuable in screening and diagnostic studies; the fourth topic is the Delphi technique and is typically used to establish a consensus opinion amongst experts in a given area, for example, the identification of the most important indicators of competent performance in final year chiropractic students; the fifth chapter describes a well-established method for prioritising the views of a group of people (quite often service users) by using a system of forced choice decisions; the sixth chapter describes three commonly used techniques of assessing the reliability of clinicians' judgements or measures – Cohen's Kappa, Inter/Intra-class Correlation Coefficients and Bland and Altman's Agreement Test – which are typically used to determine the reliability of instruments and raters. The final chapter describes the process of conducting systematic reviews of research literature, as a first stage in deciding on the best available evidence for use in practice. Each technique will be described separately.

Chapter 19

Attitude scales

CHAPTER CONTENTS

ATTITUDES AND SOME GENERAL POINTS ABOUT THEIR MEASUREMENT

Attitudes and attitude measurement are areas that have generated extraordinary interest for decades. They have particular relevance for the health care context, especially health education and promotion, since it is assumed that attitudes give rise to related outcome behaviours, and that if the attitude can be changed, then so too will the resulting behaviour. A classic example is smoking. If a health education campaign aims to make attitudes towards smoking more negative, it might be expected that actual smoking behaviour will also diminish over time. However, this does not necessarily happen, largely because attitudes, the relationship between attitudes and behaviour and the measurement of attitudes are all very complex. It might be useful to elaborate briefly on this statement.

An attitude to any given topic is a product of the individual's beliefs, feelings and behaviour, all of which can be either unchangeable or alternatively, rapidly modified by life experiences. In other words, attitudes can be highly stable or highly unstable in different circumstances. However, it would be possible to misclassify an attitude as stable, when in fact, the attitude measure is not sensitive enough to pick up any change. Conversely, an attitude could be deemed to have changed as a result of a health education campaign, when, in reality, the attitude measure is unreliable. For example, it may be that the researcher is interested in following through a patient's attitude to named practitioner care, and has formulated the following hypothesis:

H₁ Patients' attitudes towards care delivery from a named clinical therapist become more positive following experience of this type of service provision.

In order to test this hypothesis, it would be necessary to test the attitudes of a group of patients *before* receiving treatment from a named clinical therapist and again *after* treatment, using an attitude scale.

Alternatively, it is conceivable that the researcher is interested in the attitudes of different patient groups to treatment by a named clinical therapist and has constructed the following hypothesis:

H₁ Patients undergoing clinical therapy treatment for potentially embarrassing or sensitive problems are more negative towards the concept of the named clinical therapist than are patients whose treatment is not for embarrassing or sensitive conditions.

To test this hypothesis, the researcher might select a group of patients undergoing specific continence treatment and a further group who are receiving treatment to increase hip mobility. Attitude scales are administered to both groups to see whether there is any difference in attitude between them.

If either of these studies is to reveal useful data it is essential that the attitude scale is sufficiently **sensitive** to pick up any changes before and after an intervention (Hypothesis 1) or any differences between patient groups (Hypothesis 2). Sensitivity can be achieved through ensuring that the attitude scale is **reliable,** in that it measures the same attitude each time it is used and that it is **valid,** in that it measures what it is meant to measure. For example, it would be of no value at all if the attitude scale developed for the above examples measured attitudes towards the named clinical therapist concept on the first occasion it was used, but recorded opinions about the hospital service generally on the next. The scale would be similarly useless if it measured death anxiety in the subject group, i.e. it didn't measure what it was intended to measure. Obviously any

comparisons over time or across groups would be rendered nonsense by such an invalid and unreliable instrument.

The second point about attitude scales relates to the range and complexity of attitudes. An individual's attitude to any given topic is likely to be governed by a vast range of related issues. If we refer back to the examples given above, a patient's attitude towards the concept of the named therapist will be influenced by how much s/he likes the therapist in question, how much improvement is being made, the general ambience of the department, pain levels during treatment, etc. Consequently, if the researcher is to measure attitudes towards the named therapist concept, a range of issues relating to this must be covered in the attitude scale.

Attitude scales can be beset by response bias, too. In other words, some respondents will deliberately distort their answers in order to conceal their real views, or to present themselves in the best light or to please (or displease) the researcher. The section on constant errors explains ways in which some sources of response bias can be eliminated by the design of the research study.

One final point is worthy of note in relation to attitude scales. While there are a number of proprietary attitude scales available commercially, these may be either very expensive or restricted to use only by psychologists. Moreover, their content is not always sufficiently specific or directly appropriate for use in certain circumstances. These factors mean that for the majority of attitude research, it is much better to construct a customised scale that has direct relevance to the research topic under investigation. While this may sound daunting, it is not particularly difficult, providing the basic principles of test design and construction are followed. The science of psychological testing is known as **psychometrics,** and it is founded upon some basic principles, which will be outlined before proceeding with specific details about attitude test construction. Do note, however, that the following guidelines are basic principles only. More sophisticated tests would demand elaborate preliminary data collection and statistical analysis. For further information on this, the reader is referred to Beech & Harding (1990), Oppenheim (2000) and Rust & Golombok (2008).

THE BASIC PRINCIPLES OF PSYCHOLOGICAL TEST CONSTRUCTION: PSYCHOMETRICS

A good attitude scale, like any other test of a psychological attribute, should be both reliable and valid. These concepts are defined as follows.

Reliability refers to the fact that a test should measure exactly the same quality or attribute each time it is used. To take a rather extreme and facile example, there would be little point in using some weighing scales if they measured grams on one occasion, metres on another and volume on another. To be of use, weighing scales must always measure weight. Similarly with attitude scales, they should not assess attitudes to one topic on the first use, to another topic on the second use, intelligence on the third, motivation on the fourth, etc.

Validity refers to the idea that a test should measure what it is intended to measure. There are three main forms of validity.

Face validity simply asks the question: 'does the test *look* as though it is measuring what it is meant to measure?' An attitude scale about nuclear armaments that requires the respondent to define words or calculate mathematical formulae does not have much face validity or credibility. Face validity has an important PR function – respondents are more likely to complete questionnaires that look as though they are credible measures of the topic under investigation.

Construct validity refers to the concept that a test should assess the *theory* under investigation. Therefore, an attitude scale that is intended to measure patients' attitudes to being treated by a named therapist should reflect the theoretical assumptions that underlie this; for example, the whole notion of the named carer was driven by the fundamental idea that continuity of named carer fosters a patient–therapist relationship whereby the best level of care can be provided in the context of professional responsibility, mutual respect and trust. These ideas were derived from a considerable body of theoretical evidence relating to professional and long-term relationships. Establishing construct validity for an attitude scale would typically involve the researcher undertaking a thorough literature review of the theory that pertains to the topic being researched, in order to identify the key theoretical points.

Content validity refers to the notion that the theoretical concepts on which the test is founded should give rise to a range of observable and measurable behaviours which must be covered by the test. Using the above example again, the named therapist idea should produce measurable observable behaviours such as greater compliance with regimens, more non-task specific interpersonal contact, greater confidence, etc. A good test of attitudes towards the named therapist should cover a wide range of observable, quantifiable behaviours/outcomes that would be expected to spring from the underlying theory. These outcome measures should follow logically from the literature reviewed for the construct validity stage, as well as from personal and professional experience. It is also often worthwhile conducting informal interviews with appropriate people to establish their perspectives concerning which observable measures would be relevant for inclusion in the scale.

Once the scale has been developed along these lines, the scale's construct and content validity can be assessed by generating and testing hypotheses. For example, using the present example, it would be predicted that patients whose attitudes towards the named therapist system of care delivery were positive would also be more satisfied with their treatment and be more compliant with exercise routines. To test this experimentally, we would compare a group of positive-attitude patients with a group of negative-attitude patients on exercise compliance and satisfaction with treatment. If we found the expected differences, this would lend both content and construct validity to the attitude scale.

A fourth type of validity, **predictive validity** is the most difficult of the psychometric principles to attain. Attitude scales should have some capacity to predict future behaviour, although for a range of reasons people do not always behave in ways that are consistent with their attitudes. If the scale has predictive validity, it should be possible to forecast an individual's behaviour on the basis of their responses to the scale. In the present example, we would anticipate that patients with positive attitudes towards the named carer initiative, would, if given the choice in the future, select named care in preference to randomly allocated care. If this hypothesis was supported, the scale would have some predictive validity. Once again, this attribute would be assessed experimentally, through the formulation and testing of relevant hypotheses.

Key Concepts

Attitude scales, like other tests of psychological attributes, should be **reliable** and **valid**.

  Reliability means that the test should measure the same quality every time it is used.

  Validity means that the test should measure what it is intended to measure.

  There are four types of validity:

- **Face validity** – does the test look as though it is measuring what it is supposed to?
- **Construct validity** – does the test measure the theory relating to the topic under investigation?
- **Content validity** – does the test measure a full range of behaviours that would be expected to emerge from the theory?
- **Predictive validity** – does the test predict future behaviour?

THE ATTITUDE SCALE: A GENERAL OVERVIEW

As has already been mentioned, attitude scales are a frequently used tool in health care research, as a means by which opinions about service delivery, ethical issues, changes in working practices and locations, new equipment, etc. can be ascertained in an *objective and quantifiable manner.* An attitude scale typically consists of a set of slightly contentious statements, and the respondent is asked to indicate the degree to which they agree or disagree with them. The strength of agreement or disagreement can be measured in a number of ways, but one of the most commonly used methods is a **five-point ordinal scale,** called a **Likert** scale. This is usually in the following form:

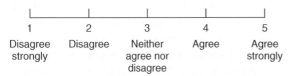

It should be noted that, because the scale is ordinal, it is not possible to say that someone who scores at 4 feels twice as strongly as someone who scores at 2 (see section on levels of measurement, Chapter 4). That having been said, many researchers ignore this data limitation.

High scores on an attitude scale are usually taken to be indicative of a positive attitude towards the topic under investigation, although this can be reversed if appropriate (i.e. high scores = negative attitudes). From this brief discussion of the basic principles of psychometrics and their application to attitude measurement, it can be seen that the construction of a good attitude scale is heavily dependent upon many of the research design rules and statistical procedures that have been discussed throughout this text. Despite the apparent complexity that attaches to these psychometric rules, the construction of an attitude scale is, in fact, reasonably straightforward. Too often, though, researchers in their quest to establish the attitudes of a specified target group, ignore the basic principles of psychometrics and simply construct a questionnaire comprising issues that they assume are crucial to the issue under investigation. This is then distributed to their chosen sample and the responses are used to guide subsequent health care planning and provision. Inevitably, a poor quality questionnaire may mislead and misinform, and in the context of health care, this may have serious implications for service delivery and patient care.

Key Concepts

- Attitude scales are intended to measure attitudes in an objective and quantifiable way.
- They comprise a set of slightly contentious statements, usually presented in questionnaire format.
- Respondents are asked to indicate the degree to which they agree or disagree with each statement.
- Subjects' answers are commonly recorded on a five-point ordinal scale, known as a Likert scale.
- High scores on an attitude scale usually indicate positive attitudes towards the topic in question.

CONSTRUCTING AN ATTITUDE SCALE

Let us take as our topic for research the issue of complementary medicine. The raised profile of complementary medicine and the burgeoning body of research that attests to its value means that it must increasingly be considered as a valid alternative to conventional medicine in the treatment of many conditions. Resistance to change and the desire to protect professional territorial boundaries has meant that the routine incorporation of complementary techniques within a total care package has not yet been realised. Let us further assume, though, that you are working in a visionary primary health care team, where there is a move to include complementary medicine as a treatment option in the practice. Before the practice goes to the expense of appointing complementary care practitioners to conduct a number of sessions per week, and making space and resources available to them, it is important to see whether the attitudes of patients towards complementary health care are sufficiently positive to merit its inclusion within the practice, and moreover, whether some types of patients are more positively disposed to this type of provision. If some groups hold more positive attitudes than others, it would make logical sense to target these patients with the option of complementary health care. It would be important, then, to develop a measuring instrument that can reliably identify the attitudes of patients towards complementary medicine and discriminate between individuals or groups of patients. The following stages are intended to guide the researcher in the development of tailored attitude scales for a range of health care problems.

1. CREATING AN ITEM POOL

To develop a preliminary set of attitude statements, it is necessary to think up a large number (about 25–30) of fairly contentious statements that are positive about complementary medicine, and a similar number that are negative about it. In order to do this, it is advisable for the researcher to read around the topic first, and to interview a number of people about their thoughts on the issue. This initial spadework provides a guide to the major points that must be covered by the attitude scale, as well as suggesting the variety of views subsumed under each major heading, all of which must be reflected in the instrument.

The initial item pool is enhanced if a number of researchers independently create their own statements in the first instance, which can then be discussed, compared and shared. This approach guarantees that a full range of perspectives and facets on the topic is covered.

Ensuring that the pool of attitude statements reflects available theory and research on complementary medicine contributes initial construct validity. By interviewing relevant personnel and developing a wide range of items that measure appropriate outcome behaviours, you achieve some preliminary content validity for the scale.

When creating the items, it is important to bear in mind the following guidelines:

- Avoid factual statements, e.g. 'acupuncture originated in China'.
- Avoid statements that almost everyone would agree or disagree with, e.g. 'the aim of complementary medicine is to make people better'.
- Include as many aspects, topics and themes as possible that relate to the topic.
- Make sure that only one thought is contained in a statement.
- Do not use double negatives.
- Use simple concepts, grammar and language.
- Ensure that the statements are short and easily comprehensible.
- Make sure that the statements are slightly contentious, e.g. 'all primary health care teams should be obliged to have a complementary health care specialist'.

Taking our sample research topic, you might come up with the following positive statements. (Note that only four have been provided here; in practice, between 25 and 30 positive statements should be constructed initially.)

- Complementary medicine is always a preferable alternative to conventional medicine because it is more natural.
- Complementary medicine should always be a treatment option provided by the NHS.

- Only bigoted people disapprove of complementary medicine.
- Complementary medicine is much more effective than formal medicine in the treatment of most medical complaints.

Similarly, a comparable number of statements that reflect negative views about complementary medicine must be created. (Again, for reasons of space, only four are suggested here.)

- Complementary medicine succeeds only because it taps into people's most primitive and superstitious instincts.
- Practitioners of complementary medicine are insufficiently qualified, and so do more harm than good.
- Complementary medicine has no scientific basis to it whatsoever.
- There is no sound evidence to suggest that complementary medicine has any beneficial impact.

2. REFINING THE ITEM POOL

Obviously if four or five researchers have independently produced their own 50–60 preliminary item pool, not only will there be a huge item bank at this stage, but there will also be a considerable degree of overlap. Hence the next stage involves getting together with the co-researchers, or with another person, if you're working on your own, to sift through the initial item bank to eliminate duplicate statements and any item that violates any of the above rules.

This process should yield a draft attitude scale that consists of about 20 positive statements and 20 negative ones (it doesn't matter, though, if you have slightly fewer or more statements at this stage). The items should be randomly ordered in the scale, so that positive and negative items are interspersed.

3. SCORING THE ITEMS

Because it is the convention to make high scores representative of a positive attitude towards the topic being studied, statements that display a favourable view of complementary medicine should be scored highly, while those that reflect an unfavourable opinion should be scored low. To score the items using this convention, first go through each statement, indicating with a '+' if the statement is positively disposed towards complementary medicine and with a '−' if it is negatively disposed. If any item is ambiguous, eliminate it.

For every statement marked with a '+' attach the following scoring key:

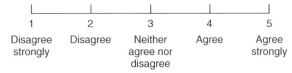

1	2	3	4	5
Disagree strongly	Disagree	Neither agree nor disagree	Agree	Agree strongly

For each of the negatively keyed items, reverse the scoring system:

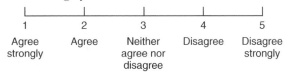

1	2	3	4	5
Agree strongly	Agree	Neither agree nor disagree	Disagree	Disagree strongly

You therefore end up with a set of attitude statements, each of which has its own scoring key, determined by whether it is positively or negatively disposed towards complementary medicine.

4. TESTING OUT THE DRAFT SCALE

You now need to test out the first draft of the questionnaire by administering it to a sample of people, ideally around 80–100. In fact, this is not always possible, for a host of practical reasons, so try to get as many people as you can, but certainly no fewer than 20–25. The subjects do not need to be members of your target group (in this case, patients at a primary health care centre), nor do they have to resemble them in any key characteristics (i.e. they do not have to be patients of any sort). Consequently, you could conduct this stage of the scale's development with a group of nurses, at a parent–teacher committee meeting, or even in the street. However, this step is part of the reliability-testing procedure, which is intended to establish whether your scale measures the same attitude each time it is used. Consequently, you will need to ask the same group of people to complete the questionnaire again in the near future, to find out whether their attitudes remain similar over a 1–2-week period. Therefore, you need to ensure that you know how and where you can contact the same individuals again, so that they can re-do the scale. You also must make sure that each respondent has some identification on their completed questionnaire.

When you administer the scale for the first time, it is essential that the procedure adopted is the same for each person. Obviously, if you tell one person nothing about the purpose of the measure, another that you want evidence to set up a complementary health care clinic and another that you want to block the proposal to establish such a clinic, you will clearly run the risk of distorting the responses from your sample. While this is an extreme example of how the researcher can influence the answers, it nevertheless illustrates that it is important to standardise any instructions that participants are given, so that everyone has exactly the same information. The best way to standardise this part of the procedure is to write an explanatory note, outlining the purpose of the scale (if this is appropriate and does not distort the data set; see section on constant errors, Chapter 8) and providing instructions for completion of the instrument. This can be read to the participants, or given to them to read. So for example, in this case, the instructions might be:

> I am researching people's attitudes to complementary medicine. By this is meant the following health care treatments: osteopathy, chiropractic, reflexology, acupuncture, aromatherapy, herbalism and other techniques of Chinese medicine. The following questionnaire contains x number of statements about complementary medicine. For each statement, I would like you to indicate whether you agree strongly, agree, neither agree nor disagree, disagree or disagree strongly. Please indicate for each statement your level of agreement/disagreement by putting a ring around the relevant number.

When each person has completed the questionnaire, ask whether they would be prepared to complete the questionnaire again in 1–2 weeks' time. If they agree, take down their name and contact details and ensure that the scale they have just completed is labelled '1', so that you know that this is the first measure of their attitudes. Obviously, the next time they complete the questionnaire, it should be labelled '2'.

5. ITEM ANALYSIS

Once you have collected a minimum of 20–25 completed attitude scales, you need to identify which statements are the 'best' – that is, which statements are the most sensitive and have the greatest power to discriminate between different strengths of attitude. To do this, add up the scores for all items to give a total score for each respondent. The higher the total score, the more positive the respondent is towards the issue of complementary medicine, and conversely, the lower the score, the more negatively disposed the respondent.

The total scores for the sample should be set out from the lowest to the highest, and the median score identified (see Chapter 5). You now take the top 33% of the scores and the bottom 33% of the scores, or if the scores are grouped together in a clearer and more distinctive pattern, take the cluster of top scores and the cluster of bottom scores. It is essential that whichever approach you adopt, you have equal numbers of high and low scores. The mid-range scores can be discarded.

Imagine we obtained the following data set:

27 28 28 30 31 31 33/44 46 47
47 47 48 52 54 58 64 66/87 88
91 97 98 101 103

There is a clear low-scoring group (27–33) with seven scores in it and a clear high-scoring group with seven scores (87–103). In this case, it would make sense to select these two clusters, even though they represent only 28% of the total number of scores, rather than 33%. Remember that, whatever protocol you adopt, you must ensure that you have equal numbers of high and low scores. Discard the middle range scores.

Now set out a scoring sheet with the headings 'low scorers' and 'high scorers' clearly labelled as in Table 19.1.

Taking attitude statement 1 (item number 1) count up how many low scorers recorded scores of 4 or 5 for this item and enter the number in the appropriate column. Then count up how many of the high scoring group provided scores of 4 or 5 on this item and make a note of this in the correct column. Then repeat the process with each of the remaining attitude statements. You

Table 19.1

Item number	Number of low scorers	Number of high scorers
1		
2		
3		
4		
:		
:		
:		
etc		

Table 19.2

Item number	Number of low scorers	Number of high scorers
1	3	6
2	4	4
3	2	6
4	4	3
:		
:		
:		
45	0	5

should end up with a scoring sheet something like that shown in Table 19.2.

This procedure is intended to establish which items in the preliminary questionnaire are discriminating, sensitive items. We would expect that low-scoring respondents should report low scores on individual items, while high scorers should record high scores on those items. If there is little difference between the high- and low-scoring groups in terms of the number of high scores recorded for any given item, then we can conclude that the item is not sensitive or discriminating. To ascertain which items are discriminating, we now need to look at the frequencies noted in the table for each group. If the numbers are equal or almost equal for the low-scoring and high-scoring groups, then the item is not discriminating between the two groups and can be eliminated. In the data set in Table 19.2, items 2 and 4 are obviously not sensitive and can be discarded. On the other hand, where there is a clear difference in the frequency of high scores between the groups, with the high-scoring group recording a greater frequency, the item is sensi-

tive and should be retained. Items 1, 3 and 45 above come into this category. Sometimes the frequencies are not as clear cut as in the example above, and you will have to decide what you consider to be a big enough difference in frequencies to warrant inclusion in the final scale. Bear in mind, though, firstly that the finished scale should be around 15 items long and secondly, that if your initial subject sample is big enough, there will be little difficulty in obtaining a sufficient number of clearly discriminating items.

Selecting just those statements that demonstrate a significant difference between the high and low scorers, you should now have a reduced scale with around 15 items in it (although anything between 12 and 25 would be fine). This process of item analysis contributes to the scale's validity.

6. ESTABLISHING RELIABILITY

To ensure that our attitude scale measures attitudes towards complementary medicine in a consistent and reliable way, it is essential that you re-test as many of the original participants as possible, using the refined version of your scale. If your test is reliable, we would expect there to be a high level of agreement between each subject's pair of scores; in other words, if the scale is measuring the same attitude each time it is used, then we would anticipate that the subjects would record similar scores on both testings.

To check the scale's reliability, between 1 and 2 weeks after the initial administration of the questionnaire, contact everyone who took part originally and give them the reduced scale. Try not to leave the re-testing much longer than this, because it is quite conceivable that their attitudes to complementary medicine may have changed anyway over an extended period of time; under these circumstances, we might assume that our test was unreliable, when in fact, it was simply reflecting genuine changes in view. Also, the longer you leave the re-testing, the more difficult it will be to track down your original subject sample.

Collect as many completed scales from this group as you can, making sure that each respond-

Table 19.3

Subject	Test 1	Test 2
1	65	59
2	42	47
3	73	68
4 etc.	52	54

ent uses the same identifier as before, enabling you to compare their two sets of responses. When you have a reasonable return (around 20 people), you will need to take the following steps.

- Taking each subject's first questionnaire, calculate the total score *only* for the items that were retained, i.e. if 19 statements were retained after the item analysis, just add up the scores for the same 19 items from the first questionnaire.
- Enter this score on a scoring sheet as shown in Table 19.3.
- To see whether there is any agreement or correlation between the first and second set of scores, the Spearman test has to be performed (see pp. 237–240). If you obtain a significant correlation, then you can conclude that your scale has test–retest reliability.

7. CONFIRMING CONSTRUCT VALIDITY

If your reduced scale is valid (i.e. it measures what it is intended to measure) it should have the capacity to discriminate between groups of people that we would expect to differ in attitudes to complementary medicine. For example, it might be predicted that people who have previously successfully used complementary medicine would have a more positive attitude than those who have not. Therefore to assess the scale's construct validity, you need to do the following.

- Select a group of people who have been successfully treated using complementary medicine, and a group who have never used it. Aim for 20–25 people per group.
- Administer your test to each group.
- Calculate the total score for each subject.

- Compare the scores of the two groups, using the Mann–Whitney U test (see pp. 205–208). If there is a significant difference between the groups in the direction predicted (more positive attitudes among the users of complementary medicine), then you can claim that your scale has construct validity.

8. ESTABLISHING PREDICTIVE VALIDITY

This is the most difficult of all the psychometric criteria to fulfil because it essentially involves the prediction of individual or group behaviour. Undoubtedly, there are many politicians, health educators, military strategists, manufacturers of goods and the like who would be delighted if there was a straightforward relationship between attitudes and behaviour, since it would take the guesswork out of their jobs. However, there are so many influences on the way in which people behave that it is notoriously hard to anticipate behaviour even when stated attitudes are strong and unambiguous. Therefore you should not worry too much if your scale has little or no predictive validity – indeed, many widely used published tests cannot claim to possess much of this attribute either.

Nonetheless, if your scale can predict behaviour, even to a limited extent, then its value increases significantly. In order to test this, it is essential that we generate some hypotheses about the outcome behaviours that we could expect from positively and negatively disposed people. For example, it is conceivable that patients who are strongly in favour of complementary medicine would be more likely to opt for these alternative treatment options, if given a choice. We can formulate the following hypothesis:

H_1 Patients who are positively disposed towards complementary medicine are more likely, when given the option, to choose this form of treatment than are people who are negatively disposed towards it.

To test this hypothesis, you would need to take the following steps:

- Survey the patients in the health centre, using the refined questionnaire. This will also provide you with the index of patient views that was one of the original aims of the study.

- From the results, identify the highest scorers (the most positively disposed) and the lowest scorers (the most negatively disposed).
- Assuming that complementary therapists are employed for some sessions each week, ask the GPs to keep a record: (a) of those patients who are offered these sessions and choose to attend; and (b) of those patients who are offered the sessions, but do not attend.
- You now need to compare the attitudes of these two groups to see whether the hypothesis is supported. To do this, record the attitude scores obtained from the survey, of each patient who selects complementary therapy; do the same for those patients who opt for conventional treatments.
- Compare the two data sets using a Mann–Whitney U test. If the scale has predictive validity, the complementary medicine group should have significantly higher attitude scores than the conventional treatment group. In other words, the scale has the capacity to predict future behaviour.

A good attitude scale (or indeed any measure of some psychological attribute) should be reliable and valid. If your scale falls at these hurdles (excepting the predictive validity criterion), then it is of little worth and you should start again.

Remember, that if health outcomes are in any way dependent upon the data obtained from your test, then you must ensure that it meets the requirements for a psychometrically sound measuring instrument.

FURTHER READING

Beech JR, Harding L (Eds) 1990 Testing people: a practical guide to psychometrics. NFER Nelson, Windsor

Bradburn N, Sudman, S, Wansink B 2004 Asking questions: the definitive guide to questionnaire design. Jossey Bass, NY

De Vellis RF 2003 Scale developemnt: theory and applications, 2nd edition. Sage. London

Krosnick JA, Fabrigar LR 2005.Questionnaire design fro attitudes measurement in social and psychological research. Oxford, OUP

McGaghie W, Van Horn L, Fitzgibbon M et al Development of a measure of attitude toward nutrition in patient care. American Journal of Preventive Medicine 20(1), 15–20. Online. Available http://linkinghub.elsevier.com/retrieve/pii/S0749379700002646 5 January 2009

Oppenheim A 2000 Questionnaire design and attitude measurement. Continuum, London

Parahoo K 2006 Nursing reseach: principles, proces and issues, 2nd edition. Palgrave Macmillan, Basingstoke

Peat J 2002 Health science research: a handbook of quantitative methods. Sage, London

Robson C 2002 Real world research: a resource for social scientists and practitioner-researchers, 2nd edition. Wiley Blackwell, London

Rust J, Golombok S 1989 Modern psychomtrics: the science of psychological assessment. Routledge, London

Schuman H, Presser S 1996 Questions and answers in attitude surveys: experiemnts on question form, wording and context. Sage, London

Chapter 20

Repertory grid analysis

INTRODUCTION

Repertory grid analysis derives from a theory of personality, called Personal Construct Theory, which was developed in the 1950s by George Kelly (Kelly 1955). In essence, the theory proposes that there is no single objective truth about the world; instead, Kelly suggested that individuals interpret events, objects and situations in ways that are specifically meaningful to themselves, personally. Kelly contended that people are actively engaged in trying to make sense out of everyday events, so that they can predict events and situations and then respond appropriately to them. From this very short synopsis of the theory, it is clearly apparent that Kelly's view is essentially experimental, portraying people as scientists who formulate cause–effect hypotheses about their world in order to predict future situations. The theory is, of course, much more detailed than this, and for the interested reader who wishes to pursue it further, there are a number of excellent texts available, a selection of which is presented in the reading list at the end of this chapter.

What is of special relevance to the present book is the method that Kelly developed to assess how individuals make interpretations of their world. This technique is called **repertory grid analysis** and it has an enormous range of applications, in education, personality testing, counselling, occupational psychology and health.

Kelly argued that individuals attempted to make sense of the events in their world by evaluating these events along a finite number of dimensions. The events could be people, ideas, objects, organisations, jobs, social situations, occurrences, etc., and are called **elements.** The interpretative dimensions which are used to make sense of the elements are known as constructs. These constructs are bipolar, that is, they use polar adjectives to describe the elements. Therefore, an element such as a hospital chief executive could be described by a subject along the constructs kind/unkind, or happy/sad or good/bad. Alternatively, bipolar phrases can be used, for example, 'makes me feel optimistic/makes me feel pessimistic'. Because of its adaptability and flexibility, a number of variations on repertory grid analysis have been developed since Kelly's original ideas; however, they all share these two concepts of elements and constructs.

THE APPLICATION OF REPERTORY GRID ANALYSIS TO HEALTH CARE RESEARCH

Repertory grid analysis has particular relevance to health care provision not only because of the flexibility that is inherent within the technique, thus allowing it to be adapted for use in just about any situation, but also because the process is an indirect or opaque one. There are two main advantages of this: first, opacity prevents response bias, simply because it is difficult for participants literally to 'see through' what is being asked of them; consequently they cannot easily predict exactly what the researcher requires and modify their answers accordingly. Second, the indirectness of the method allows the reporting of deeper, more fundamental feelings and viewpoints than would normally be obtained by other data collection exercises. This means that the real source of problems and perspectives can be accessed. A further advantage of the technique includes the richness and extent of the data it generates.

The downside of the approach is that it is time consuming because it is usually undertaken as an experimenter-led activity with individual participants. Also, some subjects find it very difficult

to describe their world in terms of bipolar dimensions. These problems notwithstanding, the technique is an invaluable one for researchers to have in their toolbox.

Some examples of the research areas that could be investigated using repertory grid analysis are:

- identifying those aspects of a health care professional's role that generate most job satisfaction and those that generate least
- establishing the personal and professional qualities of the competent and incompetent therapist
- identifying the critical features of a good therapeutic relationship
- defining the attributes of an outpatient clinic that contribute to patient wellbeing
- investigating the perceptions held by each individual in a multidisciplinary health care team of other co-members, as a first stage in team building
- changes in workforce perception of a hospital culture, following organisational development interventions (using a before–after design).

Key Concepts

- Repertory grid analysis is based on Kelly's (1955) Personal Construct Theory.
- The theory proposes that individuals attempt to make sense of their world by describing it in terms of bipolar adjectives, called **constructs.**
- The events and objects that are described in this way are called **elements.**
- The technique that is used to find out how someone perceives his/her world is called **repertory grid analysis.**
- This technique provides a lot of rich data, it has the capacity to avoid deliberate response distortion and it can be successfully applied to a wide range of research settings, including health care.

BASIC PRINCIPLES OF THE TECHNIQUE

In order to illustrate the basic technique, an example will be used. Let us imagine that we are concerned with the high staff turnover rate in a back-pain clinic. Exit interviews with departing staff have so far thrown no light on the reasons why so many therapists are leaving, although personnel tensions are suspected. As turnover continues to increase, it becomes apparent that not only is staff morale dropping, but patient care is also being compromised. If we could identify the fundamental problems attached to the relevant staff, it is conceivable that some interventions could be made that would reduce the drop-out rate. The repertory grid technique would be ideal in such a situation, because it can access underlying feelings and thoughts about salient issues in a way that most other methods cannot. It would clearly be interpersonally difficult, even at an exit interview, to vilify ex-colleagues openly. The repertory grid, with its indirect approach to information exchange, might overcome this problem.

COLLECTING THE DATA

The researcher decides that he/she will ask each departing member of staff to undertake a repertory grid analysis before leaving. The following protocol is adopted (note again that the repertory grid procedure has many forms; the present one is simply a suggestion):

The therapist is asked to identify eight people in the back-pain clinic who are particularly significant, for either positive or negative reasons. (Note that it is not essential to use eight elements – you can use any number. It is worth noting though, that some participants may find the task very difficult and in such cases, the number of elements required should be reduced accordingly.) These are the elements in the grid and they are written across the top of a sheet of paper. Let's imagine that your subject has come up with the following elements:

1 chief executive of the hospital
2 line manager
3 patient A
4 colleague A
5 colleague B
6 clinic administrator
7 consultant
8 patient services manager.

Under the elements, draw up a matrix for the number of elements you have elicited from your subject, assuming that you will obtain an equal number of constructs. While it is not essential to have an equal number of constructs as elements, it does make the analysis easier. In the present example, we have elicited eight elements and on this basis we would try to elicit eight constructs. Consequently, we need to draw up a 8×8 grid matrix (Figure 20.1).

Randomly place three circles in each row, as shown in Figure 20.1.

Taking the first line, ask the subject to look at the three elements with circles underneath them (in this case elements 1, 4 and 5) and to think about how any two of these three elements are the same as each other, but different from the third. The subject might come up with 'obsessional/relaxed'.

This forms the first bipolar construct and it should be recorded alongside the first row. Ask the subject to identify which end of the construct s/he considers to be negative. In this case, let us assume the subject says 'obsessional'.

Ask the subject to look at all the elements identified at the top of the grid and to give each of them a score out of 10, along the dimension obsessional/relaxed, using a score of 1 to mean the most negative end of the construct (in this case, obsessional), and 10 for the positive end (in this case relaxed). Consequently, every element will receive a score somewhere between 1 and 10, according to how the subject assesses it on the obsessional/relaxed dimension.

Repeat the process for each of the eight rows in the grid, asking the subject in each case to focus on the elements identified by the circles below them, and to consider how any two of the three elements are similar to each other but different from the third. *It is important to note that factual differences between the elements should not be used. For example, do not permit the subject to say that two of the elements are male and one is female, or that two are administrators and the third is a clinician. The constructs should represent a psychological attribute.*

When the subject has completed all eight rows in the above way, you should have eight bipolar constructs. Each element should have a score between 1 and 10 on each of the constructs. Let's imagine we obtain the following bipolar constructs:

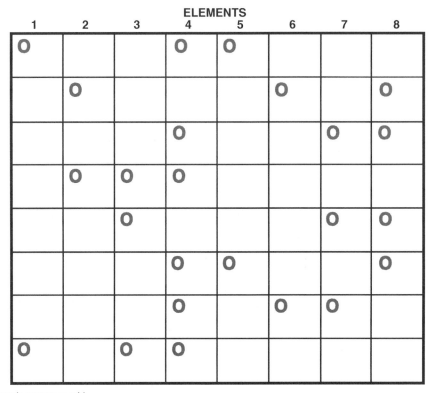

Figure 20.1   Sample repertory grid.

obsessional / relaxed
arrogant / humble
unintelligent / intelligent
rigid / flexible
slapdash / fastidious
critical / supportive
demanding / reasonable
emotionally closed / emotionally open

The negative end of each construct, as it applies in this context, is indicated by italics above.

Key Concepts

- There are many ways of conducting a repertory grid analysis, but they all involve asking the subject to rate the elements along a set of bipolar constructs.
- In the method described here, the subject is asked to identify a number of significant events/people/objects which constitute the elements.

- The subject is then asked to consider three randomly chosen elements from the set and state how any two are the same as each other but different from the third; factual descriptions are not acceptable.
- The way in which these three elements are described relative to each other comprises the first bipolar construct.
- The subject is asked to give each of the elements along this dimension a score between 1 and 10, with 1 representing the negative aspect of the dimension and 10 the positive end, as defined by the subject.
- The process is repeated until the same number of constructs has been elicited as there are elements and each element has been scored along each construct.

INTERPRETING THE GRID

You will see that the bipolar constructs are not necessarily obvious opposites, but this isn't too important. It is also apparent that some of the constructs are quite similar to one another; for example 'rigid' and 'obsessional' have similar meanings, as do 'relaxed' and 'flexible'. This would suggest that this subject is perceiving her working world in terms of a small number of related constructs. This is a very important aspect of repertory grid analysis. Some people have complex, highly differentiated views of the world and consequently use a large number of quite different constructs to describe it. Other people have a more unified perception, and so employ constructs that are semantically similar.

We now need to establish whether or how the constructs relate to each other at a deeper level – in other words which are the core underlying constructs and which the surface constructs. In the present example, we now need to find out which of these eight constructs is related in the mind of the respondent.

Let's imagine we obtained the scores shown in Table 20.1.

It should be pointed out that there are a number of very sophisticated computer programs available that will analyse grids in great detail. For example, the *Grid Analysis Package* (GAP) is capable of analysing individual grids, before/after paired comparisons, groups of grids, etc. Since, however, there is a danger of losing sight of the real issues under the mound of data these packages generate, individual,

manual analysis is often recommended. The following stages are one simple way of interpreting a completed matrix, so that an intuitive grasp of the participant's world view can be ascertained. It is called entailment analysis (Gaines & Shaw 1980, adapted by Barwell 1998).

To see how this subject's view of the world relates in terms of the underlying constructs, it is now necessary to recode the responses, using the following protocol:

- all scores in the matrix that come between 1 and 5 are now recoded 1
- all scores in the matrix that come between 6 and 10 are now recoded 0.

These recoded scores are entered into the matrix as in Table 20.2.

Now focusing on just those elements that have a recoded value of 1, look at the first construct and list all the elements with a code of 1 by the construct obsessional/relaxed. In this case, we have elements 1, 2, 3, 4, 6, 7 and 8. These are identified in bold type in Table 20.2.

Repeat the procedure for each construct in turn. Table 20.2 shows the finished product.

Entailment analysis

The principle underlying the next step is to see which construct(s) incorporate or entail the others. The ones that incorporate other constructs can be considered to be the **source constructs,**

Table 20.1   Scores out of 10 for each construct

Chief executive	Line manager	Patient A	Colleague A	Colleague B	Clinic administrator	Consultant	Patient services manager	
				Elements				
1	2	3	4	5	6	7	8	Constructs
3	1	5	5	8	2	4	3	Obessional/relaxed
4	2	7	5	6	3	2	2	Arrogant/humble
9	3	3	7	6	6	7	7	Unintelligent/intelligent
4	2	6	8	5	3	1	2	Rigid/flexible
8	2	6	6	5	2	8	2	Slapdash/fastidious
6	1	4	5	9	1	1	2	Critical/supportive
3	1	5	8	5	2	1	2	Demanding/reasonable
5	1	8	5	5	2	3	10	Emotionally closed/ emotionally open

Table 20.2   Matrix of Table 20.1 with recoded scores

Chief executive	Line manager	Patient A	Colleague A	Colleague B	Clinic administrator	Consultant	Patient services manager	Constructs
1	2	3	4	5	6	7	8	
1	1	1	1	0	1	1	1	Obsessional/relaxed: 1, 2, 3, 4, 6, 7, 8
1	1	0	1	0	1	1	1	Arrogant/humble: 1, 2, 4, 6, 7, 8
0	1	1	0	0	0	0	0	Unintelligent/intelligent: 2, 3
1	1	0	0	1	1	1	1	Rigid/flexible: 1, 2, 5, 6, 7, 8
0	1	0	0	1	1	0	1	Slapdash/fastidious: 2, 5, 6, 8
0	1	1	1	0	1	1	1	Critical/supportive: 2, 3, 4, 6, 7, 8
1	1	1	0	1	1	1	1	Demanding/reasonable: 1, 2, 3, 5, 6, 7, 8
1	1	0	1	1	1	1	0	Emotionally closed/ emotionally open: 1, 2, 4, 5, 6, 7

The columns are labelled under the heading **Elements**.

from which the others emerge. We do this by constructing a diagram, and for the following steps you will need a large sheet of paper.

- First identify the construct that has the fewest number of elements listed by it. This is a surface construct that will have emerged from a deeper source construct. In this case, it is construct 3, which includes the elements 2 and 3. Turning your paper in landscape orientation, write 'Construct 3' on the extreme left, with the elements in brackets by the side, as shown in Figure 20.2.
- Now focus on the constructs with the next fewest number of elements. In this case, it is construct 5 (elements 2, 5, 6 and 8). You now have to ask yourself whether *all* the elements attached to construct 3 are also included in those attached to construct 5. Since construct 3 has elements 2 and 3, and construct 5 has 2, 5, 6 and 8, there is only partial overlap and therefore we cannot conclude that construct 5 incorporates construct 3. Construct 5 must therefore be incorporated by a different

source construct. So you now have to write 'Construct 5' with its attached elements underneath Construct 3 and a little way to the right across the page as shown in Figure 20.3.
- Now take the constructs that have the *next* fewest number of attached elements. Here they are construct 2 (elements 1, 2, 4, 6, 7 and 8), construct 4 (elements 1, 2, 5, 6, 7 and 8), construct 6 (elements 2, 3, 4, 6, 7 and 8) and construct 8 (elements 1, 2, 4, 5, 6 and 7). We now have to see which of these *totally* incorporates either of the earlier two constructs.
- We find that construct 6 (elements 2, 3, 4, 6, 7 and 8) alone contains all the elements attached to construct 3 (elements 2 and 3) and so we draw a link between these two (see Figure 20.4). Construct 4 (elements 1, 2, 5, 6, 7 and 8) contains all the elements associated with construct 5 (elements 2, 5, 6 and 8). A line is now drawn between these (Figure 20.4). Note that as we deal with increasing numbers of elements, we move

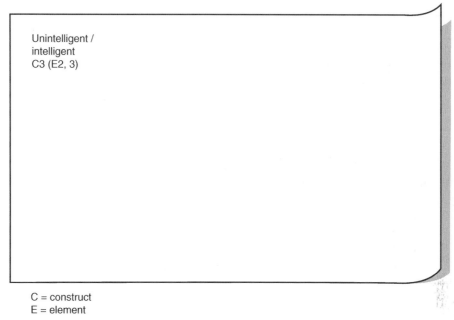

Unintelligent /
intelligent
C3 (E2, 3)

C = construct
E = element

Figure 20.2   Entailment analysis (i).

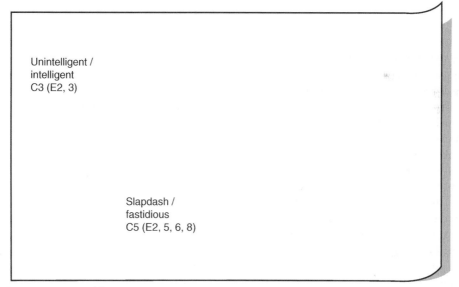

Unintelligent /
intelligent
C3 (E2, 3)

Slapdash /
fastidious
C5 (E2, 5, 6, 8)

Figure 20.3   Entailment analysis (ii).

across the page. This gives the effect of branching.

- It can be seen from this, then, that constructs 4 and 6 are source constructs for 3 and 5. Constructs 2 and 8 do not totally incorporate the earlier surface constructs and therefore must be considered to be independent or *orphan* constructs. These are arranged at the bottom of the page as in Figure 20.4.

- Now we look at the constructs that contain the next fewest number of elements; here it is construct 1 (elements 1, 2, 3, 4, 6, 7 and 8)

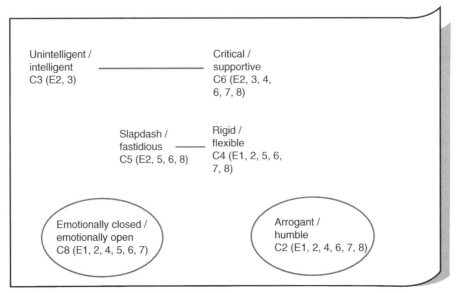

Figure 20.4   Entailment analysis (iii).

and construct 7 (elements 1, 2, 3, 5, 6, 7 and 8). We now need to see whether either of these incorporates fully the constructs identified in the previous stage (constructs 4 and 6). As construct 1 contains all the elements of construct 6, we draw a line between these two, again moving across the page, as in Figure 20.5. Construct 7 contains all the elements associated with construct 4, so we draw a line between these two (Figure 20.5).

- We now have a clearer idea about how the constructs link to each other, and which source constructs (extreme right of page) give rise through the intermediate constructs (middle of the page) to the surface constructs (left of the page). What we have here are two **source constructs** (1 and 7), two **intermediate constructs** (6 and 4) and two **surface constructs** (3 and 5). There are also two **orphan constructs** that do not subsume anything (2 and 8). This subject, then, perceives her world of work in terms of the constructs obsessional/relaxed, demanding/reasonable, arrogant/humble and emotionally closed/emotionally open. The key people at work are therefore

described in this person's mind along these basic dimensions. However, what we do not yet know is the strength of the link between each of these constructs and that is where some statistical analysis comes in.

- We need to compute a correlation coefficient to assess the degree of association between each of the constructs that are linked, in other words between:

construct 3 and construct 6
construct 6 and construct 1
construct 5 and construct 4
construct 4 and construct 7

Looking back to Table 20.1, where each element had been given a score between 1 and 10 on each construct, we need to calculate a Pearson product moment correlation coefficient on the data attaching to each pair of constructs identified above. To give one worked example, we take the first linked pair of constructs, 3 and 6, and the row of scores applying to each. Calling construct 3 'variable A' and construct 6 'variable B', we follow steps 1–9 for calculating the Pearson test (Chapter 17, pp. 240–243), leading to Table 20.3. We end up with:

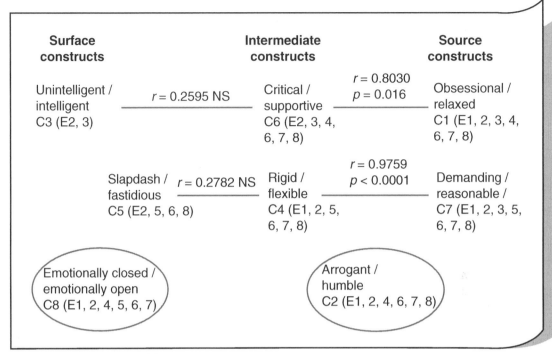

Figure 20.5   Entailment analysis (iv).

Table 20.3

Variable *A* Construct 3	Variable *B* Construct 6	*A* × *B*	*A²*	*B²*
9	6	54	81	36
3	1	3	9	1
3	4	12	9	16
7	5	35	49	25
6	9	54	36	81
6	1	6	36	1
7	1	7	49	1
7	2	14	49	4
Σ*A* = 48	Σ*B* = 29	Σ(*A*×*B*) = 185	Σ*A²* = 318	Σ*B²* = 165

$$r = \frac{8(185)-(48\times 29)}{\sqrt{[(8\times 318)-2304][(8\times 165)-841]}}$$

$$= \frac{1480-1392}{\sqrt{[2544-2304][1320-841]}}$$

$$= \frac{88}{\sqrt{240\times 479}}$$

$$= \frac{88}{339.058}$$

$$= 0.2595 \ (\text{not significant})$$

This correlation coefficient is entered along the line between constructs 3 and 6, on Figure 20.5. The correlations between each pair of linked constructs are calculated in the same way and the results entered along the relevant linkage line as shown in Figure 20.5.

We can see then that there is a significant correlation between the source construct 1 and intermediate construct 6, but that there is only a weak link between 6 and surface construct 3. Similarly, source construct 7 and intermediate construct 4 are significantly correlated, but the relevant

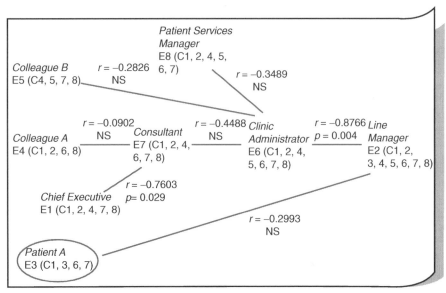

Figure 20.6   Entailment analysis for elements.

surface construct 5 has only a weak link. This suggests that the dimensions obsessional/relaxed and critical/supportive are closely linked as descriptors, and demanding/reasonable is closely linked with rigid/flexible. Intelligent/unintelligent has a weaker connection with its source dimension, as does slapdash/fastidious. This subject then sees her colleagues principally along the dimensions obsessional/relaxed, demanding/reasonable, and the two orphan dimensions arrogant/humble and emotionally closed/emotionally open.

To see how the elements are related as source and surface elements, the procedure is repeated, by turning Table 20.2 through 90°, and performing the same entailment process, but this time counting how many constructs each element has in common. The results are shown in Figure 20.6.

This linkage suggests that the line manager, who has all the negative ends of all the constructs (remember, the recode of 1 was allocated to the scores that reflected the negative descriptor) is the apparent source of most of the dissatisfaction in the unit. The clinic administrator, the consultant and the patient services manager also cause some of the difficulties, with the chief executive and then the two colleagues and patient A being relatively unproblematic. It would seem then,

that the immediate colleagues and the identified patient cause the subject least difficulties, but that the line manager is the major problem within this clinic.

If we inspect the two entailment analyses together, we can see that the negative ends of all the main constructs apply to the source element (the line manager, thus confirming that there appear to be major difficulties with this person, who is perceived to be obsessional and demanding (as well as possessing the negative poles of the intermediate and surface constructs that spring from these), arrogant and emotionally closed. The clinic administrator, the patient services manager and consultant, also cause difficulties for the departing subject, because they possess many of the negative descriptors the subject uses to describe her world of work. Colleagues, the chief executive and the patient are construed more positively, so we might conclude that the reason for this subject's departure does not lie primarily with these people. The repertory grid has provided some insight as to the nature of the problem, at least for this subject, relating to the work environment of the back-pain clinic. If repertory grids are performed on other departing staff and yield similar results, then there would be a clear case for strategic intervention to improve the working culture of the clinic and so prevent more staff from leaving. The repertory grid analysis has provided a depth and richness of data about the real issues surrounding this work situation, in a way that other, more transparent techniques might not.

ACKNOWLEDGEMENT

My sincere thanks are due to Dr Fred Barwell, whose knowledge of statistics and his capacity to explain them enabled the adaptation of entailment analysis for use here.

> ### Key Concepts
>
> - To make sense of the repertory grid results, it is to see how the constructs are related to one another in the subject's mind
> - The relationship between the constructs can be determined by undertaking an entailment analysis which shows how each construct relates to the others. This gives rise to a picture of source and surface constructs.
> - If correlation coefficients on the scores associated with the linked constructs are performed using a Pearson product moment correlation coefficient, the strength of the links can be assessed.

> - The same procedures can be applied to the analysis of the elements; this allows the researcher to identify how the salient aspects of the subject's world relate to each other.

FURTHER READING

Bannister D, Fransella F 1990 Inquiring man. Penguin, Harmondsworth

Barwell F 1998. Personal communication

Butler R 2008 Reflections in personal construct theory. John Wiley & Sons, Chichester

Butt T 2008 George Kelly: the psychology of personal constructs (mindshapers). Palgrave Macmillan, London

Cohen L, Mannion L 2007 Research methods in education, 6th edition. Croom Helm, London

Cross V 1998 Begging to differ? Clinicians' and academics' views on desirable attributes for physiotherapy students on clinical placement. Assessment and Evaluation in Higher Education 23(3):295–311

Fransella F 2005 The essential handbook of personal construct theory. Wiley Blackwell, Chichester

Fransella F, Bannister D, Bell R 2003 A manual for repertory grid technique, 2nd edition. Wiley Blackwell, Chichester

Gaines BR, Shaw M 1980 New directions in the analysis and interaction elicitation of personal construct systems. International Journal of Man-Machine Studies 13(1): 81–116

Jancowicz D 2003 The easy guide to repertory grids. Wiley Blackwell, Chichester

Kelly G 1955 The psychology of personal constructs, Vols 1 and 2. Norton, New York

Chapter 21

Using statistics in diagnostic and screening tests: Receiver Operating Characteristics

CHAPTER CONTENTS

INTRODUCTION

Receiver Operating Characteristics (ROC) have their origins in signal detection theory, used during World War II by signal operators who were engaged in trying to interpret the information on radar screens. Their task was a difficult one, because of the level of interference; consequently, the signal operators first had to decide whether or not they had seen a blip on the screen and then they had to decide whether the blip represented an enemy or allied ship. Clearly, their decision determined the subsequent actions i.e. to attack or not. Accuracy at each level of decision-making was therefore crucial to avoid either attacking friendly ships or not attacking enemy ones. It was not until about 40 years ago that the relevance of ROC to clinical decision-making became apparent.

In health care, ROC is used in diagnostic testing, to establish whether or not someone has a particular disease or condition (e.g. diabetes, prostate cancer, sarcoma, etc.), as well as in screening, to determine whether someone is at risk of getting a disease, or has asymptomatic early stages of a condition (e.g. screening all neonates for PKU, or all women of a certain age for cervical cancer). As therapists' autonomy and scope of practice continue to increase, so too, will the pressure for some diagnostic skills (e.g. the Red Flag system) and for screening decisions. The triage nurse is a typical example. While some diagnoses and screening assessments may be straightforward, there will be many situations in which decision-making may be much more complex, for example, when conditions have similar presenting symptoms making diagnosis or referral difficult, or when further tests carry a risk to the patient, or whether a patient can be safely discharged from hospital, with only minimal risk of relapse or complications. In such instances, the therapist will want to be confident that the decisions taken are accurate, since errors may compromise the patient's welfare. It is in situations such as these that ROC analysis has value. I should point out that although this may look like a complex and lengthy process, the calculations are surprisingly easy, once the concepts are understood.

Let's illustrate ROC analysis with an example. A therapist working in an obstetrics and gynaecology unit is concerned about the number of women presenting for the 6-week postnatal check-up with severe perineal morbidity, which has resulted in stress incontinence. The therapist wonders whether there would be any way of screening women immediately after birth to assess whether they are at risk of developing stress incontinence. If a valid risk scale could be developed that would identify those women most likely to develop problems, then additional post-natal support and specialist exercise regimes could be offered. The task, then, is to develop a valid risk-assessment scale that, with reasonable accuracy, could spot those women most at risk from stress incontinence.

The first stage in this process is to undertake a thorough thematic review of the literature, to see what factors are associated with postnatal stress incontinence. (It should also be pointed out that multiple and logistic regression analyses described by Pallant (2007) are very useful starting points for developing a risk assessment scale, in that they both identify the best predictors of a given outcome – in this case, stress incontinence. However, these sorts of regression analyses require a computer and relevant software package, such as SPSS and so are outside the scope of this book; Pallant (2007) has a very useful guide to these procedures). Let us further imagine that the thematic review yielded 10 factors that have been shown to be associated with postpartum stress incontinence (remember that this is all hypothetical):

- mother's age
- parity
- length of first stage of labour
- third degree tears or episiotomy
- size of the baby
- maternal weight gain during pregnancy
- use of epidural analgesia during labour
- pre-natal stress incontinence
- assisted vaginal delivery (forceps or ventouse)
- chronic constipation.

The therapist then draws up a risk scale, which we will call the Stress Incontinence Scale or SIS:

1. Age – if >35 years, score 1 ☐
2. parity – if >2 previous deliveries, score 1 ☐
3. first stage of labour – if >20 hours, score 1 ☐
4. 3rd degree tears or episiotomy – if yes to either, score 1 ☐
5. size of baby – if >4.5 kg, score 1. ☐
6. weight gain during pregnancy – if >15 kg, score 1 ☐
7. use of epidural analgesia – if yes, score 1 ☐
8. pre-natal stress incontinence – if yes, score 1 ☐
9. assisted vaginal delivery – if forceps or ventouse, score 1 ☐
10. chronic constipation – if yes, score 1 ☐
TOTAL ☐

The maximum score a woman could obtain would be 10, indicating a very high risk of postnatal stress incontinence, while the lowest score would be 0, indicating a minimum risk of stress incontinence. To establish whether this scale has any value, it must first be tested on a group of women who have actually presented with stress incontinence at the 6-week postnatal check-up and a further group of women who have not, to see whether the scale reveals any difference between the groups' scores. This will indicate whether the test has any power to discriminate between these groups, and therefore, whether it will have any accuracy in identifying women most likely to develop stress incontinence. The way in which this is done using a ROC protocol follows some key stages, which will be explained step by step below. However, some key concepts that relate to ROC will be explained.

SOME KEY CONCEPTS THAT RELATE TO DIAGNOSTIC AND SCREENING TESTS

The first point to note is that a good diagnostic or screening test is one that:

- *Correctly* identifies all those people *with* the risk factors (or with the disease); in our case, a high SIS score will correspond with a high risk of developing stress incontinence. The people correctly identified to have the risk or disease are called **true positives** (TP)
- *Correctly* identifies all those people *without* the risk factors (or the disease); in our case, a low SIS score will correspond with a low risk of developing stress incontinence. The people who are correctly identified as not having the risk/disease are called **true negatives** (TN)

However, diagnostic and screening tests are very rarely absolutely accurate, in that:

- some people with the risk/disease might be missed; in our case, the SIS scores might be low, but these women go on to develop stress incontinence. The people who are at risk or who have the disease but who are not picked up are called **false negatives** (FN), i.e. they're classified as not having the problem, when, in fact, they do have it. These are similar to the Type II errors discussed on p. 110 in that Type II errors occur when the hypothesis is classed as not having been supported by the data, when it has.
- some people without the risk/disease will be identified as having the risk/disease; in our case, the SIS scores may be high, but the women do not go on to develop stress incontinence. The people who don't actually have the risk /disease, but who have been identified as having it are called **false positives** (FP); i.e. they're classified as having the disease when, in fact, they don't. These are similar to the Type I errors discussed on p. 110, in that Type I errors are those when the hypothesis is said to

have been supported by the data, when it hasn't.

Clearly a good diagnostic or screening test will have high rates of true positives and true negatives, and low rates of false positives and false negatives. The false classifications may have serious implications for the patients, in that people classed as false negatives may miss out on further investigations or treatment, while those classed as false positives may end up having investigations and treatment they don't need. Depending on the clinical problem in question, these incorrect classifications may have serious consequences for the patients. These four classifications are essential to ROC and are represented in Table 21.1 below:

Table 21.1 Possible outcomes of diagnostic and screening tests

Negative results	Positive results
False negatives: Patient does have the risk/disease, but the test does not pick it up. This would lead to an incorrect decision not to refer for further investigations or treatment	True positives: Patient does have the risk/ disease, and the test picks it up. This would lead to a correct decision to refer for further investigations or treatment
True negatives: Patient does not have the risk/disease, and the test is negative. This would lead to a correct decision not to refer for further investigations or treatment	False positives: Patient does not have the risk/ disease, but the test says they do. This would lead to an incorrect decision to refer for further investigations or treatment

The second point to note is the capacity of a diagnostic or screening test to *correctly* identify those people who *do* have the risk/disease; this is called '**sensitivity**'. Therefore, sensitivity is the ability of a test to identify people with the risk/ disease. The capacity of a test to *correctly* identify those people who *do not* have the risk/disease is called '**specificity**'. Therefore, specificity is the ability of a test to identify the normal. Obviously, a test with high sensitivity and high specificity is a good test.

Key Concepts

- ROC analysis is used in diagnostic and screening tests to identify people who either have a condition or who are at risk of developing it.
- Diagnostic and screening tests should be able to:
  - correctly identify those people who have the condition/risk ; these are known as true positives
  - correctly identify those people who do not have the condition/risk; these are known as true negatives.
- The ability of a diagnostic or screening test to correctly identify people with the condition/risk is known as sensitivity.
- The ability of a diagnostic or screening test to correctly identify people without the condition/risk is known as specificity.
- Diagnostic and screening tests are rarely perfectly accurate; therefore:
  - some people might be identified as not having the condition/risk when, in fact, they do; these are known as false negatives and/or
  - some people might be identified as having the disease when, in fact, they don't; these are known as false positives.
- A good diagnostic or screening test will have high numbers of true positives and true negatives, and hence high sensitivity and high specificity; a good test will also have low numbers of false positives and false negatives.

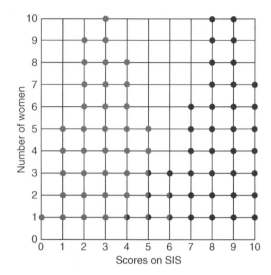

● Women with stress incontinence

● Women without stress incontinence

Figure 21.1   Hypothetical results on SIS scale from women with stress incontinence and women without.

CALCULATING THE SENSITIVITY AND SPECIFICITY OF A DIAGNOSTIC OR SCREENING TEST

To establish whether a test is sensitive and specific, the number of people falling into each of the four cells in Figure 21.1 must first be counted up. *Test sensitivity* is then measured by:

$$\frac{\text{Number of true positives}}{\text{Number of true positives} + \text{number oft rue negatives}}$$

while *test specificity* is measured by:

$$\frac{\text{number of true negatives}}{\text{number of true negatives} + \text{number of false positives}}$$

AN EXAMPLE OF THE USE OF ROC ANALYSIS IN A CLINICAL SETTING

If we apply these concepts to our example of risk assessment of stress incontinence using the SIS, they may become clearer. In order to evaluate our risk scale, we need to use it with women known to have stress incontinence and with women known not to have it, to see whether there are any differences in their scores on the SIS. For ease of demonstration, we will use the SIS with 40 women who have stress incontinence and 40 who haven't. In reality, a test would be developed on many more than this. When selecting your sample it is essential that you include an appropriate range of participants on your variables: for example, a range of ages; a range of parity; women with severe stress incontinence, moderate stress incontinence, mild stress incontinence and no stress incontinence; range of neonatal birth weights, etc., otherwise it would be easy to ensure the success of your instrument by only selecting those who are most likely to respond in the required way. Bearing in mind the maximum risk score a woman could obtain is 10, and the minimum 0, we get the following (hypothetical) results (Table 21.2):

Table 21.2   Hypothetical scores on SIS scale

Score on SIS	Number of women without incontinence recording this score	Number of women with incontinence recording this score
0	1	0
1	5	0
2	9	0
3	10	0
4	8	1
5	5	3
6	2	3
7	0	6
8	0	10
9	0	10
10	0	7
TOTAL	40	40

These findings can be plotted on a graph, with the SIS scores along the X (horizontal) axis and the number of women achieving each score along the Y (vertical) axis. The graph is presented in Figure 21.1. (Please note that instead of the usual frequency polygon or histogram, I have plotted each participant as a dot to make the subsequent explanations clearer).

While the graph suggests that there is a marked difference between the scores of the two groups, this should be tested using the Mann–Whitney U test (do not use the unrelated t-test here, even if the data are interval/ratio). Comparing the individual scores of the 40 women with stress incontinence with those of the 40 without, using a Mann–Whitney to see whether there are significant differences in the scores, the following results are obtained:

$$U = 27.5, n_1 = 40, n_2 = 40, p < 0.005 \text{ for a}$$
1-tailed hypothesis.

(As our Mann–Whitney U tables only go up to $n_1 = 20$, $n_2 = 20$, I have had to extrapolate.) This means that there is a significant difference in SIS scores between the women with stress incontinence and those without. If you were to get non-significant results at this stage, proceeding with the ROC analysis would have questionable value. As it is, the significant results mean that we can proceed with the ROC analysis.

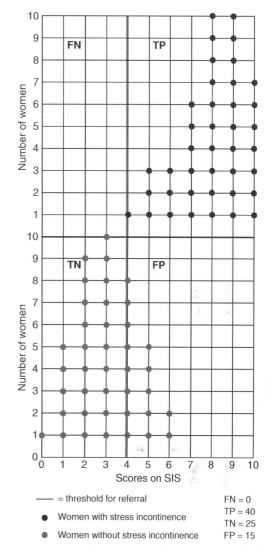

= threshold for referral

● Women with stress incontinence

● Women without stress incontinence

FN = 0
TP = 40
TN = 25
FP = 15

Figure 21.2   Hypothetical results on SIS scale showing true positives, true negatives, false positives and false negatives when the threshold for referral is set at 4.

The graph presented in Figure 21.1 must now be interpreted. From this we can see that all women who have stress incontinence score between 4 and 10 on the SIS, with the majority getting 8 or 9. The women who do not have stress incontinence all score between 0 and 6, with the majority getting 2 or 3. In other words, the test looks as though it is differentiating between the two groups of women, but there is an overlap in the scores of 4, 5 and 6, since some women who have stress incontinence and some who don't all record scores of 4, 5 and 6. On this basis, at what point would we refer a woman for further support and exercises?

DECIDING ON THE THRESHOLD FOR REFERRAL/TREATMENT

If we said all women with scores of 4 and above, this would mean that from our sample, all the women who do get stress incontinence would get help, but 15 women who do not develop stress incontinence will be unnecessarily referred (these are the false positives – the non-stress incontinence women scoring 4, 5 and 6). The cut-off point for is called the **threshold**. This can be illustrated with an adapted graph – see Figure 21.2. Remember that:

True positive = TP   False positive = FP
False negative = FN   True negative = TN

We might want to adjust this threshold, because of the high number of women being referred for unnecessary treatment. With a revised threshold of 5, the graph now looks like this (Figure 21.3):

Likewise, the threshold can be moved up to 6, with the following results (Figure 21.4)

If on the other hand, we said that only women scoring 7 and above would get referred, then none of the women who don't get stress incontinence will get unnecessary intervention, but 7 women who do get stress incontinence will not be referred for further help (these are the false negatives – the stress incontinence women scoring 4, 5 and 6 on the SIS). The true positives, true negatives, false positives and false negatives are shown as Figure 21.5.

By setting the threshold at different points, we can alter the sensitivity and specificity of the test. Therefore, at what threshold should we decide to refer? In order to answer this, we must remember that a good test should have high sensitivity (i.e. can correctly identify all those people who are at risk or have the disease) and high specificity (i.e. can correctly identify all those people who do not have the risk/disease). Both sensitivity and specificity are scored on a scale of 0–1.0, (though these scores can be converted to %); using the formulae above, with the closer the scores to 1.0, the better the sensitivity and specificity. We can

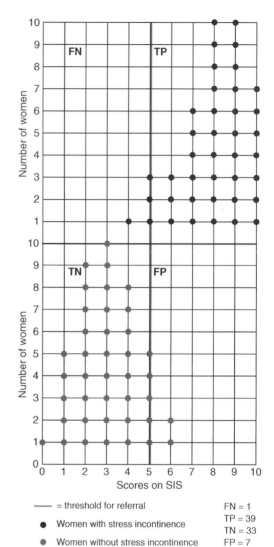

Figure 21.3 Hypothetical results on SIS scale showing true positives, true negatives, false positives and false negatives when the threshold for referral is set at 5.

calculate these values for each of the possible referral points on our scale.

CALCULATING SENSITIVITY AND SPECIFICITY FOR THE SIS

If we want to ensure that we capture *all* the women at risk of developing stress incontinence, then we would set the threshold, at 4, since this would mean we didn't miss anyone. In other words, if we want a high sensitivity rate, then all women who get 4+ on the SIS will get further

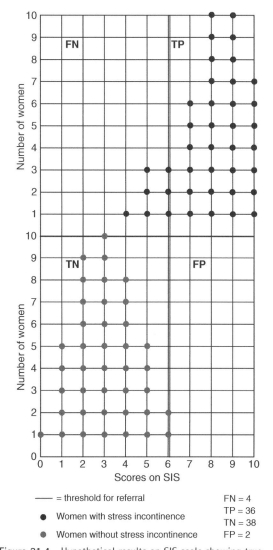

Figure 21.4   Hypothetical results on SIS scale showing true positives, true negatives, false positives and false negatives when the threshold for referral is set at 6.

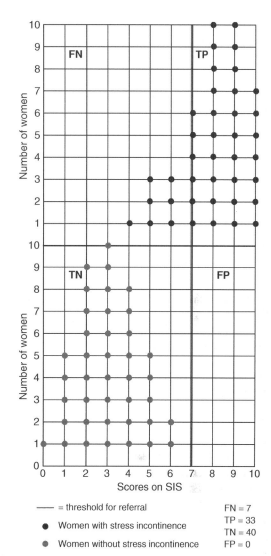

Figure 21.5   Hypothetical results on SIS scale showing true positives, true negatives, false positives and false negatives when the threshold for referral is set at 7.

intervention, even though some of these might not need it. Therefore, we need to use the figures from Figure 21.2 in our calculations.

The sensitivity score with a threshold of 4 is:

$$\text{Sensitivity} = \frac{\text{TP}}{\text{TP} + \text{FN}}$$

$$= \frac{40}{40 - 0}$$

$$= 1.0 \, (100\%)$$

Therefore, with a threshold for referral of 4, the SIS sensitivity score is perfect.

Using the following formula to calculate specificity:

$$\text{Specificity} = \frac{\text{TN}}{\text{TN} + \text{FP}}$$

$$= \frac{25}{25 + 15}$$

$$= 0.63 \, (63\%)$$

Therefore, the threshold of 4 gives a much lower and rather unsatisfactory specificity score of 0.63. This means that 0.37 or 37% of women may get unnecessarily referred for treatment they don't need, which may be very wasteful of time and resources.

If we move the threshold for referral up to 5 and using the figures from Figure 21.3, then the sensitivity score becomes:

$$\frac{39}{39+1}$$

$$=0.98\,(98\%)$$

And the specificity score becomes:

$$\frac{33}{33+8}$$

$$=0.83\,(83\%)$$

This threshold means that there is a slight drop in sensitivity and a significant rise in specificity.

If we move the threshold to 6 and using the figures from Figure 21.4, then sensitivity becomes:

$$\frac{36}{36+4}$$

$$=0.90\,(90\%)$$

And specificity becomes

$$\frac{38}{38+2}$$

$$=0.95\,(95\%)$$

Therefore, if the threshold for referral is moved to an SIS score of 6, then sensitivity drops to 90%, but specificity rise to 95%.

And finally, if the threshold for referral for treatment is set at an SIS score of 7, and using the figures from Figure 21.5, then sensitivity becomes:

$$\frac{33}{33+7}$$

$$=0.83\,(83\%)$$

And specificity becomes:

$$\frac{40}{40+0}$$

$$=1.0\,(100\%)$$

Table 21.3 Sensitivity and specificity scores for various thresholds on SIS

Threshold for referral on SIS	Sensitivity	Specificity
4	1.0	0.63
5	0.98	0.80
6	0.90	0.95
7	0.83	1.0

Table 21.3 summarises these results.

You can see from this that by changing the threshold for referral you can adjust the sensitivity and specificity scores of a test, and with them, the number of people who are referred for treatment. However, as the test does not have perfect sensitivity *and* specificity, then there will have to be a trade-off about whether you overlook people who need treatment but don't get it (i.e. the false negatives) or whether you send people for treatment even though some may not need it (false positives). Where you set your threshold will depend on the consequences of having the disease and not being treated, or on the consequences of having treatment for a disease the patient doesn't have. Clearly, then, the decision is very dependent on the clinical situation. For some clinical situations, it is better to have a high sensitivity rate, so that everyone who needs an intervention or treatment gets it. An example of this is the routine blood test for PKU given to all neonates. While only a very small number will actually have the condition, the test is so straightforward and non-invasive that it is better to ensure that every baby with the disease is picked up, so that they can be treated. For other clinical conditions, it may be better to have a high specificity rate, in order to avoid giving an intervention to people who don't need it. Treatments that are invasive, risky or costly would suggest that a high specificity might be desirable – *but it will depend on the condition being studied*. The final decision about the threshold will be based on extensive research, best evidence and expert opinion, but where there is no clear case for high sensitivity rather than high specificity and vice versa, then a formula called Youden's Index can be used to decide the threshold.

YOUDEN'S INDEX FOR CALCULATING THE SUITABILITY OF THRESHOLDS

Youden's Index is expressed as J and is calculated using the sensitivity and specificity values for our test. The closer Youden's Index J is to 1.0 the better the selected threshold. Youden's index formula is:

$$J = sensitivity + specificity - 1$$

Therefore, taking our four sensitivity and specificity values above, we can calculate four values for J:

1. Threshold of 4

$$J = 1.0 + 0.63 - 1$$

$$= 0.63$$

2. Threshold of 5

$$J = 0.98 + 0.83 - 1$$

$$= 0.81$$

3. Threshold of 6

$$J = 0.9 + 0.95 - 1$$

$$= 0.85$$

4. Threshold of 7

$$J = 0.83 + 1.0 - 1$$

$$= 0.83$$

For our test, then, it would seem that the highest Youden's Index of 0.85 comes from sensitivity value of 0.9 and a specificity value of 0.85, which are associated with a threshold for referral of 6 on our SIS. Therefore, any women who scored 6 and above would be targeted for further intervention.

THE ROC GRAPH

We can further assess the performance of our SIS by plotting the sensitivity and specificity scores on a ROC graph. By calculating the area under the line, we can derive a measure of the test's performance. The area under the line is called the AUROC (Area Under Receiver Operating Characteristics) curve – the greater the area under the line, the better the test. To plot our sensitivity

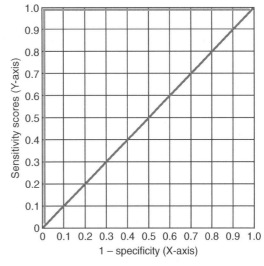

—— A perfect test with 100% performance accuracy
—— A poor test with only a 50:50 chance of accuracy

Figure 21.6   AUROC curves demonstrating a test with poor diagnostic/screening performance and a test with perfect diagnostic/screening performance.

and specificity scores, we need to use a 10×10 cell graph like Figure 21.6 (because both sensitivity and specificity are measured from 0–1.0 in units of 0.1)

The X axis represents the false positive scores calculated as 1 – specificity, while the Y axis represents the sensitivity scores. A test which had no diagnostic or screening function would be represented by a straight diagonal line, indicated by the dotted line in Figure 21.6; the area under the diagonal line would be 50% or 0.5, suggesting that the test's ability to identify patients at risk or with a disease is 50:50 or chance. A perfect test would be indicated by a line that went straight up the vertical or Y axis from the point where both sensitivity and 1 – specificity scores equal 0, and then horizontally across the top of the graph to the top right hand corner (where sensitivity and 1 – specificity scores both equal 1.0) – indicated by a grey line. The area under the line of the perfect test is 1.0 or 100%, suggesting that it has perfect capacity to identify people with the risk/disease. Obviously the vast majority of tests do not come near this, but the closer the area under the line comes to 1.0, the better the test.

Table 21.4 Values of sensitivity and 1 – specificity for plotting on ROC curve

Sensitivity	Specificity	1 – Specificity
0.00		0.00
0.83	1.00	0.00
0.90	0.95	0.05
0.98	0.83	0.17
1.0	0.63	0.37
1.00		1.00

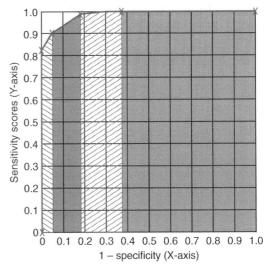

Figure 21.7 AUROC curve for SIS performance.

To calculate our AUROC value, we first need to plot each pair of sensitivity and 1 – specificity scores we obtained. In addition, we need to ensure that we also plot additional values of

$$\text{sensitivity} = 0, \ 1-\text{specificity} = 0$$

and

$$\text{sensitivity} = 1.0, \ 1-\text{specificity} = 1.0$$

to ensure that our plotted line starts at the bottom left hand corner and finishes at the top right hand corner. These values have been added to Table 21.4.

Taking our sensitivity and 1 – specificity results shown in Table 21.4, we need to plot each pair of values. The graph or ROC line is presented in Figure 21.7. The convention is to join the plots using a series of straight lines, rather than a curved one.

To calculate the area under the ROC curve, you can either count the number of squares under it, or more properly and accurately, you can use the following system, which allows you to calculate the area beneath each pair of dots on the graph: The areas you need to calculate are represented as: downward sloping dotted line; pale blue; upward sloping dotted line; dark blue in Figure 21.7.

To calculate each area:

a) the difference between the two relevant 1 – specificity scores must be computed, i.e.

$$\left(1-\text{specificity}_1\right)-\left(1-\text{specificity}_2\right)$$

(NB: ignore any minus signs in the results.)
b) the two relevant sensitivity scores must be added together and the results divided by 2, i.e.:

$$\frac{\text{sensitivity}_1+\text{sensitivity}_2}{2}$$

c) And the results from these two calculations are then multiplied together, i.e.:

$$[(1-\text{specificity}_1)-(1-\text{specificity}_2)]\times$$
$$\frac{\text{sensitivity}_1+\text{sensitivity}_2}{2}$$

Calculation c) is the area under the two points on the curve.

1. Taking the first pair of points on the graph ((downward sloping dotted line) underneath) where the first point represents sensitivity = 0.83, 1 – specificity = 0, and the second point represents sensitivity = 0.9 and 1 – specificity = 0.05, then calculation a) is

$$0.05-0 = 0.05 \ \text{(ignore minus sign)}$$

Calculation b) is

$$\frac{0.9+0.83}{2} = \frac{1.73}{2} = 0.865$$

Calculation c) is

$$0.05\times0.865 = 0.043$$

2. Taking the second pair of points on the graph (coloured pale blue underneath) (i.e. the second point represents sensitivity = 0.9, 1 – specificity = 0.05, while the third point

represents sensitivity = 0.98 and 1 − specificity = 0.17), then

Calculation a) is

$$0.05 - 0.17 = 0.12 \text{ (ignore minus sign)}$$

Calculation b) is

$$\frac{0.9 + 0.98}{2} = \frac{1.88}{2} = 0.94$$

Calculation c) is

$$0.12 \times 0.94 = 0.113$$

3. Taking the third pair of points on the graph (upward sloping dotted line) (i.e. the first point represents sensitivity = 0.98, 1 − specificity = 0.17, while the second point represents sensitivity = 1.0 and 1 − specificity = 0.37), then

Calculation a) is

$$0.17 - 0.37 = 0.20 \text{ (ignore minus sign)}$$

Calculation b) is

$$\frac{0.98 + 1.0}{2} = \frac{1.98}{2} = 0.99$$

Calculation c) is

$$0.2 \times 0.99 = 0.198$$

4. Taking the fourth pair of points on the graph (coloured dark blue underneath) (i.e. the first point represents sensitivity = 1.0, 1 − specificity = 0.37, while the second point represents sensitivity = 1.0 and 1 − specificity = 0), then

Calculation a)

$$1.0 - 0.37 = 0.63$$

Calculation b) is

$$\frac{1.0 + 1.0}{2} = \frac{2.0}{2} = 1.0$$

Calculation c) is

$$0.63 \times 1.00 = 0.63$$

Then add together these four values:

$$0.043 + 0.113 + 0.198 + 0.63 = 0.984$$

INTERPRETING THE AUROC SCORE

The value of 0.984 can be interpreted as the probability that a woman who develops postnatal stress incontinence has a higher SIS score than one who doesn't. Because of the high AUROC value, our test would appear to have some value as a screening tool for postnatal stress incontinence. As a rough index for deciding on the performance of a test, the following interpretations of the AUROC are usually used:

0.9–1.0 = excellent
0.8–0.9 = good
0.7–0.8 = fair
0.6–0.7 = poor
0.5–0.6 = fail

On this basis, the SIS would be classified as excellent.

However, there are further questions that need to be asked of diagnostic or screening tool – in this case, the SIS:

1. If a patient gets a positive score on the test, what is the likelihood that s/he has the condition? (In our case, if a woman records a high SIS score, what is the chance that she will get stress incontinence?) This is the test's capacity to predict true positives.

To answer this question, a value called the **positive predictive value** (PPV) must be calculated for the test. Using the hypothetical data for the SIS and the selected threshold of 6, the PPV is computed by the following formula:

$$\frac{\text{number of true positives}}{\text{number of true positives} + \text{number of false negatives}}$$

Using the data in Figure 21.5 that relate to the threshold of 6, our values can be substituted:

$$\frac{36}{36 + 2}$$

Therefore, our PPV = 0.95

The higher the PPV, the better the sensitivity of the test, and the better the chosen threshold, since together they have a greater capacity to identify women at risk of stress incontinence.

2. If a patient gets a negative result on a diagnostic or screening test, what is the likelihood that s/he does not have the condition? (In our case, what is the chance of a woman obtaining low SIS scores not developing stress incontinence?) This is the test's capacity to predict true negatives.

This question is answered by calculating the **negative predictive value** (NPV). The formula for this is:

$$\frac{\text{number of true negatives}}{\text{number of true negatives} + \text{number of false negatives}}$$

Using our data for the chosen threshold (Figure 21.4 above) we get the following results:

$$\frac{38}{38 + 4}$$

Therefore our NPV = 0.91

The higher the NPV the better the specificity of the test and the chosen threshold, since together they indicate that that the test has a high chance of correctly identifying those patients who don't have the risk/condition.

3. How accurate is the test overall? In other words – what is the proportion of test results that have accurately identified:

those with the risk/condition
those without the risk/condition

In our example, this means how good is the SIS at correctly predicting those at risk from developing stress incontinence *and* those not at risk. This is the test's capacity to correctly predict the true positives and the true negatives and is known as the test's **accuracy**.

The question is answered by the following formula:

$$\frac{\text{Number of TPs} + \text{number of TNs}}{\text{Number of TP} + \text{number of TNs} + \text{number of FPs} + \text{number of FNs}}$$

Using the data from Figure 21.5, our values can be substituted thus:

$$\frac{36 + 38}{36 + 38 + 2 + 4}$$

Therefore, the overall accuracy of the SIS is 0.93. For a life-threatening condition, this accuracy level may be too low, and the test may need to be reconsidered or perhaps used in conjunction with others.

4. How much more likely is it that a patient who has the risk/condition will test positive, in comparison with a patient who does not have the risk/condition? (For the SIS, the question is how much more likely is it that a woman who develops stress incontinence gets high SIS scores, compared with a woman who does not develop stress incontinence?)

Clearly, it is highly desirable that a diagnostic or screening test will be more likely to pick out those patients who either have a disease or who are at risk. This is known as the **likelihood ratio-positive** or LR+. Using the data in Figure 21.4, we can calculate the LR+ by taking the sensitivity score for our selected threshold of 6 and dividing it by 1 – specificity, i.e.:

$$LR+ = \frac{\text{sensitivity}}{1 - \text{specificity}}$$

Taking the specificity and sensitivity scores from Table 21.4. then:

$$LR+ = \frac{0.90}{1 - 0.95}$$

$$= 18$$

The LR+ can be interpreted as meaning that a high SIS score is 18 times more likely for a patient who develops stress incontinence than for one who doesn't. Clearly, the higher the LR+, the better the test is at identifying people with the risk/condition.

5. How much more likely is it that a negative test result will be found in a patient who doesn't have the risk/condition compared with one who does? (In our example, how much more likely are low SIS scores to be found in women without stress incontinence than in women with stress incontinence?)

A good test will be more likely to return negative test results for a patient who doesn't have the risk/condition than for a patient who does. This is called the likelihood ratio-negative or LR–. It is calculated using the following formula:

$$LR- = \frac{1-\text{sensitivity}}{\text{specificity}}$$

For our figures from Table 21.4 and the threshold of 6:

$$LR- = \frac{1-0.90}{0.95}$$

$$= 0.12$$

This figure can be interpreted to mean that the test is 0.12 times more likely to show negative results for a patient who actually has the disease, and hence, the lower this figure the better.

To summarise, then. A good diagnostic or screening test will have:

- high sensitivity (correctly identifying people with the risk/condition)
- high specificity (correctly identifying people without the risk/condition)
- a high PPV (a high probability that someone who has tested positive for the risk/condition actually has it)
- a high NPV (a high probability that someone who has tested negative for the risk/condition does not have it)
- a high overall accuracy level (the proportion of results that correctly identify both those people with the risk/condition *and* those without)
- a high LR+ (a greater likelihood of getting a positive test result for someone who actually does have the risk/condition, than for someone who doesn't)
- A low LR– (a lower likelihood of getting negative results on a test for someone who does have the risk/condition than for someone who doesn't).

There are a few further points to make about ROC analyses. First, the prevalence of a condition will influence some of the above factors. While sensitivity and specificity are not much affected by the rarity of a disease, the PPV and

NPV scores are. With a rare condition, the probability of a high scorer actually having the condition drops. This means that any test developed for use with a rare condition will not be of much value as a screening tool, because the chances of someone who scores positive on the test actually having the disease is reduced. For this reason, disease-specific diagnostic tests may have limited use as a screening test for the general population.

Second, while the development of a screening or diagnostic test may be relatively straightforward, to have any use at all, it *must* be tested against established gold standard measures, such as an established test or screening device. For example, the PSA (prostate-specific antigen) test to screen for prostate cancer would have had to be checked against other established gold standard tests, such as transrectal ultrasonography to establish its accuracy; similarly, the Triple test or Bart's test in early pregnancy is used as a screening tool to assess for Down's syndrome. Its accuracy would first have to have been assessed against the results of amniocentesis tests, before it was considered to be sufficiently accurate as a first-stage screening device. In our example, we might want to check the performance of the SIS against a set of results from a urodynamics clinic. It is important to ensure that every woman who is tested in the urodynamics clinic is also tested on the SIS, and vice versa.

Finally, you will need to consider the usability of your test. For example, if different people use the test, do they get similar scores? If one person uses the new test on the same person on several different occasions and without any significant change in the patient's condition, are the results similar? (These are issues of inter-rater and intra-rater reliability and will be covered in Chapter 23). And if your test is shown to be a reliable and valid diagnostic or screening tool, with good ratings on all the key attributes, would it be of any value in practice? Is it any better than the existing tests? Is it too cumbersome or time-consuming to use? Is the test acceptable to the patients and to the staff who have to use it? Is it too costly to use? Does it have any real value in identifying a clinical problem?

Key Concepts

- The cut-off point for referring someone for further investigations or treatment is called the threshold.
- The threshold can be adjusted to provide the most suitable sensitivity and specificity levels for the clinical problem in question; where there is no obvious choice about the threshold, Youden's Index can be used instead.
- The performance of a diagnostic or screening test can be assessed by plotting the sensitivity and 1 – specificity scores on a graph and calculating the area under the graph.
- The area under the graph is called the AUROC and the greater the area, the better the performance of the test.
- A diagnostic or screening test should also have:
  - a high PPV (the probability that someone who has tested positive actually has the risk/condition)
  - a high NPV (the probability that someone who has tested negative does not have the risk/condition
  - a high accuracy level (the proportion of results that correctly identify those people with and without the risk/condition)
  - a high LR+ (a higher likelihood of obtaining a positive test result from someone who actually has the risk/condition, than from someone who doesn't)
  - a low LR- (a lower likelihood of getting negative results on a test from someone who does have the risk/condition than for someone who doesn't).

10 STEPS IN UNDERTAKING A ROC ANALYSIS

1. Develop a diagnostic/screening test from clinical data, a thematic review of the literature, etc.
2. Use your scale with a group of people known to have the risk/condition and a group of people known not to have it; ensure that you include a wide range of people in each group so as not to bias the results in favour of the test.

3. Plot the scores from each group on a graph to establish where the overlapping scores lie.
4. Calculate the TP, TN, FP. and FN scores for every score where the scores of the two groups overlap
5. Calculate the sensitivity and specificity scores for every score where the scores of the two groups overlap
6. Decide on your threshold for referral; this will involve a decision about whether sensitivity is more important than specificity and vice versa.
7. If no there is no obvious threshold, use Youden's Index to establish the best cut-off
8. Plot your sensitivity and 1 – specificity scores on a ROC curve and calculate the area under the curve.
9. Calculate the PPV, NPV, overall Accuracy, LR+ and LR- scores
10. Test your scale against a known gold-standard measure, ensuring everyone who is tested on the gold-standard also receives your test and vice versa.

FURTHER READING

Altman DG, Bland JM 1994 Diagnostic tests 1: sensitivity and specificity. BMJ 308:1552

Altman DG, Bland JM 1994 Diagnostic tests 3: receiver operating characteristics plots. BMJ 309:118

Anthony D 1996 Receiver operating characteristics analysis: an overview. Nurse Researcher 4(2):75–88

Anthony D 1999 Understanding advanced statistics. Churchill Livingstone, Edinburgh

Bewick V, Cheek L, Ball J 2007 Statistics review 13: receiver operating characteristic curves. Critical Care 8:502–512. Online. Available http://ccforum.com/content/8/6/508 5 January 2009

Greenhalgh S, Selfe J 2006 Red flags: a guide to identifying serious pathology of the spine. Churchill Livingstone/Elsevier, Edinburgh

Greenhalgh T 1997 How to read a paper: papers that report diagnostic or screening tests. BMJ 315:540–543

MedCalc – Statistical Software http://www.medcalc.be/manual/roc.php 5 January 2009

Pallant J 2007 SPSS Survival Manual, 2nd Edition. Buckingham, Open University Press

University of Nebraska Medical Center http://gim.unmc.edu/dxtests/roc3.htm 5 January 2009

Chapter 22

Capturing expert opinion: the Delphi technique

CHAPTER CONTENTS

INTRODUCTION

The principal aim of the Delphi technique is to arrive at a consensus of professional opinion on any given topic. The method is particularly useful when decisions have to be made where there is either too much information or too little, or where there is contradictory evidence. Typical examples in the health care arena might be:

- the identification of core competencies to be achieved at the end of preregistration training of manual therapists
- the prioritising of research topics for funding
- the core skills to be evaluated on clinical placements
- the role of the clinical educator
- clinical risk factors likely to occur if staffing levels are reduced.

In all these situations, there may be inadequate published or empirical information to inform the decision-making process, and so the opinions of relevant experts in each of these areas would be sought using the Delphi method, as one means by which relevant professional expertise and experience can be synthesised and used to arrive at an informed decision. While committee meetings and focus groups may also have this purpose, their outcomes are heavily dependent on the group interactions that take place, with the most powerful, vociferous or influential person often dictating the discussion and conclusion. The Delphi technique, on the other hand, uses an individual postal survey approach, which targets relevant experts in the field. This avoids the bias that can be introduced by the interplay between group members at a meeting, and often elicits a more honest and therefore valuable, set of responses.

In essence, the Delphi approach involves identifying expert professionals in the field of investigation; they are then sent a survey form, the purpose of which is to investigate their views on the topic being researched. This might involve either:

- inviting the experts to provide their opinions on the topic in an unstructured free-response format, or
- the researcher outlining a perspective on the topic, or the central issues under investigation and asking the expert panel to express their level of agreement with these, usually using a numerical rating scale.

The completed survey form is returned to the researcher, who examines the replies, compiles a list of the viewpoints most endorsed by the experts and then redistributes this reduced list to the same panel. The experts are asked to rank order the items on the list, in order of the importance they attach to each and their responses are returned again to the researcher, for further distillation. The procedure is repeated several times until a shortlist of items is obtained that has the agreement of the entire expert panel.

Agreement in a Delphi study, then, takes two forms: first, the experts' agreement with the issues under investigation; and second, the agreement between the panel members. At all times, the responses are anonymous and confidential, thereby avoiding the interpersonal influences that occur in face-to-face meetings.

THE DELPHI TECHNIQUE IN PRACTICE

To illustrate the Delphi technique in practice, let us take as our example the identification of manual therapy research topics to be prioritised for funding. Since there are always fewer resources than there are research proposals, let us further imagine that the members of a regional research and development (R & D) panel have decided that they will try to agree on a set of

research priorities that the region should adopt over the next 5 years. In order to arrive at a list of topics that will reflect the various therapy professions and health needs of the region, the panel decides to seek the opinions of the key professionals in the areas, using a Delphi approach. The following stages are adopted.

Stage 1

The R & D panel identifies all the manual therapy experts in the region. These include all the most senior clinical personnel, heads of clinical services and departments, clinical managers, heads of training and education centres, regional managers with particular responsibility for strategic planning and development of the manual therapies, etc.

Stage 2

A letter is written to each expert, outlining the problem – namely, that the regional R & D panel wishes to identify the key research priorities to be targeted over the next 5 years and is therefore seeking the opinions of a range of senior professionals about the topics to be included. The expert is then invited to identify as many research topics as s/he wishes, that are perceived to be important to manual therapy research over this period. The completed form is then returned to the R & D panel for analysis.

Stage 3

When a sufficient number of survey forms are returned, the panel analyses the responses, in order to identify the most frequently cited research topics. Let's imagine that the following topics are suggested:

1. Improving communication with terminally ill patients.
2. A randomised controlled trial on three different approaches to the alleviation of back pain.
3. Counselling disabled people regarding psychosexual problems.
4. Encouraging manual therapists to use research findings to inform their practice.
5. Standardising the core competencies required of newly qualified chiropractors.
6. Investigation of staff turnover rates in care of the elderly.

7. Training initiatives in physiotherapy.
8. Development of a core curriculum for osteopathy students.
9. Empirical assessment of the role of reflexology in the treatment of multiple sclerosis patients.
10. Impact of improved communication on patient compliance with exercise regimes.
11. Embedding research into routine clinical practice.
12. Evaluation of three different approaches to increasing reflective practice among newly qualified manual therapists.
13. Comparison of transcutaneous electrical nerve stimulation (TENS) with standard drug analgesia in reducing pain in patients with spinal problems.
14. The impact of a post-registration counselling course for manual therapists for counselling the chronically sick.
15. An evaluation of a social skills training package for communication among manual therapists.
16. Stress and stress-related illness in qualified manual therapists.
17. Investigation of the reasons for high absenteeism rates in an outpatient physiotherapy clinic.
18. A comparison of the value of the hospital-at-home service vs hospital management of laminectomy patients.
19. The value of research groups in enhancing the scientific basis of manual therapy practice.
20. The relative value of written vs oral communication in explaining the exercise regime for stress incontinence.

Stage 4

Clearly, with a large expert panel and the option to cite as many topics as they desire, the initial pool of research areas will be considerably larger than this one, but for the reasons of space, only this small number will be used for illustration purposes. Closer inspection of the 20 subjects listed above suggests that they fall under the following broad headings:

- communication issues (items 1, 10, 15, 20)
- clinical management of back problems (items 2, 13, 18)

- the research/practice divide (items 4, 11, 12, 19)
- training (items 5, 7, 8)
- counselling in clinical practice (items 3 and 14)
- occupational issues (items 6, 16 and 17)
- advanced clinical issues (item 9).

These preliminary findings suggest that communication issues and the research/practice divide are each quoted four times; clinical management of back pain, training and occupational issues are all cited three times, with counselling and advanced clinical issues being named twice and once respectively.

Stage 5

Although the accuracy of these headings is not always double-checked during the Delphi procedure, this is clearly a sensible precaution to take wherever possible. Accuracy can be checked in the following ways.

The first method is to ask another researcher familiar with the area to classify the original topics under generic headings. If this is done as a single-blind procedure (see pp. 105–106), such that this researcher undertakes this task independently and without any knowledge of the headings used by other researchers, then the percentage degree of overlap can be easily assessed. For example, using the current example, we have classified the original responses into seven overarching headings: communication, back pain, counselling, the research/practice divide, training, occupational issues and advanced clinical practice. The next person who is asked to classify the topics might come up with:

- information giving and communication (items 1, 10, 15, 20)
- advanced clinical issues (items 2, 9, 13, 18)
- evidence-based practice (items 4, 11, 12, 19)
- staffing (items 6, 16, 17)
- training (items 5, 7, 8, 14)
- counselling and psychosocial issues (item 3).

This researcher has come up with six categories of which three are identical to the first classification, in that they use similar titles and include the same original topics. These include: staffing/occupational issues, research/evidence-based care and communication/information exchange. These three categories, then, account for 11 (55%) of the topics supplied in the first round. However, advanced clinical issues and the management of back pain have been conflated under a single heading and a counselling topic (item 14) has been regrouped under training. Despite this, there is a high degree of agreement about the groupings, in that of the 20 topics supplied, only two (items 9 and 14) have been placed in different categories by this researcher. This means that 18 out of 20 items were similarly classified, indicating 90% agreement between the two researchers. While there is no officially recommended cut-off point for concluding that independent categorisations are in agreement, anything in excess of 70% would seem reasonable, especially where there is a large original item pool that has to be classified. It should be noted that some researchers select much lower cut-off points, some as low as 51%.

An alternative method of establishing suitable category headings (of particular use when personal qualities or adjectives are elicited in the first round) is for the researcher to use *Roget's Thesaurus* to cross-check semantically similar words and place them in groups with appropriate titles.

Stage 6

The panel now has to decide which topics to select for the next round. In essence the decision in the current example rests on two factors:

- whether to restrict the research priorities just to those that were quoted three or four times, or to include the areas that were quoted once or twice as well, and
- whether to accept the first or second classification, or alternatively to find a compromise position between the two.

Since there are once again no recommended guidelines for making decisions about these points, the researcher would have to settle upon his/her own strategy. In the present case, let us imagine that the panel decides to exclude only the research topic that was quoted once and to use the first classification. The panel then drafts another letter to the members of the original panel informing them that the following research topics emerged as the most frequently cited areas for targeting over the next 5 years:

1. communication
2. counselling in clinical practice
3. the clinical management of back pain
4. the research/practice divide
5. occupational issues
6. training initiatives.

(Notice that these topics have been rearranged so that they do not appear in the order of most frequently cited; this should reduce possible response bias in this current round.) It should be emphasised that the interval between administering the first and second round of the Delphi should not exceed 8 weeks.

Stage 7

The experts are now asked to rank these topics in order of perceived importance to the region's research policy over the next 5 years, giving a rank of 1 to the most important, a rank of 2 to the next most, and so on. The completed forms are returned to the R & D panel for further analysis and reduction. (Only 11 respondents will be used here; more would normally be expected.)

Stage 8

The results shown in Table 22.1 are obtained.

To assess the degree of agreement among the expert panel, a Kendall coefficient of concordance must be performed on the rankings. Because there are 6 items to be ranked, the first version of the Kendall (presented on pp. 243–246) is required. The following results are obtained:

$$W = \frac{742.84}{\frac{1}{12}11^2\left(6^3 - 6\right)}$$

$$= 0.352$$

$$S = 742.84$$

$$n = 11$$

$$N = 6$$

$$p < 0.01$$

There is, therefore, a significant level of agreement among the 11 experts who responded to the second round.

Table 22.1 Experts' ranking of importance of research topics. **1** communication; **2** counselling in clinical practice; **3** the clinical management of back pain; **4** the research/practice divide; **5** occupational issues; **6** training initiatives.

Subject	Topic					
	1	2	3	4	5	6
1	2	3	1	6	4	5
2	6	4	3	5	2	1
3	4	3	1	6	5	2
4	3	6	2	5	6	1
5	3	1	5	4	6	2
6	6	1	2	5	3	4
7	1	2	3	5	4	6
8	2	4	1	6	5	3
9	1	2	4	5	3	6
10	4	3	2	5	6	1
11	3	1	2	6	5	4

Stage 9

In order to find out which topics are generally agreed to be most important, the rank totals for each topic must be added up. The topic with the smallest rank total would be considered to be the most important, the one with the next smallest, the next most important and so on. On this basis, we find the following rank totals:

Topic 1 = 35
Topic 2 = 30
Topic 3 = 26
Topic 4 = 58
Topic 5 = 49
Topic 6 = 35

This means that the topics have the following order of importance:

1.	clinical management of back pain	rank total = 26
2.	counselling in clinical practice	rank total = 30
3 and 4.	{communication, training initiatives}	rank total = 35
5.	occupational issues	rank total = 49
6.	research/practice divide	rank total = 58

Although the Kendall has been used here, it is possible to define agreement using techniques of descriptive statistics. In this case, the scores would be recorded from the lowest to the highest, and then plotted on a graph. The least frequently occurring responses (usually the bottom 25%), would be eliminated.

Stage 10

These items are then re-presented to the original expert witnesses in the above order of importance. The list is clearly stated to be a group response, with which the respondent is free to agree or disagree. The experts are invited to re-rank the items, with the option of changing their previous assessment in view of the group response.

Stage 11

On receipt of a sufficient number of responses, the re-ranked items are subjected to another Kendall coefficient of concordance test. If there is a high level of agreement on this round, the Delphi can be stopped; if there is insufficient consensus, further rounds (using stages 9–11) may be repeated until the researcher is satisfied that there is adequate accord.

Stage 12

Let us imagine that a further round of the Delphi produces the following rank-ordered list, with a p value <0.01:

- clinical management of back pain
- communication issues
- occupational issues
- research/theory divide
- training
- counselling.

The R & D panel may now decide that this is an adequate level of agreement and so terminate the Delphi. The above rankings will now be accepted as the research priorities for the region over the next 5 years.

ADVANTAGES OF THE DELPHI TECHNIQUE

- Because the Delphi is an anonymous process, it encourages answers that are unbiased and free from peer group and top-down pressures. It also allows well-informed, but less dominant, inhibited individuals to express an opinion, something that is often difficult in an open meeting. As a result, the data obtained may be considered to be more honest than that found using comparable methods.
- The approach uses postal surveys, which means that it is relatively cheap.
- The postal method also means that participants' responses are uncontaminated by interviewer pressure.
- The method allows for the collection of large quantities of data from a wide range of experts, who may have diverse backgrounds. It would be impossible, for various practical and financial reasons, to elicit the same level and amount of data from interviews or meetings.
- The method, because it taps into a range of expert opinions, ensures that it has content validity (see chapter on Attitude measures).
- It is a highly flexible technique that can be adapted to a range of professional and subject disciplines.

DISADVANTAGES OF THE DELPHI TECHNIQUE

The technique has been criticised for its lack of scientific rigour; in particular, the following points have been made in this regard.

SAMPLING

There are no recommended inclusion criteria for selection of the expert panel; expert in this context may be taken to mean anyone who has risen to a certain position of seniority or notoriety in the profession. Consequently, a Delphi study concerned with some form of clinical intervention would need to include specialist clinicians practising in the area, as a starting point. To this cohort may be added managers with a special clinical responsibility and academics who had a research interest in the field.

Also, because a wide range of expert opinion is sought, the total population of experts in a given area is usually targeted, for example, *all* manual therapists above a certain grade. Consequently, in these circumstances, representative sampling may be neither possible nor appropriate.

The size of the expert panel is also open to debate. Beretta (1996) notes that Delphi studies have been undertaken with as few as ten experts, or as many as 1685. The generalisability of the findings may be compromised, however, if the selection criteria cannot be justified or demonstrated to be associated with a genuine population.

RELIABILITY AND VALIDITY

Reliability of results is a major problem with the Delphi technique. Establishing reliable categories after the first round may be problematic and there are no well-defined guidelines for achieving this. Some semantic juggling is often required to ensure that some agreement regarding categories is reached by the people classifying first-round responses.

Attrition, and the relatively little attention paid to an individual's changes in response from one round to the next may also affect reliability and validity.

EXPERIMENTER BIAS EFFECTS

While there is no potential for interviewer pressure, the researcher has enormous potential to influence results, at the following points.

- Deciding the point at which consensus is reached. For most Delphi studies, consensus is not defined at the outset, but rather is decided in a totally arbitrary way, once the data have been analysed.
- Excluding outlying views, which may eliminate valuable, if minority, perspectives.
- Classifying the first-round responses under broader headings can involve some arbitrary assumptions and decisions; moreover, these categories can reflect the researcher's personal agenda, values and aims.

Although this is not a problem of *experimenter* bias, because the technique employs *expert* opinion, it has the capacity for undue influence on more junior members of a workforce, who may be reluctant to challenge the findings. This is particularly the case in hierarchical organisations, like the health service.

CONCLUSION

Providing a justifiable and sound methodology is adopted for a Delphi study, the results can provide a useful data base from which future health care decisions and strategies can be developed. The technique is invaluable in a wide range of health care debates where there is inadequate or conflicting available evidence to inform the decision-making process.

Key Concepts

- The Delphi technique is a valuable method of obtaining a consensus opinion from a panel of experts on any topic on which there is either insufficient evidence or contradictory evidence.
- The technique involves a series of postal surveys that use questionnaires to elicit experts' opinions on a specific topic.
- The first questionnaire aims to get a response to a broad subject area; the next questionnaire presents a synopsis of these findings and seeks the experts' level of agreement with this.
- Subsequent rounds present further syntheses of the preceding rounds, each one inviting the experts to express the extent of their agreement/ disagreement with the distilled data set.
- When an adequate level of consensus has been reached (often after several rounds), the results are used as a basis for future health care planning and decision making.
- Although the technique has many advantages, it also has some methodological flaws, most of which relate to the absence of any definitions to guide sampling or consensus levels.

FURTHER READING

Baker J 2006 How expert are the experts? An exploration of the concept of 'expert' within Delphi panel technique. Online. Available http://www.nurseresearcher. rcnpublishing.co.uk/resources/archive/GetArticleById. asp?ArticleId=6160

Beech B 2005 The Delphi approach: recent applications in health care. Online. Available http://www. nurseresearcher.rcnpublishing.co.uk/resources/archive/ GetArticleById.asp?ArticleId=6164

Beretta R 1996 A critical review of the Delphi technique. Nurse Researcher 3 (4):79–89

Cantrill JA, Sibbald B, Buetow S 1996 The Delphi and nominal group techniques in health services research. International Journal of Pharmaceutical Practice 4 (2):67–74

Hardy DJ, O'Brien AP, Gaskin CJ et al 2004 Practical applications of the Delphi technique in a bicultural mental health nursing study in New Zealand. Journal of Advanced Nursing 46 (1):95–109

Jones J, Hunter D 1995 Consensus methods for medical and health care research. BMJ 311:376–380

McKenna HP 1994 The Delphi technique: a worthwhile approach for nursing? Journal of Advanced Nursing 19:1221–1225

Mead D, Moseley L 2005 The use of Delphi as a research approach. Online. Available http://www. nurseresearcher.rcnpublishing.co.uk/resources/archive/ GetArticleById.asp?ArticleId=6162

Moseley L, Mead D 2005 Considerations in using the Delphi approach: design, questions and answers. Online. Available http://www.nurseresearcher.rcnpublishing. co.uk/resources/archive/GetArticleById. asp?ArticleId=6163

Walker A 1994 A Delphi study of research priorities in the clinical practice of physiotherapy. Physiotherapy 80 (4):205–207

Walker A, Selfe J 1996 The Delphi method: a useful tool for the allied health researcher. International Journal of Therapy and Rehabilitation 3 (12):677–681

Watson R, McKenna H, Cowman S, Keady J 2008 Nursing research: designs and methods. Churchill Livingstone, Edinburgh

www.emeraldinsight.com/Insight/html/Output/ Published/EmeraldFullTextArticle/Pdf/0250170103_ref. html (this is an excellent source of other Delphi references) Emerald Insight Publishers

Chapter 23

Capturing the user voice: Thurstone's paired comparison technique

INTRODUCTION

The technique described in this chapter uses correlations to assess agreement in applied research projects. Thurstone's paired comparison technique is particularly valuable in service planning or re-organisation, when decisions have to be made about the delivery of care within a context of resource and other practical constraints.

THURSTONE'S PAIRED COMPARISON TECHNIQUE (TPCT)

It is notoriously difficult to get useful information about priorities for service planning just by asking respondents to rank order a set of items according to the importance they ascribe to them, because after around six rankings, it becomes increasingly difficult for respondents to differentiate between the items' importance. As a consequence, the rankings may become random and meaningless and of little help in informing decision-making. Thurstone's methodology – a long established technique, dating back to 1927 – compensates for this difficulty in making meaningful distinctions between items, by ensuring that respondents are forced into making a series of choices between pairs of options. The format is questionnaire-based and the result is a finely tuned ranking of the choices which is both useful and relatively free of the sort of response bias that affects other ranking procedures. It has a particular value in service planning and design, for instance when there is a resource restriction on what can be incorporated, and when the user voice is important in establishing preferences in service planning. Some examples of where this method might be useful are:

- What do users consider to be the most important features of a new family planning service? Issues for consideration might be locality, confidentiality, walk-in service, female staff, opening hours, convenience of access, range of facilities, doctors and clinical nurse specialists available, range of other services available, etc. To ask users to simply rank order these in order of preference might lead to a database distorted by the difficulties of making differentiated and considered choices among so many features.
- Would patients prefer a therapist-led outpatient clinic or a consultant-led one? Again, simply to ask this question may mean that patients have not given due consideration to all the relevant issues, such as waiting times, local provision, length of consultation, expertise, convenience, prescribing authority, referral problems, etc.

In both cases, the Thurstone approach would be a valuable research approach. There are many ways in which this method can be made more sophisticated, for instance, by weighting the importance of the rankings, or by weighting the importance of the respondents' disagreement between the rankings, but the variant described here will focus on the technique in its simplest form. Let's take an example to see how it works in practice.

Imagine you are charged with the responsibility of revising the undergraduate speech and language therapy curriculum. (Here, you might either be a member of staff responsible for updating the curriculum or you might be a student rep who has to collect the views of other undergraduates, in order to inform the changes; for either role, the paired comparison method will work well.) You will first need to identify the amendments to the course that could be made, which might relate to either the mode of delivery or the content. This information can be gathered in a number of ways – a thematic review of: profes-

sional policy documents, available research evidence, the findings from focus groups held with staff and students, interviews, the comments on the course evaluation forms, the minutes of the staff-student committees, the contents of a suggestion box or a combination of any of the above. Let's suppose that we have used the course evaluation forms, the suggestions box and the available research evidence relating to undergraduate speech and language therapy education. You distil the information from these sources of information (using an established thematic review process, such as Attride-Stirling, 2001) and obtain the following recurring topics (please note that for the purposes of space and brevity, only six topics will be used in the illustration; more can easily be included):

1. Problem-based learning (PBL).
2. Increase in web-based learning (WBL).
3. Replacing at least half the unseen exams with seen exams (E).
4. More supervised small-group work (SGW).
5. An increase in the psycho-social content of the course (PSC).
6. A move from 1-day per week clinical visits to block placements (CP).

The items have been abbreviated, so that they can fit into the questionnaire set out below. Clearly, these course amendments will have resource implications, so a staff–student committee decides that when the results come in, only the three top-rated points will be incorporated for the forthcoming year, with the option of including the rest at a later point. It is decided that all three undergraduate years will be asked to make a priority assessment of the six proposed amendments, using the Thurstone Paired Comparison Technique (TPCT). To do this, each of the six items has to be paired with every other, so that the respondent has to make repeated choices between one feature over the other in each pairing, for example:

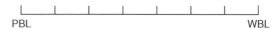

PBL   WBL

The respondent is instructed to put a mark according to how far s/he favours PBL over WBL or vice versa. You can see that this is an 8-point scale, which means that a mid-point 'don't know' option is not available and in consequence, the respondent is made to choose one item over the other. It is important to note, too, that the points along the scale are equidistant and that they are unlabelled, except for the ends. Both items on the scale get a score. So supposing that the respondent had responded with the following:

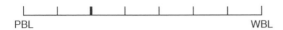

PBL   WBL

This would mean that s/he had a preference of PBL over WBL. The method of scoring will be dealt with later.

The key feature of the TPCT is the fact that the respondent is forced to choose between every possible pairing of the items included in the study. Therefore, to ensure that every item gets paired with every other item, you will need to set out the range of possible pairings like this

One way of checking whether you have all the possible combinations included is to use the following formula:

Item 1 will be paired with the total number of items to be paired minus 1, i.e.:

$$\text{item } 1 = 6 - 1$$
$$= 5 \text{ pairings}$$

Item 2 will be paired with the total minus 2

$$\text{Item } 2 = 6 - 2$$
$$= 4 \text{ pairings}$$

Item 3 will be paired with the total minus 3

$$\text{Item } 3 = 6 - 3$$
$$= 3 \text{ pairings}$$

Item 4 will be paired with the total minus 4

$$\text{Item } 4 = 6 - 4$$
$$= 2 \text{ pairings}$$

Item 5 will be paired with the total minus 5

$$\text{Item } 5 = 6 - 5 \text{ pairings}$$
$$= 1 \text{ pairing}$$

Item 6 will be paired with the total minus 6

$$\text{Item } 6 = 6 - 6$$
$$= 0 \text{ pairings}$$

Add up all the pairings to get the total number of paired items or questions in your TPCT questionnaire:

Table 23.1 Total possible pairings of items in the TPCT

Item	paired with	Item
1		2
1		3
1		4
1		5
1		6
2		3
2		4
2		5
2		6
3		4
3		5
3		6
4		5
4		6
5		6

$$5 + 4 + 3 + 2 + 1 + 0 = 15$$

Therefore, our TPCT questionnaire will have 15 paired item questions, with each item appearing five times (count the number of 1s, 2s, 3s, 4s, 5s, and 6s appearing in Table 23.1 to check)

It is important to make sure that these paired items are randomly distributed throughout the questionnaire to avoid clustering items together. It is also important that each item appears exactly the same number of times throughout the questionnaire and a similar number of times on the left-hand side of the scale as on the right. This will clearly offset response bias. Therefore, for our questionnaire, we might set out the paired items like this:

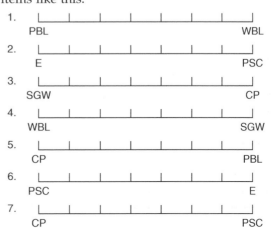

1.   PBL   WBL

2.   E   PSC

3.   SGW   CP

4.   WBL   SGW

5.   CP   PBL

6.   PSC   E

7.   CP   PSC

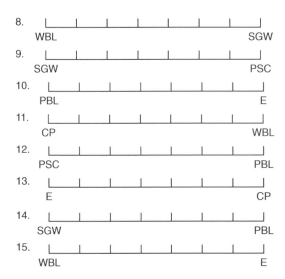

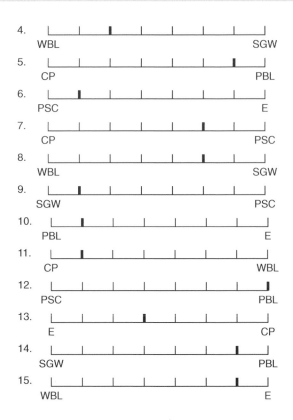

For each question, the respondent has to indicate which aspect of the curriculum change s/he would prefer, by putting a mark at one of the points, thus forcing a choice between each possible pair of items. The closer to one end the mark is, the greater the preference for it. The questionnaire should be accompanied by a covering sheet explaining its purpose, what each item means and what was required of the respondent with respect to completing the questionnaire; an example showing a hypothetical completed question would also be useful as a guide and to avoid incorrect completion. In addition, some questions about the respondent's biographical details, which did not include any identifier, but which collected relevant data such as year of study, age, gender etc. would also be helpful. The questionnaire would then be distributed and (hopefully) returned. We now have to score the responses.

SCORING

For each respondent, their total scores for each item have to be calculated. Let's imagine that the first respondent scored the paired items like this:

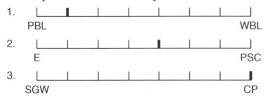

Every question will get two scores – one for each of the paired items. For example, to score question 1 (PBL vs WBL) both PBL and WBL will get a score. To obtain the PBL score, start from the PBL side, and count the number of marked intervals to the respondent's reply; here the PBL score would be 2, because the respondent has shown a distinct preference for PBL and has marked the second point in from the left. To find the WBL score for question 1, start from the WBL side and count the number of marks to the reply; here the WBL score would be 7. Therefore, for question 1, PBL scores 2, and WBL scores 7, showing a clear preference for PBL over WBL. These scores need to be recorded and an easy way is to make a table like Table 23.2 for each participant, with the items across the top and the questions down the side. Every score for every question can then be logged on the table for this participant. For questions 2 and 3, repeat the process. Therefore, for question 2, we get a score for E of 5, and for PSC of 4; for question 3, we get a score of 8 for SGW and for CP of 1, etc. Enter these scores into the table (see Table 23.2). Note that the lower the score for an item, the stronger the preference.

As each of our items appears five times (see Table 23.2), the maximum score an item could achieve would be $5 \times 8 = 40$, and the minimum would be $5 \times 1 = 5$. The lower the score an item has the greater the respondent's preference for it. Calculate each respondent's scores for each of the 6 items in the same way and enter the final totals in a table like this (for ease of illustration and economy of space only 10 participants are shown in Table 23.3).

The focus of interest here is to establish whether the respondents identify the same priorities for change; we are not interested in how close the respondents' actual scores were, but simply whether they agreed on which are the top priorities for change. To establish whether there

Table 23.2 Hypothetical scores for a single respondent completing the TPCT

Question	PBL	WBL	E	PSC	SGW	CP
1	2	7				
2			5	4		
3					8	1
4		3			6	
5	2					7
6			7	2		
7				3		6
8		6			3	
9				7	2	
10	2		7			
11		7				2
12	1			8		
13			4			5
14	2				7	
15		7	2			
Total	9	30	25	24	26	21

Table 23.3 All respondents' scores on hypothetical TPCT (ranks in brackets)

Participant	PBL	WBL	E	PSC	SGW	CP
1	15 (2)	22 (3.5)	33 (5)	22 (3.5)	38 (6)	12 (1)
2	28 (3)	18 (2)	36 (6)	30 (4)	33 (5)	17 (1)
3	19 (1)	30 (5)	29 (4)	26 (3)	35 (6)	21 (2)
4	13 (1)	25 (4)	31 (6)	19 (2.5)	30 (5)	19 (2.5)
5	18 (1)	24 (3)	33 (4.5)	33 (4.5)	36 (6)	22 (2)
6	25 (3)	20 (2)	34 (5)	27 (4)	38 (6)	18 (1)
7	23 (3)	19 (1)	24 (4)	26 (5)	29 (6)	20 (2)
8	15 (1)	30 (5)	30 (5)	29 (3)	30 (5)	21 (2)
9	19 (1.5)	25 (4)	26 (5)	19 (1.5)	32 (6)	23 (3)
10	20 (2)	27 (4)	28 (5.5)	22 (3)	28 (5.5)	13 (1)
Total						
Rank total	195 (18.5)	240 (33.5)	304 (50.0)	253 (34.0)	329 (56.5)	186 (17.5)

is any agreement within the group of respondents about the preferred changes to the curriculum, a Kendall Coefficient of Concordance formula 1 must be calculated (see Chapter 17). This formula is the correct one for any study where seven or fewer items are being ranked; here we have six items. First, we must rank order each participant's scores for the items; therefore, going across each row of the table (Table 23.3), assign the ranks (see ranks in brackets). Using our values from the above table in the Kendall 1 formula:

$$W = \frac{s}{\frac{1}{12}n^2(N^3 - N)}$$

$$= \frac{1269}{0.083 \times 100(216 - 6)}$$

$$= 0.73$$

where

$s = 1269$

$n = 10$

$N = 6$

$p < 0.01$

This means that there is significant agreement within the group about those aspects of the curriculum that they would like to see introduced. Taking the rank totals, it can be seen that the group's preferences are for:

1. CP (a change to block clinical placements)
2. PBL (problem based learning)
3. WBL (more web-based learning)
4. PSC (an increase in the psycho-social content of the curriculum)
5. E (a change to more see exams)
6. SGW (more small group work).

If there are limited resources to implement the changes, then just the first three might be targeted for amendment. This technique is useful in eliciting this information, as it allows informed decisions to be made, avoids response bias and allows – in theory at least – the relatively impartial rank ordering of a set of items. It is also quick to complete and very suited to research situations where user involvement in service planning is of interest.

Key Concepts

- The Thurstone paired comparison technique is a method of eliciting preferences and priorities, through a system of forced choice comparisons.
- It is a questionnaire-based method, which involves identifying the key themes in a given area and then pairing each theme with every other theme
- The respondent is required to indicate a preference for one theme over the other, in each question; there is no mid-point 'don't know' option
- In its simplest form, the results are ranked and participants' agreement between the ranking calculated using the Kendall Coefficient of Concordance
- If there is agreement within the sample, then the rank-ordered priorities can be used to inform service planning, etc.

FURTHER READING

Attride-Stirling J 2001 Thematic networks: an analytic tool for qualitative research. Qualitative Research 1(3): 385–405

http://www.socialresearchmethods.net/kb/scalthur.php (Web Centre for Social Research Methods)

McKenna S, Hunt SM, Mcewen J 1981 Weighting the seriousness and perceived health problems using Thurstone's method of paired comparison. International Journal of Epidemiology 10(1):93–97

Prieto L, Alonso J 2000 Exploring health preferences in sociodemographic and health-related groups through the paired comparison of the items of the Nottingham Health Profile. Journal of Epidemiology and Community Health 54:537–543

Thurstone LL 1927 A law of comparative judgement. Psychological Review 34:237–286

Van Wijk AJ, Hoogstraten J 2004 Paired comparisons of sensory pain adjectives. European Journal of Pain 8(4):293–297

Chapter 24

Capturing the clinician's view: reliability measures

INTRODUCTION

Clinical therapists undertake numerous measures in the course of their work: for example, equipment readings; treatment outcome measures; patient assessments; baseline measures against which treatment effectiveness can be based; risk assessments, etc. In order to evaluate whether these measures have any value in the clinical setting, it is important to measure the reliability of the measures themselves, and the reliability of the therapists taking the measurements. Reliability here is defined as the consistency or repeatability of a measure. No piece of equipment, measuring device or rater is 100% reliable and therefore there will always be some degree of measurement error. How much error can be tolerated will depend on the study and the clinical situation. However, when reliability is high, it suggests that there is little variation in the repeated measurements, and therefore the researcher can have confidence in a set of measures. Where reliability is low, this suggests wide variation in the measurements, meaning that it would be doubtful whether the measures could be reproduced and that there would be little confidence in the measures taken.

Of particular interest to the therapist are two forms of reliability:

- **Intra-rater reliability** – the degree of consistency of a set of measures taken by the same rater; for example, a dietician might use callipers to measure skinfold thickness of a group of liver transplant patients over a period of several weeks to see whether there is any improvement in nutritional status. It would be essential that the therapist's measurements are reliable so that any problems can be quickly identified and progress reliably assessed.

- **Inter-rater reliability** – the degree of consistency in the measures taken by two or more raters. For example, the physiotherapists in a sports injury clinic might use the universal goniometer to measure knee flexion in post-meniscectomy patients. In these circumstances, it would be important that any of the physiotherapists can measure any of the patients using the goniometer, without significant errors in the readings.

The choice of reliability measure depends on the design and assumptions of your study (which we will come to later) and on the level of measurement used in the study. Where nominal data are collected, then Cohen's Kappa should be used to measure the agreement; where ordinal data are collected, then weighted Kappa can be used (Davies and Fleiss 1982; Haas 1991); where interval/ratio data have been collected, then an appropriate interclass correlation coefficient (ICC) can be used. It should be noted that weighted Kappa requires a weighting to be given to the importance of any disagreement between the raters and this will obviously vary according to the sort of study that is being conducted. Cohen (1968) recommends that these weightings are decided in advance by a committee of experts, which makes this test rather a complex one for many researchers to use in practice. In this chapter, we will look at the reliability tests for nominal data (Cohen's Kappa), and for interval/ratio data (ICC).

COHEN'S KAPPA

While the majority of reliability studies conducted by clinical therapists will typically involve the use of interval/ratio data, sometimes there is a need to see whether there is any agreement between nominal data sets. Therefore, this sort of design would be used when the researcher wants

to establish whether there is any agreement between *two* raters, when *nominal* data have been used. There are several examples of where this sort of study might be encountered, for example:

- You might want to assess the risk of your elderly patients suffering a fall following a stroke. You might rate each patient as either 'at risk' or 'not at risk' (nominal data) and then ask another health care professional to make the same, but independent, assessment of these patients. You then need to see what level of agreement there is between the two sets of risk assessments.
- You are marking the portfolio assignments for students on a speech and language therapy course. The mark is either 'pass' or 'fail' (nominal data). All assignments have to second-marked blind and so the other marker makes the same pass/fail judgements. You need to see what level of agreement there is in the assessments.
- You are undergoing the orthopaedic part of your training and have been assigned to a radiologist in order to develop your skills at interpreting X-rays. A number of X-ray plates of children with possible greenstick fractures are shown to you and you have to decide whether or not there is a fracture (nominal data). Your judgement and that of the radiologist are assessed for the level of agreement in your interpretations.

In each case, the nominal data from the two raters would be examined to assess the extent of their agreement. To do this, you would need a test called Cohen's Kappa or κ. Let's take an example.

You are working in an orthopaedic hospital, to which a lot of patients are referred for hip problems, and who are likely to need hip replacements. Many of these patients are over 80 and a general anaesthetic would be risky. Therefore, the hospital policy is to treat as many of these patients as possible using conservative interventions. However, you need to decide for which patients conservative intervention would be suitable, and which patients would be better suited to surgery. To ensure that this initial assessment is as accurate as possible, you recruit another therapist to make an independent assessment of

Table 24.1 Raters' data for assessing suitability of patients for conservative intervention

Patient	Therapist 1's scores	Therapist 2's scores
1	1	1
2	1	1
3	1	1
4	1	0
5	0	0
6	1	1
7	0	0
8	0	0
9	0	0
10	1	0
11	1	1
12	1	1
13	1	1
14	1	1
15	0	0
16	1	0
17	0	1
18	0	1
19	1	1
20	1	1
21	1	0
22	1	1
23	1	1
24	0	1
25	0	0

all the over-80s. Both you and the other therapist assess 25 patients as either:

suitable for conservative intervention

or

not suitable for conservative intervention

This is a nominal classification, with two independent raters, and your aim is to establish whether you and the other therapist agree about which patients are suitable for conservative intervention. Therefore, this design is suitable for Cohen's Kappa test. You get the results shown in Table 24.1:

Where 1 = suitable for conservative intervention
0 = not suitable for conservative intervention

(It doesn't matter how you label these evaluations, e.g. √ could mean suitable and X could mean not suitable, or vice versa.)

You now need to

1. Count up all the patients for whom both you and the other therapist were in agreement about the suitability for conservative intervention: i.e. you both scored 1. Here this number is 12 (and is the number in cell D in Table 24.3).
2. Count up all the patients for whom both you and the other therapist agreed would not be suitable for conservative intervention: i.e. you both scored 0. Here this number is 6 (and is the number in cell A in Table 24.3).
3. Count up all the patients therapist 1 said would be suitable for conservative intervention, but therapist 2 said would not: i.e. therapist 1 scored 1 and therapist 2 scored 0. Here this number is 4 (and is the number in cell B in Table 24.3).
4. Count up all the patients therapist 1 said would not be suitable for conservative intervention, but for whom therapist 2 said would be suitable: i.e. therapist 1 scored 0 and therapist 2 scored 1. Here this number is 3 (and is the number in cell C in Table 24.3).

(If you add up all these values you should get the same as the number of patients – here this is 25.)

Note that calculations 1 and 2 indicate the agreements between the raters, while calculations 3 and 4 indicate the disagreements.

The first stage in the calculation of Kappa involves taking the total number of agreements between the two raters and dividing this by the total number of judgements overall. This value is called P_0.

$$\frac{\text{total number of agreements}}{\text{total number of judgements}}$$

If we substitute our figures, then

$$\frac{12+6}{25}$$

$$P_0 = 0.72$$

You now need to calculate a second value, called P_c. To do this, you need to set the four values derived from the four calculations above into a 2×2 table like Table 24.2.

Table 24.2 2 × 2 table format for Kappa calculations

A therapist 1 scored 0 therapist 2 scored 0	B therapist 1 scored 1 therapist 2 scored 0
C therapist 1 scored 0 therapist 2 scored 1	D therapist 1 scored 1 therapist 2 scored 1

The cells should be set out in this way, with the top left hand cell (A) representing the number of agreements between the two raters of the patients' unsuitability for conservative intervention. In other words, the top left-hand cell must represent Rater 1's assessment of unsuitability and Rater 2's assessment of unsuitability (Table 24.2).

Table 24.3 2 × 2 table showing raters' hypothetical data

		Rater 1	
		Unsuitable	Suitable
Rater 2	Unsuitable	A 6	B 4
	Suitable	C 3	D 12

You now need to add up the values of cell A + cell B, which we will call R1

$$R1 = 10$$

the values of cell C + cell D, which we will call R2

$$R2 = 15$$

the values of cell A + cell C, which we will call C1

$$C1 = 9$$

the values of cell B + cell D, which we will call C2

$$C2 = 16$$

(R simply stands for Row, while C stands for Column)

To calculate P_c, you also need the value of N, which is the number of patients, i.e. 25.

Using the following formula:

$$P_c = \frac{1}{N}\left[\left(\frac{R1 \times C1}{N}\right) + \left(\frac{R2 \times C2}{N}\right)\right]$$

Insert our values like this:

$$P_c = \frac{1}{25}\left[\left(\frac{10 \times 9}{25}\right) + \left(\frac{15 \times 16}{25}\right)\right]$$
$$= \frac{1}{25}\left[\left(\frac{90}{25}\right) + \left(\frac{240}{25}\right)\right]$$
$$= 0.04[3.6 + 9.6]$$
$$= 0.04 \times 13.2$$
$$P_c = 0.53$$

You now need to use the values of P_0 and P_c to calculate Kappa or κ. Kappa is a correlation coefficient of agreement and will range from a value of 0 to 1. The formula is:

$$\kappa = \frac{P_0 - P_c}{1 - P_c}$$
$$= \frac{0.72 - 0.53}{0.47}$$
$$\kappa = 0.404$$

To interpret this result as a measure of agreement, we need to look at the following recommendations from Everitt (1992) and Landis and Koch (1977)

0.0–0.20 = poor agreement
0.21–0.40 = fair agreement
0.41–0.60 = moderate agreement
0.60–0.80 = substantial agreement
0.81–1.0 = almost perfect agreement

This means that you and the other therapist show only fair agreement about who is suitable for conservative intervention. It is worth noting that some researchers simply calculate the value for P_0 and use this as an index of agreement. In our example, P_0 gave us a percentage agreement of 72% or 0.72, which is considerably higher than our κ value. This would be very misleading and might result in some dangerous assumptions about the reliability of the therapists' ratings, with the consequent problems for the patients. Therefore, it is important to calculate kappa if you want to undertake the sort of study that is looking for agreement between two raters, and which uses two nominal categories.

INTERCLASS CORRELATION COEFFICIENTS

Despite the importance of reliability ratings in clinical therapy, there is no universally agreed method of assessing inter- and intra-rater reliability when interval/ratio data are used. A whole range of methods have been used in the literature involving both tests of differences (e.g. *t*-tests, ANOVAS, etc.), and correlational tests (e.g. the Pearson test). However, on their own, each is an insufficient measure of reliability (see Bruton et al, 2000 and Rankin and Stokes, 1998 for a review of this). For example, many studies have used a correlation coefficient, such as the Pearson test (see Chapter 17), to assess the relationship between two sets of scores; however, while this will tell the researcher about whether there is a relationship or association between the data sets, it will provide no information about the *closeness* of these ratings, that is the *degree* to which the raters agree. The correlational examples used so far in this text have been concerned to find out whether two sets of data co-vary; they have not been interested in the degree of closeness of the data sets. The degree of closeness of ratings, however, is something that is of particular relevance for the clinical therapist, since accuracy between raters' measurements is essential in many aspects of their work. Let's take an example to illustrate this. Suppose you are responsible for a specialist clinical module as part of an undergraduate OT course on which you teach. A new member of staff has been appointed, who is new to teaching. As part of her duties, she will be second marking a set of assignments for your module. To ensure that the new member of staff is marking to the standards required in the department, you decide that you will assess her marks against the first marker's to see whether their marks agree. This would merit an inter-rater reliability test. Let's suppose the marks obtained for the 15 students taking the module are as in Table 24.4.

Table 24.4   Hypothetical data from two markers

Student	Marker 1 (%)	Marker 2 (%)
1	34	14
2	66	46
3	83	63
4	64	44
5	78	58
6	75	55
7	55	35
8	60	40
9	62	42
10	67	47
11	74	54
12	76	56
13	64	44
14	65	45
15	77	57

If a Pearson test is used to calculate whether there is any association or correlation between the two sets of marks, the results would be $r = +1.00, p < 0.000$ (you might want to check this). However, while the two sets of marks are perfectly correlated (+1.00), the second marker is always 20% lower than the first marker. Thus, the marks correlate perfectly, but the difference between the two sets of marks is considerable – in other words, the markers don't *agree*. The consequences of this would be substantial; assuming a 50% pass mark, students 2, 4, 7, 8, 9, 10, 13 and 14 would be passed by Marker 1, but failed by Marker 2. This should illustrate why a correlation coefficient is an insufficient measure of inter-rater reliability. We will return to this example later.

Although a correlation coefficient is clearly *not* a good measure of reliability, it was noted earlier that there is no universally agreed technique for undertaking reliability assessments; all have their advantages and disadvantages. What some researchers are inclining to, however, is the use of two or more reliability measures. For example, Rankin and Stokes (1998) recommend the use of interclass correlations (ICC) together with the Bland and Altman Agreement tests, although they summarise the advantages and disadvantages of these approaches too. Taking this advice, this chapter will cover these approaches. Before we look at these measures, it is important to consider the different types of designs and assumptions that can be used in these sorts of reliability studies.

There are many situations when a researcher might want to make a reliability check, and each requires a different formula. Two common examples are as follows.

- A situation where a new make of goniometer is purchased. To establish how reliable the readings are, a study is conducted in which five therapists assess the shoulder movement of a group of patients with whiplash injuries. The reliability of these ratings would be assumed to apply to *any* set of therapists who used the appliance. In other words, the reliability of this study would be assumed to apply universally to any therapists using the goniometer. This sort of study would be particularly relevant when the reliability of a machine, or other measurement device, is the focus of interest. Here the emphasis is on the question – does this machine or measuring device give reliable readings *irrespective of who is using it*?
- A second common situation focuses on the question – *are these particular raters reliable*, irrespective of when and where they are conducting the readings? Here the interest is in the particular people undertaking the measurements. One illustration might be an outpatient clinic, run by two clinical therapists, both of whom are responsible for taking pre-operative measures of the patients. If the two therapists are reliable in their assessments, then they can be used interchangeably to take the measures, thereby releasing the other therapist to do something else.

There are many variations of these two common designs, for example, whether the therapist(s) take just one reading from a group of patients, or a series of readings, over a number of days or weeks. However, these designs are beyond the scope of this text and the reader is referred to the references cited at the end of this chapter for further information on how to go about undertaking this sort of reliability analysis. In this chapter, we will concentrate on Example 2 above, where our interest is on the reliability of two particular raters. We are not assuming that any other set of raters will produce similar results, but rather that these two raters will produce similar measurements whenever and wherever they take them.

Before we proceed, it is important to note that the two examples outlined above illustrate examples of the different designs and assumptions in reliability testing, which in turn will determine how the ICC is calculated. However, all ICCs use ANOVA results in their calculations, but the type of ANOVA used is also determined by the design and assumptions underpinning the study. If the focus of interest is the generalisability of a set of ratings (Example 1) then a random-effects ANOVA model is needed. If the focus of interest is the reliability of specified raters (like Example 2 above), then a fixed-effects ANOVA model is used. It might be helpful to explain these ideas.

If a researcher is comparing the effect of three different antibiotic doses on the reduction of infection in elderly patients, the following design might be used:

Group 1	Group 2	Group 3
500 mg erythromycin per day	1000 mg erythromycin per day	1500 mg erythromycin per day

The three groups might be compared after 10 days to see whether there are any differences between them in infection levels, depending on antibiotic dosage. The data would be analysed using a 1-way ANOVA for different subject designs (see Chapter 16, pp. 226–230), because we have three different groups, each receiving a different intervention. Let's imagine that the results suggest that there is a difference in infection between all three groups, with the heavier dosage being associated with the lowest residual infection. Assuming that this study has been well designed, we would be able to infer that whenever these three dosage levels of erythromycin were used with similar groups of elderly patients, the results would be similar. In other words, the treatments are fixed at 500 mg, 1000 mg and 1500 mg, and whenever these treatment levels are used, then the outcomes would be comparable. We would not be assuming that the dosage levels can be varied randomly, and the same outcomes obtained – this would make nonsense of the research and all clinical trials. Therefore, we call this a fixed-effects model, because the treatments or interventions are fixed or constant (Gelman, 2005).

This fixed-effects model is analogous to Example 2 above, where our interest is only in the two raters concerned. If we think about each rater as a treatment or drugs dosage, then whenever these raters use the measuring device then similar reliability results will be obtained. Therefore, when a researcher conducts a reliability study where the focus of interest is in two (or more) fixed raters, then a fixed-effects ANOVA is used. This is the model that has already been described in this book.

On the other hand, if the issue of concern is whether a measuring device can be used by anyone, and still give reliable results, then the underlying assumptions change. To undertake a study of this kind, a number of therapists might use the measuring device, and their results would be assumed to be similar to any other group of therapists using the device. The raters are not fixed, therefore, but can be anyone randomly selected to take the measures. This would be akin to giving random amounts of erythromycin rather than the three sets of dosages used in the study, in the hope that the same results will obtain (Gelman, 2005). Because the reliability measurements taken in this sort of study are assumed to be similar to those taken by any randomly-selected group of raters, this sort of ICC requires a random-effects ANOVA in the formula. This is beyond the scope of the text, and the reader would be strongly advised to use SPSS in these circumstances. So, for instance, if you wanted to assess the reliability of a new model of vibrameter for measuring peripheral neuropathy in patients with diabetes, you might take a group of 10 therapists and ask them to assess a group of patients with diabetes mellitus on 10 successive occasions. Here your focus of interest is whether this instrument is a reliable one for use in this way, irrespective of which therapists are using it – in other words, would the findings from your study generalise to any other therapist in this context. This assumption means that a random-effects ANOVA is required and you would need to use SPSS. To do this, you will need to go into:

Analyse
 Scale
  Reliability
   Statistics
    Model

When you click on Model, you will need to select the appropriate ANOVA model for your study, which will depend on how you have designed your study.

The worked ICC example that will be described here will be based on the second example described above, where specific identified (or fixed) raters are the focus of interest. Consequently, a fixed-effect ANOVA like that described in Chapter 16 can be used.

Before we look at how the ICC works in practice, you should note that Bruton et al (2000) suggest that:

1. the number of measurements x the number of raters should be 25 or more (e.g. 5 raters × 5 measurements each, or 3 raters × 9 measurements each, etc.)
2. the ICC, which will always be somewhere between 0 (no agreement) and 1 (complete agreement), should be at least 0.6 to be of any clinical value (Chinn, 1991).

To illustrate the use of the ICC, let's return to the example provided earlier, of a new lecturer and her marking. Rather than having her mark consistently 20% lower than the first marker, let's assume instead that the marks in Table 24.5 are obtained for the 15 students doing that assignment. We have two raters, each taking 15 measurements, which means that we can fulfil condition 1 above. We are also only interested in the level of agreement between these two markers – no one else – and because each marker is marking 15 different scripts (one each from 15 different students) we are not interested in whether there is any intra-rater reliability. Had the raters been repeatedly assessing 1 student on 15 occasions, then we might well have been keen to know whether each marker agreed with her own marks (i.e. intra-rater reliability). However, as it is, the 15 students will produce different quality assignments and we would not expect that there would be any similarity between the assignment marks for the group. Therefore, the

Table 24.5   Revised marks awarded by two markers on an assignment

Student	Marker 1 (%)	Marker 2 (%)
1	24	30
2	56	50
3	73	68
4	54	55
5	68	70
6	65	60
7	45	50
8	50	45
9	52	45
10	57	60
11	64	69
12	66	60
13	54	59
14	55	56
15	67	60

analysis will simply be based on the agreement between these two markers. The revised data are presented in Table 24.5

As ICCs require some of the calculations that are obtained when computing ANOVAS, an ANOVA is the first stage in the ICC calculations. (Normally, when just two separate groups using interval/ratio data are being compared, then an unrelated (independent) t-test would be used; however, the ICC demands aspects of the ANOVA calculation, which means that this is the test of choice here). If we analyse the two sets of marks from Table 24.5 using a 1-way ANOVA for unrelated designs, we would get the following results (Table 24.6). (Remember, each marker must be thought of as a 'group'.)

Table 24.6   ANOVA results for first and second markers

	Sums of squares	df	Mean square	F	Significance
Between groups variation	5.633	1	5.633	0.044	NS
Error variation	3571.733	28	127.562		
Total	3577.367	29			

To obtain the ICC for these marks, we use the following formula (from Anthony 1999)

$$r_i = \frac{(m \times SS_{error}) - SS_{tot}}{(m-1)SS_{tot}}$$

Where
r_i = the inter-rater reliability coefficient (ICC), which will be between 0 and 1

m = the number of raters
= 2 (because we have two markers)

SS_{error} = the sums of squares for the error calculation in the ANOVA
= 3571.733 (from Table 24.6)

SS_{tot} = the sums of squares calculation for the total
= 3577.367 (from Table 24.6)

Substituting these values we get

$$r_i = \frac{(2 \times 3571.733) - 3577.367}{(2-1)3577.367}$$
$$= \frac{7143.466 - 3577.367}{3577.367}$$
$$r_i = 0.997$$

Using the recommended level of >0.6 to indicate useful agreement, this ICC value suggests that the markers show a high level of consistency between their marks. However, if we are to follow Rankin and Stokes' (1998) recommendations, we now need to do a Bland and Altman agreement test to supplement this result, since the ICC on its own is not considered to be sufficient.

Before we do this though, let's return to the marks in Table 24.4, where the second marker was consistently marking 20% lower that the first marker, in order to demonstrate the inadequacy of simply using a correlational test in these circumstances. The Pearson test yielded a perfect positive correlation of +1.00, although there was no agreement between the two sets of marks. To confirm how misleading a correlation coefficient would be if used in reliability studies, the data in this table will be used in an ICC calculation. The

ANOVA table for the data is as shown in Table 24.7.

Table 24.7 ANOVA results for first and second markers based on data from Table 24.4

	Sums of squares	df	Mean square	F	Significance
Between groups variation	3000.000	1	3000.000	21.007	0.000
Variation due to error	3998.667	28	142.810		
Total	6998.667	29			

$$r_i = \frac{(2 \times 3998.667) - 6998.667}{(2-1)6998.667}$$

$$= 0.143$$

This level of agreement is not nearly high enough to be useful (i.e. it is significantly less than the 0.6 recommended by Chinn, 1991), and yet the Pearson test provided a perfect positive correlation. This should demonstrate clearly that a standard correlation coefficient like the Spearman or Pearson will not provide a measure of the closeness of any agreement between two sets of scores.

BLAND AND ALTMAN AGREEMENT TEST

As noted earlier, no single rater reliability measure is considered sufficient on its own, and one recommended practice (Rankin and Stokes 1998) is the use of an ICC together with the Bland and Altman Agreement test (BAAT). This is, in essence, a graphical representation of the data that are to be checked for reliability. Now that the appropriate ICC has been calculated on our hypothetical data set, we now have to present graphically some of the descriptive statistics relating to these data.

1. The first stage in this process is the calculation of the differences between each pair of marks. Using the data from Table 24.5, we get the following difference scores (Table 24.8; remember to put the + or

Table 24.8 Marks awarded by two markers on an assignment: first stage in the Bland and Altman Agreement test

Student	Marker 1 (%)	Marker 2 (%)	d	Average
1	24	30	−6	27
2	56	50	+6	53
3	73	68	+5	70.5
4	54	55	−1	54.5
5	68	70	−2	69
6	65	60	+5	62.5
7	45	50	−5	47.5
8	50	45	+5	47.5
9	52	45	+7	48.5
10	57	60	−3	58.5
11	64	69	−5	66.5
12	66	60	+6	63
13	54	59	−5	56.5
14	55	56	−1	55.5
15	67	60	+7	63.5

– signs in front of each as appropriate). Enter these in the column entitled 'd'.
2. Next take each pair of marks and calculate their average. Enter these means in the last column (entitled 'Average').
3. Calculate the standard deviation of the difference scores (i.e. all the figures in the column labelled 'd'). The SD for our d scores is 5.069.
4. The BAAT involves plotting the measurement error, by plotting each difference score against the relevant mean score on a graph (i.e. for student 1, −6 vs 27; for student 2, +6 vs 53; for student 3, +5 vs 70.5, etc.), with the aim of identifying how many scores fall within 2 SDs of the d scores either side of the mean. Therefore, to construct your graph, along the Y (vertical) axis you need to plot intervals that are appropriate for ±2 SDs either side of the mean. Here, our SD is 5.069, which means that

$$+2 \text{ SDs} = +10.138$$

and

$$-2 \text{ SDs} = -10.138.$$

5. Therefore, our Y axis must have intervals running from −10.138 through 0 to +10.138

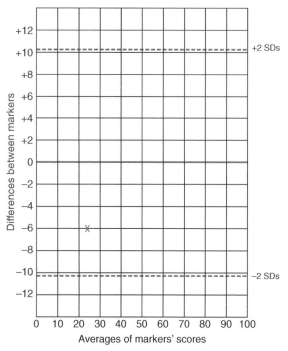

Figure 24.1 Format of graph for Bland and Altman's Agreement test, showing 2 SDs above and below mean.

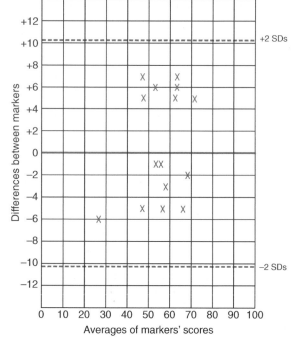

Figure 24.2 Bland and Altman's Agreement test for markers' assignment marks.

– see Figure 24.1. Draw a horizontal line across the middle of your graph to represent the mean, which we will label 0; then draw horizontal lines at +10.138 and –10.138. This is shown in Figure 24.1. You now have a line representing the mean and 2 SDs either side of it.

6. Along the X (horizontal) axis should be intervals representing the range of mean scores, as presented in the 'Average' column in Table 24.8. Our mean scores run from 27 to 70.5, so appropriate interval sizes should be used to reflect this range. Again, these can be seen in Figure 24.1.

7. Taking the first difference and mean, (–6 and 27), plot these on the graph. This first point can be seen on Figure 24.1. Continue in this way until all 15 differences and means have been plotted. Our results are shown in Figure 24.2.

Bland and Altman (1986) suggest that 95% of the plotted differences should fall between +/– 2 SDs of the mean. If more than 5% of the differences fall outside these boundaries, then our measures would be deemed unreliable.

Our results plotted on a graph indicate clearly that all the marks fall within ±2 SDs either side of the mean, confirming the high reliability provided by the ICC calculation. The new lecturer's marks are in substantial agreement with those of the experienced lecturer. As long as the differences within ±2 SDs are not too important, then these two lecturers could be used interchangeably to mark this module, should staff shortages and workload make this necessary.

The BAAT affords an at-a-glance assessment of whether the measurement errors fall between 2 SDs either side of the mean; it also highlights any outliers. However, this approach can only be used with two sets of measurements – if more than two raters are used, then the data have to be transformed. According to Rankin and Stokes (1998), the methodology for doing this has not been fully described.

Key Concepts

- Reliability measures are defined as the consistency or repeatability of a set of measurements; they focus on the closeness of sets of measures.
- Inter-rater reliability refers to the degree of agreement/consistency between two or more sets of raters.
- Intra-rater reliability refers to the degree of agreement/consistency within a single rater.
- Where two raters and nominal data are used, Cohen's Kappa is used to analyse the data.
- Where two raters and ordinal data are used, then weighted kappa is the method of analysis.
- Where one or more raters are used with interval/ratio data, there is no universally agreed method of analysing the results.
- In these circumstances, ICCs and a supplementary method of reliability assessment, such as the Bland and Altman Agreement test, are often recommended.
- The ICC requires some of the ANOVA calculations, but the type of ANOVA used will depend on the assumptions and designs of the reliability study.
- It is insufficient and incorrect to use simply a correlation coefficient in this case, because the results will be misleading, in that they provide no measure of the closeness of the readings, which is essential in this sort of study.

FURTHER READING

Cohen's Kappa

Anthony D 1999 Understanding advanced statistics: a guide for nurses and health care researchers. Churchill Livingstone, Edinburgh

Cohen J 1960 A coefficient of agreement for nominal scales. Educational and Psychological Measurement 20:37–46

Everitt BS 1992 The analysis of contingency tables. Chapman & Hall, London

Landis JR, Koch GG 1977 The measurement of observer agreement for categorical data. Biometrics 33:117–129

ICC and Bland and Altman Agreement tests

Anthony D 1999 Understanding advanced statistics. Churchill Livingstone, Edinburgh

Bland JM, Altman DG 1986 Statistical methods for assessing agreement between two methods of clinical measurement. Lancet Feb 8, 307–310

Bruton A, Conway JH, Holgate ST 2000 Reliability: what is it and how is it measured? Physiotherapy 86 (2), 94–99

Chinn S 1991 Repeatability and method comparison. Thorax 46:454–456

Cohen J 1968 Weighted Kappa: nominal scale agreement with provision for scaled disagreement or partial credit. Psychological Bulletin 70:213–220

Davies M, Fleiss JL 1982 Measuring agreement for multinomial data. Biometrics 38:1047–1051

Gelman A 2005 Analysis of variance – why it is more important than ever. The Annals of Statistics 33(1):1–33

Haas M 1991 Statistical methodology for reliability studies. Journal of Manipulative Physiological Therapy 14:119–132

Hayen A, Dennis RJ, Finch CF 2007 Determining the intra- and inter-observer reliability of screening tools used in sports injury research. Journal of Science and Medicine in Sport 10:201–210

McGraw KO, Wong SP 1996 Forming inferences about some intra-class correlation coefficients. Psychological Methods 1(1):30–46

Rankin G, Stokes M 1998 Reliability of assessment tools in rehabilitation: an illustration of appropriate statistical analyses. Clinical Rehabilitation 12:187–199

Rosher B 1982 On estimation and testing of interclass correlations: the general case of multiple replicates for each variable. American Journal of Epidemiology 116(4):722–730

Shrout PE, Fleiss JL 1979 Intra-class correlations: uses in assessing rater reliability. Psychological Bulletin 86(2):420–428

Chapter 25

Undertaking systematic reviews

INTRODUCTION

Systematic reviews are an essential component of evidence-based health care. With the massive increase in published research, it is impossible for the individual practitioner to read and evaluate every publication on the topic of interest, in advance of making any decisions about whether the research findings should be incorporated into clinical practice. This is where the systematic review is useful. Defined as a 'scientific tool that can be used to summarise, appraise and communicate the results and implications of otherwise manageable quantities of research' (CRD Report 4, 1996), the systematic review can inform practice and research by objectively synthesising a comprehensive array of research studies, large and small, published and unpublished. They can also help the researcher by identifying studies relevant to his/her own area of interest, highlighting effective research methodologies and contextualising the proposed research. The systematic review can answer questions about effectiveness of interventions, cost effectiveness, diagnosis, screening, prevention and prognosis.

The systematic review differs in a number of respects from the normal narrative review typically used in the introduction to a research report or article. The most important differences are the level of objectivity and the comprehensiveness of the literature covered. The narrative review typically selects published research that is deemed relevant to the topic in question, or which makes a case for conducting a piece of research, and the author then makes a subjective assessment of its value; it is therefore, *selective* and *subjective*. The systematic review, in contrast, attempts to collect *all* the information on the topic in question (not just published papers) in a *systematic* way; the information is then judged by independent reviewers using objective criteria and guidelines; the conclusions of the review should be reproducible by other reviewers. The systematic review is therefore, *comprehensive* and *objective*. The main differences between the two types of review are presented below

DIFFERENCES BETWEEN NARRATIVE REVIEWS AND SYSTEMATIC REVIEWS (Petticrew, 2001)

Narrative reviews:

- involve a general discussion or a topic area
- do not attempt a comprehensive search of all literature, both published and unpublished
- provide no justification for the inclusion or exclusion of given studies
- overlook differences in study methodologies or quality
- when drawing conclusions, fail to differentiate between good and poor studies
- are based on the reviewer's subjective opinion.

Systematic reviews:

- specify a clear question to be answered by the review
- attempt to include all published and unpublished studies
- are explicit about the criteria for inclusion/exclusion
- use a rigorous protocol for assessing the quality of the studies to be reviewed
- weight the relevance of the studies according to their quality
- base the conclusions and recommendations on the best studies
- are relatively unbiased and objective.

The systematic reviews that are used in developing clinical/treatment guidelines and proto-

cols that are used to inform clinical practice (e.g. National Service Frameworks) have usually been funded and undertaken by teams of reviewers. However, with increasingly stringent ethical procedures, many undergraduate and postgraduate courses now offer students a choice of assignments for the research component of their courses. The options often include undertaking a piece of original research, or alternatively some other project, of which the systematic review might be an option. Therefore, systematic reviews do not have to be well funded or based on team effort – they can be conducted at many levels and with varying degrees of resource investment. The guidelines provided here are targeted at the undergraduate or postgraduate project, but the reader who is interested in conducting a funded review is referred to CRD (2001) for a comprehensive guide on how to do this. It should be noted that within the general area of systematic reviews are meta-analyses and health technology assessments (HTAs). Meta-analyses use special statistical techniques to synthesise and assess a number of studies in the same area, while HTAs consider 'the effectiveness, appropriateness, costs and broader impact of health technologies using both primary research and systematic reviews' CRD (2001). Both these variants are beyond the scope of this text.

The stages for a systematic review are as follows (each stage will be described in detail later):

1. Identifying the need for a review in a given subject area.
2. Specifying the precise topic area for the review or the review question.
3. Development of a review protocol.
4. Search strategies for identifying the relevant literature.
5. Selecting the studies for inclusion in the review.
6. Assessment of the quality of studies.
7. Extracting the data.
8. Synthesising the data.
9. Production of the report (CRD, 2001; ScHARR, 1996).

These stages apply to reviews of experimental research, diagnostic research or qualitative research. However, as this text relates primarily to experimental – or *effectiveness* – research, this will be the focus here.

1. *Identifying the need for a review in a given subject area*

   To ensure that the topic of your choice has not already been subject to a systematic review, it is essential that a thorough search of existing or ongoing systematic reviews is undertaken. If there is already a review in the area, this could be expanded or updated, but it may be better to shift your focus to another topic. The sources outlined in Chapter 10 will all be of value in this initial research process, in particular (all websites correct as of January 2009):

   - The Cochrane Library (http://www.cochrane.org)
   - This contains information about existing systematic reviews, updated reviews and ongoing reviews
   - DARE (http://www.crd.york.ac.uk/crdweb/)

   This is an abstract database and includes reviews that have not been included in the Cochrane Library, as well as from hand (as opposed to electronic) searches and from grey (unpublished) literature

   - ARIF (http://www.arif.bham.ac.uk/)
   - NICE (http://nice.org.uk)
   - National Library for health (http://www.library.nhs.uk)
   - MEDLINE
   - EMBASE see Chapter 10 for details of these
   - CINAHL

2. *Specifying the precise topic area for the review*

   The previous stage involved a preliminary review of the literature to establish whether your topic had already undergone a systematic review. Once you have established that it hasn't, you will need to be much more precise about what exactly you are interested in looking at. Therefore, this stage involves a much more detailed specification of what your review will focus on:

   - what precise clinical topic will be investigated
   - which patient or participant group will be studied – gender, age etc.
   - the exact treatment used

- the outcomes of interest; these may include *therapeutic interventions* (identification of the treatment/interventions that are likely to benefit the particular group of patients); *prevention* (identification of interventions that reduce the risk of illness); *diagnosis* (identification of the best diagnostic process for a treatable condition); or *screening* (identification of best techniques for targeting individual risks for a treatable disease)
- the sorts of study designs or relevance e.g. RCTs, diagnostic or screening tests, experimental, qualitative, etc.

Therefore, your task at this stage is to focus on these issues in order to make your review area precise, transparent, replicable by other reviewers and manageable.

If we take a hypothetical example, let's suppose that we have found that there has been no review of the use of dietary supplements in the treatment of childhood eczema. Therefore our focus will be:

- Childhood eczema – use of dietary supplements.

The review question will be:

- For pre-pubescent children suffering from non-allergic eczema, does the use of Vitamin D supplements improve the condition?
- The population: children, i.e. 2.0 years–prepubescent
- Intervention: vitamin D vs. 1% hydrocortisone
- Outcomes: reduction in severity and extent of eczematous patches
- Study Designs: RCTs/experimental trials.

3. *Development of a review protocol*

   You need to specify how the review will be conducted in order to provide yourself with a *plan* of the structured set of stages you will follow. This is akin to a research proposal for a piece of original research, in that it sets out your framework, intentions and procedure – what you are planning to do in your systematic review. The CRD (2001) recommends that the following sections are included in your review:

- background to the topic area – context, prevalence, incidence, treatment, etc.
- precise review question
- your search strategy when identifying the research to be reviewed, including the databases to be searched and the key words to be used
- study selection criteria – how you will decide on which studies will be included in your review and which will be rejected
- what data will be synthesised and interpreted.

This stage helps you to focus on the key steps in the review process and provides a plan of campaign.

4. *The search strategies used to identify the relevant literature*

It is essential that a comprehensive and thorough review of all available literature is conducted, which must include both published and unpublished research, without any restrictions on age of publication. You must also state which search words you have used in the process. Therefore this stage will include (all websites correct as of January 2009):

- Electronic searches of published databases using the sites outlined in Stage 1 and in Chapter 10
- Manual searches of journals and grey literature (unpublished work) using sites such as SIGLE (System for Information on Grey Literature, BNBRL (British National Bibliography for Report Literature http://www.bl.uk) – available from 1986 onwards, CRD (Centre for Research and Dissemination http://www.york.ac.uk/inst/crd/htadbase.htm).
- Reference lists from key articles – this is an invaluable source of information and will typically yield a considerable number of relevant references (Greenhalgh, 2005)
- Conference proceedings – available from the British Library (http://www.bl.uk) or Conference Papers Index (see references at the end of this chapter).
- Internet: this is a surprisingly valuable source of information; the following search engines are helpful.
  Copernic 2000 – http://www.copernic.com

Dogpile – http://www.dogpile.com
Northern Light Technology – http://northernlight.com
OMNI – http://www.omni.ac.uk
MedNets – http://www.mednets.com
- Registers of research e.g. National Research Register (http://www.nrr.nhs.uk).

It is essential to use unpublished as well as published research, because publication bias is well documented i.e. a tendency of journals to publish only significant results. Therefore, any review based just on published research will incline towards a conclusion of treatment effectiveness, when, in fact, the reverse may be true. You will also need to decide whether to include research which used English. Most journals are published in English, but because of publication bias, this may mean that excluding research reported in other languages may exacerbate the bias.

The search words should be specified clearly for each part of your review: i.e. the population under consideration, the condition, treatment, outcome and design. For our hypothetical review, we might use the following terms (please note these are neither exhaustive nor definitive):

Population: childhood, child
Condition: eczema, atopic dermatitis
Treatment: vitamin D, calcium, dietary supplements, hydrocortisone, anti-inflammatory agents, antipruritics, topical administration, ointment, emollient
Outcome: outcomes, results,
Design: RCTs, experiment, research design

It is useful to do a pilot search to see whether you are using the best sources and the most valuable search words. If you do a trial run, you can see whether the studies produced do, in fact, yield the sort of research you're interested in, or whether they are wide of the mark. If this latter is the case, then adjusting the search words may be useful. Librarians can be very helpful in this respect. Remember, too, that obtaining a useful article that directly relates to your chosen review topic can not only provide you with further references but will also give you a lead on the relevant search terms.

5. *Selecting studies for inclusion*

The previous stage may well generate a vast selection of research for possible inclusion. These results now need to be reduced to those studies which are most directly relevant to your review question. This reduction process must be free from bias, which will involve setting clear inclusion and exclusion criteria for selection. The reduction process should properly take place once you have retrieved all the studies produced by your search. However, the reduction process may need several iterations to refine it. For example, it may only become apparent on reading some of the articles that no systematic assessment or outcome of the treatment was made, and so these would be discarded. The process continues until your selected studies meet the criteria you have specified. The selection should also be undertaken as a 'blind' process i.e. the authors and their affiliations should be removed so that any bias accruing from the status of the researchers or their institutions can be removed (see Peters and Ceci, 1982 for a very interesting study on this). So for our example, we might use the inclusion and exclusion criteria shown in Table 25.1.

Table 25.1 Hypothetical criteria for inclusion of research studies

	Inclusion	Exclusion
Population	children who are over 2 years and also prepubescent, undergoing treatment for eczema	Other skin conditions; adolescents, babies, under 2s
Intervention	Vitamin D compared with 1% hydrocortisone	Other treatments; no comparison; a non-intervention control
Outcome	Reduction in severity and extent of eczematous patches	No systematic measurement; other outcomes, e.g. infection
Study design	RCTs	Single cases studies; non-randomised studies; other designs

Using these criteria, you and an independent reviewer should sift through these studies and decide which ones should be included and which excluded. This should further reduce selection bias. Objective assessment of the degree of agreement achieved between you and the other reviewer should be made using Cohen's Kappa – see Chapter 24 for how to do this.

So, for example, suppose your initial trawl had yielded 112 studies that met your search terms, you and the independent reviewer would need to read these and decide whether or not each one met the criteria for inclusion (Table 25.2). Let's imagine that you both agree that

83 of the studies should be included
19 of the studies should be excluded

But you think that a further 8 should be included, while the independent reviewer thinks these should be excluded and you think that 2 should be excluded, while the independent reviewer thinks these should be included.

This means that $P_0 = \dfrac{83+19}{112}$

$= 0.92$

Therefore, to calculate Kappa, the results must be set out in a 2×2 table like this:

$$P_c = \frac{1}{112}\left[\left(\frac{21\times27}{112}\right)+\left(\frac{91\times85}{112}\right)\right]$$
$$= 0.009\times(5.06+69.06)$$
$$= 0.67$$

Table 25.2 2×2 table of reviewers' agreement regarding the inclusion/exclusion of studies in a systematic review

		Reviewer 1		
		Exclude	Include	
Reviewer 2	Exclude	19	2	21
	Include	8	83	91
		27	85	

Therefore,

$$\kappa = \frac{0.92 - 0.67}{1 - 0.67}$$

$$= \frac{0.25}{0.33}$$

$$= 0.76 \ \left(\text{substantial agreement}\right)$$

In the cases where you and the other reviewer disagreed, then this must be resolved.

It is essential that the process of selecting the studies for inclusion should be clearly documented. If the initial search generates only a few RCTs, then the search should be expanded to include less rigorous designs e.g. quasi-experimental.

6. *Assessing the quality of the studies*

All the studies that have been selected for inclusion must now be thoroughly read and assessed using a set of predefined criteria, in the form of a published appraisal tool such as the following:

Verhagen at al (1998)
Moher et al (1995)
Jadad et al (1996)
Chalmers et al (1981)
Sindhu et al (1997)
Johnston et al (1995)
CRD (2001) (Appendix 2)
(All these are referenced at the end of this chapter.).

It is important to note that most of these checklists have not been rigorously developed and so they may yield quite different quality scores. It is also possible to construct your own appraisal tool that meets your requirements. There are different appraisal tools for different types of study (e.g. qualitative, experimental, etc.). Moher et al (1995) provides a bibliographic overview of these, while CRD (2001) provides examples for reviewing effectiveness studies (like our hypothetical eczema topic), test accuracy studies and economic evaluations. Irrespective of the checklist used, the primary concerns when evaluating your studies are its internal validity – in other words, its design, conduct and analysis – and its external validity – the population,

interventions and outcome measures. The quality checklist selected should be relevant to both the general methodological issues as well as the specific aspects of the review topic. Any study failing to meet the stated quality criterion should be excluded. The remaining studies can be graded or ranked for their quality. Again, this should all be done independently from the other reviewer.

7. *Extracting the data*

The purpose of this stage of the review process is to identify the relevant design aspects and the results of the selected studies, so that they can be compared and the findings synthesised into a report. To do this, you will need to design a data extraction form, which should be piloted before use. The sorts of headings to be included in your form are:

General:

● name of reviewer extracting the information (if more than one)
● bibliographic details of the study, e.g. title, authors, journal, etc.
● source of the study.

Specific:

● study design: population (type and sample size); context/setting; methodological quality; interventions/treatments; outcomes
● results: participant attrition; missing data; tests/p values; implications; effect size
● any notable difference between this study and the others should be noted.

Useful examples of data extraction forms can be found in Appendix 3 of CRD (2001). Accuracy and consistency are the lynch-pin of this stage – every study must be scrutinised without bias and using the same criteria. Try to get an independent reviewer to check your assessment or a sample of these (this does not need to be done blind). If there are any disagreements, these must be resolved by discussion or via a third independent party.

8. *Synthesising the data*

The results of the data extraction phase now need to be synthesised and summarised, so that you can get a picture of the effectiveness of the interventions and whether the effectiveness is consistent across studies. If there is any inconsistency in findings, the reasons for these discrepancies must be explored. This synthesis may be a description of the studies' similarities, differences and outcomes, or it can be a quantitative meta-analysis. This latter is outside the scope of this book, so we will focus on a qualitative summary of the studies. The purpose of a qualitative synthesis of the studies is to provide a meaningful and easily accessible summary of the design and results and is best achieved by tabulating the studies as in Table 25.3 (a fabricated example has been used).

Etc., etc.

Table 25.3 Summary table of studies selected for a systematic review of the effectiveness of Vitamin D supplements in the treatment of childhood eczema

Study	Population and sample size	Intervention	Settings	Constant errors	Outcome measures	Results	Findings/ conclusions
Jones et al 2007	6–10-year-olds $N = 785$	Vitamin D (1000 IU pd) or 1% hydrocortisone twice daily	Home	No compliance check; children with allergies not excluded	Reduction in patches measured photographically and by subjective report	Hydrocortisone more effective $p < 0.001$	1% hydrocortisone more effective than vitamin D
Smith et al 2008	5–11-year-olds $N = 235$	Vitamin D 1000 IU pd or 1% hydrocortisone twice daily	Home	Study took place in summer, when exposure to sunshine could have increased vitamin D production	Subjective response by patient and carer; mm rules for patch size; assessment of bleeding and exudate on 5-point scale	Hydrocortisone more effective $p < 0.01$	1% hydrocortisone more effective than vitamin D

The information in the table should ensure that all the key points are clearly included, and that any similarities or differences between the studies are highlighted. Where studies are similar in terms of participants, interventions, outcomes and methods, it should be possible to draw some conclusion about the overall effectiveness of the intervention in these studies. However, if the table contains studies that differ in these regards, then an overall conclusion should not be drawn. It may, in these circumstances, be possible to see whether there are any ways of subgrouping the studies, so that conclusions can be drawn for each subgroup, for example for studies using children between 2 and 5, and those using children of 5–10 years.

9. *Reporting the review*

This is the final stage of your review, and it will present a serious challenge to distil your analysis and synthesis into a manageable report, especially if a lot of studies are to be included. If you are doing a systematic review as an assignment, then the stipulated word-length must be observed; if you are planning to submit your review for publication, then follow the journal's Guidelines for Authors. It is unlikely, though, that papers for journals will exceed 5000 words, so you will need to be succinct. The review should include the following headings:

- title
- background to the review – its evidence, prevalence, data, justification, context etc

- the review question
- the review methodology – sources; search terms; quality assessment protocol; data extraction methods; synthesis procedure
- details of the studies that have been included (tabulated)
- details of the studies that have been excluded giving the reasons for exclusion (tabulated). These can be included in the Appendix.
- results – findings of the review; robustness of the conclusion
- interpretation of the results – important features of the study
- strengths and weaknesses of the review
- conclusions and implications for practice and should consider the benefits and problems of the intervention
- future research
- references – every study cited
- appendices – quality assessment and data extraction forms.

The Recommendations for Practice can be graded according to the quality of the studies, such that high quality RCTs which produced similar results would be graded more highly than studies that only covered low quality studies whose findings were diverse. For a detailed review of the possible grading systems, see CRD, Stage III, Phase 8 (2001).

Undertaking a thorough and rigorous review can be a big task, especially if your chosen topic generates a lot of research studies. The advantages and disadvantages of systematic reviews are presented below, so that you can make an at-a-glance assessment of whether your review ideas are feasible and worthwhile. If you decide to conduct a review, remember that there are many sources of help available to assist you through each stage.

ADVANTAGES OF A SYSTEMATIC REVIEW

- Comprehensive rather than selective review
- Objective
- Explicit about which studies have been included
- Unbiased
- Reproducible by other reviewers because of the objectivity and clear, systematic methodology
- Focused question
- Conclusions influenced by the quality of the studies included, rather than assuming all studies have equal value
- May generalise widely because of the comprehensive cover of studies
- Reduces a large quantity of data to a manageable amount
- Informs interventions, treatment guidelines etc.
- Carries authority
- May highlight reasons for different study outcomes.

DISADVANTAGES OF THE SYSTEMATIC REVIEW

- Results of systematic reviews may disagree with the results of large scale clinical trials
- Authority implicit in the review may be false or misguided
- Systematic reviews on the same review question may disagree with each other, because of differences in selection criteria or quality assessment protocols
- Results may be too general for the practitioner to apply in a particular setting
- Limited by the quantity and/or quality of the studies available
- Even though objective assessment measures are used, these can still be influenced by subjective opinion
- Including a diverse range of studies means that their quality is likely to be disparate
- Grey literature not always easily accessible
- May be subject to publication, selection and language bias.

Key Concepts

- The aim of the systematic review is to summarise all the available published and unpublished research evidence, in a specified area, into a manageable amount.
- Systematic reviews involve a rigorous, objective and comprehensive evaluation of all the relevant research literature.
- Conducting a systematic review involves nine stages:
  - identifying the need for a review in a specified area
  - defining the precise topic or review question
  - development of a review protocol
  - development of search strategies to identify all the relevant published and unpublished literature
  - selection of studies for inclusion in the review
  - assessment of the quality of the studies
  - extraction of the information
  - synthesis of the information
  - production of the report (Scharr 1996; CRD 2001).
- The findings from the review can be used to inform practice.

FURTHER READING

Centre for Dissemination and Reviews 2001 Undertaking systematic reviews of research on effectiveness. CRD Report 4 (2nd Ed). Online. Available http://www.york.ac.uk/inst/crd/report4.htm 12 January 2009

Chalmers TC, Smith H, Blackburn B, et al 1981 A method for assessing the quality of a randomised controlled trial. Controlled Clinical Trials 2:31–49

Conference Papers Index 2000 Bethesda, MD, Cambridge Scientific Abstracts

Greenhalgh T 2005 Effectiveness and efficiency of research methods in systematic reviews of complex evidence: an audit of primary sources. BMJ 331:1064–1065

http://www.shef.ac.uk/scharr/ir/units/systrev/reading.htm 12 January 2009 University of Sheffield School of Health and Related Research

Jadad AR, Moore RA, Carroll D et al 1996 Assessing the quality of reports of randomised controlled trials: is blinding necessary? Controlled Clinical Trials 7:1–12

Moher D, Jadad AR, Nichol G, Penman M, Tugwell P, Walsh S 1995 Assessing the quality of randomised controlled trials: an annotated bibliography of scales and checklists. Controlled Clinical Trials 16:62–73

Petticrew M 2001 Systematic reviews from astronomy to zoology – myths and misconceptions. BMJ 322:98–101

http://www.shef.ac.uk/scharr/research/publications in the 'Search for' box, type in 'Systematic Reviews'

Sindhu F, Carpenter L, Seers K 1997 Development of a tool to rate the quality assessment of randomised controlled trials using a Delphi technique. Journal of Advanced Nursing 25:1262–1268

Verhagen AP de Vet HC, de Bie RA, et al 1998 The Delphi List: a criteria list for quality assessment of randomised clinical trials for conducting systematic reviews developed by Delphi consensus. Journal of Clinical Epidemiology 51:1235–1241

Walley T 2007 Health technology assessment in England: assessment and appraisal. Medical Journal of Australia 187(5):283–285

Watson, R, McKenna H, Cowman S, Keady J 2008 Nursing research: designs and methods. Edinburgh, Churchill Livingstone.

Appendix 1

Basic mathematical principles

BRACKETS

You will not always meet with straightforward calculations in statistical tests. Many of them have quite complex formulae and it is essential to know which part of the formula should be computed first. One way of indicating which part should be dealt with first is by using brackets. Any figures or formulae contained in brackets should be calculated before anything else, or else you will get quite incorrect results. This can be illustrated by the following examples:

$$114 - (15 + 23)$$
$$= 114 - 38$$
$$= 76$$

as opposed to:

$$(114 - 15) + 23$$
$$= 99 + 23$$
$$= 122$$

Brackets can change your answer quite dramatically. Therefore, the first principle you must remember when calculating any statistical tests is:

All calculations contained in brackets must be carried out first.

However, not all formulae are as convenient as this. Some have brackets within brackets, e.g.

$$14 + [(15 \times 3) - 12]$$

In these cases, you must calculate the formula in the innermost brackets first, then go on to the formula in the next set of brackets and so on. Therefore, the above formula becomes:

$$14 + [45 - 12] = 14 + 33 = 47$$

So:

Always calculate the formula in the innermost set of brackets first and then work outwards.

ADDITION, SUBTRACTION, MULTIPLICATION AND DIVISION

Although any formula in brackets must always be calculated first, not all formulae have brackets.

Sometimes you will come across something like this:

$$12 + 19 - 7 - 4 + 8$$

In such cases, where you have a mixture of just additions and subtraction and no brackets, you simply start calculating from the left-hand side and work systematically across to the right. The importance of this principle can be illustrated by the following example:

$$72 - 34 + 9$$

If you work systematically from left to right, the answer is 47. If, however, you do the addition first, the answer is 29 – quite different and quite incorrect. So the next principle to remember is:

When you have a row of additions and subtractions only and no brackets, start the calculations at the left-hand side and work systematically across to the right.

Similarly, there will be occasions when you have a row of additions only, e.g.

$$19 + 17 + 9$$

subtractions only, e.g.

$$28 - 4 - 16$$

divisions only, e.g.

$$45 \div 3 \div 5$$

multiplications only, e.g.

$$7 \times 8 \times 14$$

While it doesn't matter too much in which order these are carried out, it is easier and less confusing if you stick to the left-to-right rule.

To recap on what has been outlined so far:

- First, carry out the calculations in brackets. If there are brackets within brackets, do the calculations in the inside brackets first.
- Second, if there are no brackets, just work from left to right.

Just one final point – sometimes you will see something like 9(12 – 2). This means 9 × (12 – 2), except that the multiplication sign between the 9 and the bracket is *assumed*.

POSITIVE AND NEGATIVE NUMBERS

It's easy to get confused over positive and negative numbers. While 40 – 20 is simple to work out, 20 – 40 starts to cause confusion. Perhaps the easiest way to overcome the problems of plus and minus numbers is to think of the left-hand figure as your 'bank' of money in a Monopoly® game. Obviously, you can add to your bank or you can take away from your bank, but both transactions will alter the resulting amount of money you have to play with. Suppose you started with £200 but then landed on your competitor's Mayfair property, which meant you owed him/her £300. You have, then £200 – £300. This means that you are £100 in the red, in other words you have –£100. Suppose now that another player landed on your Park Lane property which meant you could receive £200. Because you're already in debt to the tune of £100, half the money you're owed must go towards putting your debt right, which means that you're £100 in credit. In other words you have:

$$-£100 + £200 = +£100$$

However, it's often more expensive than this in Monopoly®. Suppose that while you are £100 in debt, you land on the Strand and owe a further £50. This means you have one debt of £100 (–£100) plus another debt of £50 (–£50). This can be expressed as:

$$(-£100) + (-£50) = -£150$$

There are, of course, many occasions when you will be either multiplying or dividing plus and minus numbers, e.g.

$$(+5) \times (-10) \text{ or } (-80) \div (+8)$$

Multiplying or dividing a mixture of plus and minus numbers always gives a minus answer. So in the examples above, the answers are –50 and –10 respectively. Multiplying or dividing with positive numbers *only* always results in positive answers, but multiplying or dividing with minus numbers only also produces a positive number. If you think about this in terms of double negatives in speech, 'I didn't do nothing' actually means 'I did something'. Similarly, double negatives in maths also mean a positive.

We can state some further mathematical principles now:

1. Adding two negative numbers results in a negative answer, e.g.

$$(-20) + (-10) = -30$$

2. Adding one plus number to a minus number is the same as taking the minus number from the plus number, e.g.

$$-24 + 6 = -18$$

$$+6 - 24 = -18$$

3. Multiplying two positive numbers always results in a positive answer.
4. Multiplying one positive number by one negative number always results in a negative answer.
5. Multiplying two negative numbers always results in a positive answer.
6. Dividing one positive number by another positive number always results in a positive answer.

7. Dividing one positive number by one negative number always results in a negative answer.
8. Dividing one negative number by another negative number always results in a positive answer.

SQUARES AND SQUARE ROOTS

Two common calculations you will have to carry out in the statistical tests are squares and square roots.

The **square** of a number is quite simply that number multiplied by itself and is expressed by a small 2, thus:

$$8^2$$

This means that you multiply 8 by 8. So whenever you see the small ^{2} to the top right of a number, you simply multiply that number by itself. The answer you will obtain will always be a positive number, since if you square +8 you multiply $+8 \times +8$ which will give you +64, while if you square −8, you multiply -8×-8 which will still give you +64, since multiplying two negative numbers always gives a positive number.

The **square root** of a number is actually the opposite of the square, in that the square root of any given number is a number which multiplied by itself gives the number you already have. It is expressed by the symbol $\sqrt{\ }$. Therefore

$$\sqrt{25} = 5, \text{ since } 5 \times 5 = 25$$

While your calculator will almost certainly have a square root function (which you should not hesitate to use), this is a good example of an occasion when you should be 'eyeballing' the result. For example, while you cannot easily work out in your head what the square root of 14 is, you do know that it must be somewhere between 3 and 4, since 3 is the square root of 9 and 4 is the square root of 16; if you come out with something larger or smaller, something has gone wrong somewhere!

In many of the formulae in this book, you will find that the square root sign extends over more than one number, e.g.

$$\sqrt{45 + 19} = \sqrt{64} = 8$$

Do make sure that you complete all the calculations under the square root symbol before computing the square root.

ROUNDING UP DECIMAL PLACES

When using decimals in fairly complicated calculations, you can often end up with a whole row of figures to the right of the decimal point. To continue your calculations with all these numbers is both cumbersome and unnecessarily accurate. Therefore, it is easier to limit the number of figures to the right of the decimal point to 2 or 3. In order to do this correctly, we do not simply chop off the excess figures, but **round them up**.

This is done by starting with the figure on the extreme right of the decimal point. If this figure is equal to 5 or larger, then the number to its immediate left is increased by 1. If the end figure is less than 5, then the number to its left remains the same, e.g.

9.14868125 becomes

9.1486813

If you wish to drop the 3, the same rule applies, so that the above decimal becomes

9.149681

If you wish to cut down the number of decimal places to 2, the process is:

9.148681 becomes

9.14868 which becomes

9.1487 which becomes

9.149 which becomes

9.15

While this process is relatively straightforward in the above example, look at the following decimal number, which we wish to round up to two places:

7.19498

Here, dropping the last number changes the 9 to a 10, and this automatically changes the 4 to 5 which in turn changes the next 9 into a 10, such that the end result is 7.2, even though we were rounding up to 2 decimal places, thus:

7.19498 becomes

7.195 which becomes

7.2

Throughout this book, the figures have been rounded to three decimal places. If you have chosen to round up to two decimal places throughout the calculations, you will find that the end result is slightly different. Don't worry about this unless there is a massive discrepancy which will probably mean that something has gone wrong somewhere in your calculations.

Appendix 2

Statistical probability tables

Table A2.1 Critical values of χ^2 at various levels of probability. For your χ^2 value to be significant at a particular probability level, it should be equal to or larger than the critical values associated with the df in your study. (Reproduced from Lindley DV, Scott WF (1995) New Cambridge Statistical Tables, 2nd edn. Cambridge University Press, with permission.)

df	Level of significance for a two-tailed test				
	0.10	0.05	0.02	0.01	0.001
1	2.71	3.84	5.41	6.64	10.83
2	4.60	5.99	7.82	9.21	13.82
3	6.25	7.82	9.84	11.34	16.27
4	7.78	9.49	11.67	13.28	18.46
5	9.24	11.07	13.39	15.09	20.52
6	10.64	12.59	15.03	16.81	22.46
7	12.02	14.07	16.62	18.48	24.32
8	13.36	15.51	18.17	20.09	26.12
9	14.68	16.92	19.68	21.67	27.88
10	15.99	18.31	21.16	23.21	29.59
11	17.28	19.68	22.62	24.72	31.26
12	18.55	21.03	24.05	26.22	32.91
13	19.81	22.36	25.47	27.69	34.53
14	21.06	23.68	26.87	29.14	36.12
15	22.31	25.00	28.26	30.58	37.70
16	23.54	26.30	29.63	32.00	39.29
17	24.77	27.59	31.00	33.41	40.75
18	25.99	28.87	32.35	34.80	42.31
19	27.20	30.14	33.69	36.19	43.82
20	28.41	31.41	35.02	37.57	45.32
21	29.62	32.67	36.34	38.93	46.80
22	30.81	33.92	37.66	40.29	48.27
23	32.01	35.17	38.97	41.64	49.73
24	33.20	36.42	40.27	42.98	51.18
25	34.38	37.65	41.57	44.31	52.62
26	35.56	38.88	42.86	45.64	54.05
27	36.74	40.11	44.14	46.97	55.48
28	37.92	41.34	45.42	48.28	56.89
29	39.09	42.56	46.69	49.59	58.30
30	40.26	43.77	47.96	50.89	59.70

NB   If you have a one-tailed hypothesis, look up your value as usual and simply halve the associated p value shown for a two-tailed hypothesis.

Table A2.2 Critical values of T (Wilcoxon test) at various levels of probability. (For your T value to be significant at a particular probability level, it should be equal to or less than critical values associated with the N in your study.) (Reproduced from Wilcoxon F, Wilcox RA (1949) Some Rapid Approximate Statistical Procedures. American Cyanamid Company, with permission.)

	Level of significance for one-tailed test					Level of significance for one-tailed test			
	0.05	0.025	0.01	0.005		0.05	0.025	0.01	0.005
	Level of significance for two-tailed test					Level of significance for two-tailed test			
N	0.10	0.05	0.02	0.01	N	0.10	0.05	0.02	0.01
5	1	–	–	–	28	130	117	102	92
6	2	1	–	–	29	141	127	111	100
7	4	2	0	–	30	152	137	120	109
8	6	4	2	0	31	163	148	130	118
9	8	6	3	2	32	175	159	141	128
10	11	8	5	3	33	188	171	151	138
11	14	11	7	5	34	201	183	162	149
12	17	14	10	7	35	214	195	174	160
13	21	17	13	10	36	228	208	186	171
14	26	21	16	13	37	242	222	198	183
15	30	25	20	16	38	256	235	211	195
16	36	30	24	19	39	271	250	224	208
17	41	35	28	23	40	287	264	238	221
18	47	40	33	28	41	303	279	252	234
19	54	46	38	32	42	319	295	267	248
20	60	52	43	37	43	336	311	281	262
21	68	59	49	43	44	353	327	297	277
22	75	66	56	49	45	371	344	313	292
23	83	73	62	55	46	389	361	329	307
24	92	81	69	61	47	408	379	345	323
25	101	90	77	68	48	427	397	362	339
26	110	98	85	76	49	446	415	380	356
27	120	107	93	84	50	466	434	398	373

Dashes in the table indicate that no decision is possible at the stated level of significance.

Table A2.3   Critical values of χ_r^2 (Friedman test) at various levels of probability. (For your χ_r^2 value to be significant at a particular probability level, it should be equal to or larger than the critical values associated with the C and N in your study.) (Reproduced from Friedman M (1937) The use of ranks to avoid the assumptions of normality implicit in the analysis of variance. Reprinted with permission from The Journal of the American Statistical Association. Copyright (1937) by the American Statistical Association. All rights reserved.)

a. Critical values for three conditions ($C = 3$)

$N=2$		$N=3$		$N=4$		$N=5$		$N=6$		$N=7$		$N=8$		$N=9$	
χ_r^2	p	χ_r^2	p	χ_r^2	p	χ_r^2	p	χ_r^2	p	χ_r^2	p	χ_r^2	p	χ_r^2	p
0	1.000	0.000	1.000	0.0	1.000	0.0	1.000	0.00	1.000	0.000	1.000	0.00	1.000	0.000	1.000
1	0.833	0.667	0.944	0.5	0.931	0.4	0.954	0.33	0.956	0.286	0.964	0.25	0.967	0.222	0.971
3	0.500	2.000	0.528	1.5	0.653	1.2	0.691	1.00	0.740	0.857	0.768	0.75	0.794	0.667	0.814
4	0.167	2.667	0.361	2.0	0.431	1.6	0.522	1.33	0.570	1.143	0.620	1.00	0.654	0.889	0.865
		4.667	0.194	3.5	0.273	2.8	0.367	2.33	0.430	2.000	0.486	1.75	0.531	1.556	0.569
		6.000	0.028	4.5	0.125	3.6	0.182	3.00	0.252	2.571	0.305	2.25	0.355	2.000	0.398
				6.0	0.069	4.8	0.124	4.00	0.184	3.429	0.237	3.00	0.285	2.667	0.328
				6.5	0.042	5.2	0.093	4.33	0.142	3.714	0.192	3.25	0.236	2.889	0.278
				8.0	0.0046	6.4	0.039	5.33	0.072	4.571	0.112	4.00	0.149	3.556	0.187
						7.6	0.024	6.33	0.052	5.429	0.085	4.75	0.120	4.222	0.154
						8.4	0.0085	7.00	0.029	6.000	0.052	5.25	0.079	4.667	0.107
						10.0	0.00077	8.33	0.012	7.143	0.027	6.25	0.047	5.556	0.069
								9.00	0.0081	7.714	0.021	6.75	0.038	6.000	0.057
								9.33	0.0055	8.000	0.016	7.00	0.030	6.222	0.048
								10.33	0.0017	8.857	0.0084	7.75	0.018	6.889	0.031
								12.00	0.00013	10.286	0.0036	9.00	0.0099	8.000	0.019
										10.571	0.0027	9.25	0.0080	8.222	0.016
										11.143	0.0012	9.75	0.0048	8.667	0.010
										12.286	0.00032	10.75	0.0024	9.556	0.0060
										14.000	0.000021	12.00	0.0011	10.667	0.0035
												12.25	0.00086	10.889	0.0029
												13.00	0.00026	11.556	0.0013
												14.25	0.000061	12.667	0.00066
												16.00	0.0000036	13.556	0.00035
														14.000	0.00020
														14.222	0.000097
														14.889	0.000054
														16.222	0.000011
														18.000	0.0000006

NB   These values are all for a two-tailed test only.

Table A2.3 (contd) Critical values of χ_r^2 (Friedman test) at various levels of probability. (For your χ_r^2 value to be significant at a particular probability level, it should be equal to or larger than the critical values associated with the C and N in your study.) (Reproduced from Friedman M (1937) The use of ranks to avoid the assumptions of normality implicit in the analysis of variance. Reprinted with permission from The Journal of the American Statistical Association. Copyright (1937) by the American Statistical Association. All rights reserved.)

b. Critical values for four conditions ($C = 4$)

$N = 2$		$N = 3$		$N = 4$			
χ_r^2	p	χ_r^2	p	χ_r^2	p	χ_r^2	p
.0	1.000	0.0	1.000	0.0	1.000	5.7	0.141
.6	0.958	0.6	0.958	0.3	0.992	6.0	0.105
1.2	0.834	1.0	0.910	0.6	0.928	6.3	0.094
1.8	0.792	1.8	0.727	0.9	0.900	6.6	0.077
2.4	0.625	2.2	0.608	1.2	0.800	6.9	0.068
3.0	0.542	2.6	0.524	1.5	0.754	7.2	0.054
3.6	0.458	3.4	0.446	1.8	0.677	7.5	0.052
4.2	0.375	3.8	0.342	2.1	0.649	7.8	0.036
4.8	0.208	4.2	0.300	2.4	0.524	8.1	0.033
5.4	0.167	5.0	0.207	2.7	0.508	8.4	0.019
6.0	0.042	5.4	0.175	3.0	0.432	8.7	0.014
		5.8	0.148	3.3	0.389	9.3	0.012
		6.6	0.075	3.6	0.355	9.6	0.0069
		7.0	0.054	3.9	0.324	9.9	0.0062
		7.4	0.033	4.5	0.242	10.2	0.0027
		8.2	0.017	4.8	0.200	10.8	0.0016
		9.0	0.0017	5.1	0.190	11.1	0.00094
				5.4	0.158	12.0	0.000072

NB These values are all for a two-tailed test only.

Table A2.4 Critical values of L (Page's L trend test) at various levels of probability. (For your L value to be significant at a particular probability level, it should be equal to or larger than the critical values associated with the C and N in your study.)(Reproduced from Page EE (1963) Ordered hypotheses for multiple treatments: a significant test for linear ranks. Reprinted with permission from The Journal of the American Statistical Association. Copyright (1963) by the American Statistical Association. All rights reserved.)

N	3	4	5	6	$p<$
			C		
			(no. of conditions)		
2	–	–	109	178	0.001
	–	60	106	173	0.01
	28	58	103	166	0.05
3	–	89	160	260	0.001
	42	87	155	252	0.01
	41	84	150	244	0.05
4	56	117	210	341	0.001
	55	114	204	331	0.01
	54	111	197	321	0.05
5	70	145	259	420	0.001
	68	141	251	409	0.01
	66	137	244	397	0.05
6	83	172	307	499	0.001
	81	167	299	486	0.01
	79	163	291	474	0.05
7	96	198	355	577	0.001
	93	193	346	563	0.01
	91	189	338	550	0.05
8	109	225	403	655	0.001
	106	220	393	640	0.01
	104	214	384	625	0.05
9	121	252	451	733	0.001
	119	246	441	717	0.01
	116	240	431	701	0.05
10	134	278	499	811	0.001
	131	272	487	793	0.01
	128	266	477	777	0.05
11	147	305	546	888	0.001
	144	298	534	869	0.01
	141	292	523	852	0.05
12	160	331	593	965	0.001
	156	324	581	946	0.01
	153	317	570	928	0.05

NB   These values are for a one-tailed test only.

Table A2.5   Critical values of *t* (related and unrelated *t*-tests) at various levels of probability. For your *t* value to be significant at a particular probability level, it should be equal to or larger than critical values associated with the df in your study. (Reproduced from Lindley DV, Scott WF (1995) New Cambridge Statistical Tables, 2nd edn. Cambridge University Press, with permission.)

df	Level of significance for one-tailed test					
	0.10	0.05	0.025	0.01	0.005	0.0005
	Level of significance for two-tailed test					
	0.20	0.10	0.05	0.02	0.01	0.001
1	3.078	6.314	12.706	31.821	63.657	636.619
2	1.886	2.920	4.303	6.965	9.925	31.598
3	1.638	2.353	3.182	4.541	5.841	12.941
4	1.533	2.132	2.776	3.747	4.604	8.610
5	1.476	2.015	2.571	3.365	4.032	6.859
6	1.440	1.943	2.447	3.143	3.707	5.959
7	1.415	1.895	2.365	2.998	3.499	5.405
8	1.397	1.860	2.306	2.896	3.355	5.041
9	1.383	1.833	2.262	2.821	3.250	4.781
10	1.372	1.812	2.228	2.764	3.169	4.587
11	1.363	1.796	2.201	2.718	3.106	4.437
12	1.356	1.782	2.179	2.681	3.055	4.318
13	1.350	1.771	2.160	2.650	3.012	4.221
14	1.345	1.761	2.145	2.624	2.977	4.140
15	1.341	1.753	2.131	2.602	2.947	4.073
16	1.337	1.746	2.120	2.583	2.921	4.015
17	1.333	1.740	2.110	2.567	2.898	3.965
18	1.330	1.734	2.101	2.552	2.878	3.922
19	1.328	1.729	2.093	2.539	2.861	3.883
20	1.325	1.725	2.086	2.528	2.845	3.850
21	1.323	1.721	2.080	2.518	2.831	3.819
22	1.321	1.717	2.074	2.508	2.819	3.792
23	1.319	1.714	2.069	2.500	2.807	3.767
24	1.318	1.711	2.064	2.492	2.797	3.745
25	1.316	1.708	2.060	2.485	2.787	3.725
26	1.315	1.706	2.056	2.479	2.779	3.707
27	1.314	1.703	2.052	2.473	2.771	3.690
28	1.313	1.701	2.048	2.467	2.763	3.674
29	1.311	1.699	2.045	2.462	2.756	3.659
30	1.310	1.697	2.042	2.457	2.750	3.646
40	1.303	1.684	2.021	2.423	2.704	3.551
60	1.296	1.671	2.000	2.390	2.660	3.460
120	1.289	1.658	1.980	2.358	2.617	3.373
∞	1.282	1.645	1.960	2.326	2.576	3.291

NB   When there is no exact df use the next lowest number, except for very large dfs (well over 120), when you should use the infinity row. This is marked ∞.

Table A2.6 Critical values of F (ANOVAS) at various levels of probability. For your F value to be significant at a particular probability level, it should be equal to or larger than the critical values associated with v_1 and v_2 in your study. (Reproduced from Lindley DV, Scott WF (1995) New Cambridge Statistical Tables, 2nd edition. Cambridge University Press, with permission.)

a. Critical value of F at $p < 0.05$

v_2	v_1											
	1	2	3	4	5	6	7	8	10	12	24	∞
1	161.4	199.5	215.7	224.6	230.2	234.0	236.8	238.9	241.9	243.9	249.0	254.3
2	18.5	19.0	19.2	19.2	19.3	19.3	19.4	19.4	19.4	19.4	19.5	19.5
3	10.13	9.55	9.28	9.12	9.01	8.94	8.89	8.85	8.79	8.74	8.64	8.53
4	7.71	6.94	6.59	6.39	6.26	6.16	6.09	6.04	5.96	5.91	5.77	5.63
5	6.61	5.79	5.41	5.19	5.05	4.95	4.88	4.82	4.74	4.68	4.53	4.36
6	5.99	5.14	4.76	4.53	4.39	4.28	4.21	4.15	4.06	4.00	3.84	3.67
7	5.59	4.74	4.35	4.12	3.97	3.87	3.79	3.73	3.64	3.57	3.41	3.23
8	5.32	4.46	4.07	3.84	3.69	3.58	3.50	3.44	3.35	3.28	3.12	2.93
9	5.12	4.26	3.86	3.63	3.48	3.37	3.29	3.23	3.14	3.07	2.90	2.71
10	4.96	4.10	3.71	3.48	3.33	3.22	3.14	3.07	2.98	2.91	2.74	2.54
11	4.84	3.98	3.59	3.36	3.20	3.09	3.01	2.95	2.85	2.79	2.61	2.40
12	4.75	3.89	3.49	3.26	3.11	3.00	2.91	2.85	2.75	2.69	2.51	2.30
13	4.67	3.81	3.41	3.18	3.03	2.92	2.83	2.77	2.67	2.60	2.42	2.21
14	4.60	3.74	3.34	3.11	2.96	2.85	2.76	2.70	2.60	2.53	2.35	2.13
15	4.54	3.68	3.29	3.06	2.90	2.79	2.71	2.64	2.54	2.48	2.29	2.07
16	4.49	3.63	3.24	3.01	2.85	2.74	2.66	2.59	2.49	2.42	2.24	2.01
17	4.45	3.59	3.20	2.96	2.81	2.70	2.61	2.55	2.45	2.38	2.19	1.96
18	4.41	3.55	3.16	2.93	2.77	2.66	2.58	2.51	2.41	2.34	2.15	1.92
19	4.38	3.52	3.13	2.90	2.74	2.63	2.54	2.48	2.38	2.31	2.11	1.88
20	4.35	3.49	3.10	2.87	2.71	2.60	2.51	2.45	2.35	2.28	2.08	1.84
21	4.32	3.47	3.07	2.84	2.68	2.57	2.49	2.42	2.32	2.25	2.05	1.81
22	4.30	3.44	3.05	2.82	2.66	2.55	2.46	2.40	2.30	2.23	2.03	1.78
23	4.28	3.42	3.03	2.80	2.64	2.53	2.44	2.37	2.27	2.20	2.00	1.76
24	4.26	3.40	3.01	2.78	2.62	2.51	2.42	2.36	2.25	2.18	1.98	1.73
25	4.24	3.39	2.99	2.76	2.60	2.49	2.40	2.34	2.24	2.16	1.96	1.71
26	4.23	3.37	2.98	2.74	2.59	2.47	2.39	2.32	2.22	2.15	1.95	1.69
27	4.21	3.35	2.96	2.73	2.57	2.46	2.37	2.31	2.20	2.13	1.93	1.67
28	4.20	3.34	2.95	2.71	2.56	2.45	2.36	2.29	2.19	2.12	1.91	1.65
29	4.18	3.33	2.93	2.70	2.55	2.43	2.35	2.28	2.18	2.10	1.90	1.64
30	4.17	3.32	2.92	2.69	2.53	2.42	2.33	2.27	2.16	2.09	1.89	1.62
32	4.15	3.29	2.90	2.67	2.51	2.40	2.31	2.24	2.14	2.07	1.86	1.59
34	4.13	3.28	2.88	2.65	2.49	2.38	2.29	2.23	2.12	2.05	1.84	1.57
36	4.11	3.26	2.87	2.63	2.48	2.36	2.28	2.21	2.11	2.03	1.82	1.55
38	4.10	3.24	2.85	2.62	2.46	2.35	2.26	2.19	2.09	2.02	1.81	1.53
40	4.08	3.23	2.84	2.61	2.45	2.34	2.25	2.18	2.08	2.00	1.79	1.51
60	4.00	3.15	2.76	2.53	2.37	2.25	2.17	2.10	1.99	1.92	1.70	1.39
120	3.92	3.07	2.68	2.45	2.29	2.18	2.09	2.02	1.91	1.83	1.61	1.25
∞	3.84	3.00	2.60	2.37	2.21	2.10	2.01	1.94	1.83	1.75	1.52	1.00

Table A2.6 (contd) Critical values of F (ANOVAs) at various levels of probability. For your F value to be significant at a particular probability level, it should be equal to or larger than the critical values associated with v_1 and v_2 in your study. (Reproduced from Lindley DV, Scott WF (1995) New Cambridge Statistical Tables, 2nd edition. Cambridge University Press, with permission.)

b. Critical value of F at $p < 0.025$

v_2	1	2	3	4	5	6	7	8	10	12	24	∞
						v_1						
1	648	800	864	900	922	937	948	957	969	977	997	1018
2	38.5	39.0	39.2	39.2	39.3	39.3	39.4	39.4	39.4	39.4	39.5	39.5
3	17.4	16.0	15.4	15.1	14.9	14.7	14.6	14.5	14.4	14.3	14.1	13.9
4	12.22	10.65	9.98	9.60	9.36	9.20	9.07	8.98	8.84	8.75	8.51	8.26
5	10.01	8.43	7.76	7.39	7.15	6.98	6.85	6.76	6.62	6.52	6.28	6.02
6	8.81	7.26	6.60	6.23	5.99	5.82	5.70	5.60	5.46	5.37	5.12	4.85
7	8.07	6.54	5.89	5.52	5.29	5.12	4.99	4.90	4.76	4.67	4.42	4.14
8	7.57	6.06	5.42	5.05	4.82	4.65	4.53	4.43	4.30	4.20	3.95	3.67
9	7.21	5.71	5.08	4.72	4.48	4.32	4.20	4.10	3.96	3.87	3.61	3.33
10	6.94	5.46	4.83	4.47	4.24	4.07	3.95	3.85	3.72	3.62	3.37	3.08
11	6.72	5.26	4.63	4.28	4.04	3.88	3.76	3.66	3.53	3.43	3.17	2.88
12	6.55	5.10	4.47	4.12	3.89	3.73	3.61	3.51	3.37	3.28	3.02	2.72
13	6.41	4.97	4.35	4.00	3.77	3.60	3.48	3.39	3.25	3.15	2.89	2.60
14	6.30	4.86	4.24	3.89	3.66	3.50	3.38	3.29	3.15	3.05	2.79	2.49
15	6.20	4.76	4.15	3.80	3.58	3.41	3.29	3.20	3.06	2.96	2.70	2.40
16	6.12	4.69	4.08	3.73	3.50	3.34	3.22	3.12	2.99	2.89	2.63	2.32
17	6.04	4.62	4.01	3.66	3.44	3.28	3.16	3.06	2.92	2.82	2.56	2.25
18	5.98	4.56	3.95	3.61	3.38	3.22	3.10	3.01	2.87	2.77	2.50	2.19
19	5.92	4.51	3.90	3.56	3.33	3.17	3.05	2.96	2.82	2.72	2.45	2.13
20	5.87	4.46	3.86	3.51	3.29	3.13	3.01	2.91	2.77	2.68	2.41	2.09
21	5.83	4.42	3.82	3.48	3.25	3.09	2.97	2.87	2.73	2.64	2.37	2.04
22	5.79	4.38	3.78	3.44	3.22	3.05	2.93	2.84	2.70	2.60	2.33	2.00
23	5.75	4.35	3.75	3.41	3.18	3.02	2.90	2.81	2.67	2.57	2.30	1.97
24	5.72	4.32	3.72	3.38	3.15	2.99	2.87	2.78	2.64	2.54	2.27	1.94
25	5.69	4.29	3.69	3.35	3.13	2.97	2.85	2.75	2.61	2.51	2.24	1.91
26	5.66	4.27	3.67	3.33	3.10	2.94	2.82	2.73	2.59	2.49	2.22	1.88
27	5.63	4.24	3.65	3.31	3.08	2.92	2.80	2.71	2.57	2.47	2.19	1.85
28	5.61	4.22	3.63	3.29	3.06	2.90	2.78	2.69	2.55	2.45	2.17	1.83
29	5.59	4.20	3.61	3.27	3.04	2.88	2.76	2.67	2.53	2.43	2.15	1.81
30	5.57	4.18	3.59	3.25	3.03	2.87	2.75	2.65	2.51	2.41	2.14	1.79
32	5.53	4.15	3.56	3.22	3.00	2.84	2.72	2.62	2.48	2.38	2.10	1.75
34	5.50	4.12	3.53	3.19	2.97	2.81	2.69	2.59	2.45	2.35	2.08	1.72
36	5.47	4.09	3.51	3.17	2.94	2.79	2.66	2.57	2.43	2.33	2.05	1.69
38	5.45	4.07	3.48	3.15	2.92	2.76	2.64	2.55	2.41	2.31	2.03	1.66
40	5.42	4.05	3.46	3.13	2.90	2.74	2.62	2.53	2.39	2.29	2.01	1.64
60	5.29	3.93	3.34	3.01	2.79	2.63	2.51	2.41	2.27	2.17	1.88	1.48
120	5.15	3.80	3.23	2.89	2.67	2.52	2.39	2.30	2.16	2.05	1.76	1.31
∞	5.02	3.69	3.12	2.79	2.57	2.41	2.29	2.19	2.05	1.94	1.64	1.00

Table A2.6 (contd) Critical values of F (ANOVAs) at various levels of probability. For your F value to be significant at a particular probability level, it should be equal to or larger than the critical values associated with v_1 and v_2 in your study. (Reproduced from Lindley DV, Scott WF (1995) New Cambridge Statistical Tables, 2nd edition. Cambridge University Press, with permission.)

c. Critical value of F at $p < 0.01$

v_2	v_1												
	1	2	3	4	5	6	7	8	10	12	24	∞
1	4052	5000	5403	5625	5764	5859	5828	5981	6056	6106	6235	6366
2	98.5	99.0	99.2	99.2	99.3	99.3	99.4	99.4	99.4	99.4	99.5	99.5
3	34.1	30.8	29.5	28.7	28.2	27.9	27.7	27.5	27.2	27.1	26.6	26.1
4	21.2	18.0	16.7	16.0	15.5	15.2	15.0	14.8	14.5	14.4	13.9	13.5
5	16.26	13.27	12.06	11.39	10.97	10.67	10.46	10.29	10.05	9.89	9.47	9.02
6	13.74	10.92	9.78	9.15	8.75	8.47	8.26	8.10	7.87	7.72	7.31	6.88
7	12.25	9.55	8.45	7.85	7.46	7.19	6.99	6.84	6.62	6.47	6.07	5.65
8	11.26	8.65	7.59	7.01	6.63	6.37	6.18	6.03	5.81	5.67	5.28	4.86
9	10.56	8.02	6.99	6.42	6.06	5.80	5.61	5.47	5.26	5.11	4.73	4.31
10	10.04	7.56	6.55	5.99	5.64	5.39	5.20	5.06	4.85	4.71	4.33	3.91
11	9.65	7.21	6.22	5.67	5.32	5.07	4.89	4.74	4.54	4.40	4.02	3.60
12	9.33	6.93	5.95	5.41	5.06	4.82	4.64	4.50	4.30	4.16	3.78	3.36
13	9.07	6.70	5.74	5.21	4.86	4.62	4.44	4.30	4.10	3.96	3.59	3.17
14	8.86	6.51	5.56	5.04	4.70	4.46	4.28	4.14	3.94	3.80	3.43	3.00
15	8.68	6.36	5.42	4.89	4.56	4.32	4.14	4.00	3.80	3.67	3.29	2.87
16	8.53	6.23	5.29	4.77	4.44	4.20	4.03	3.89	3.69	3.55	3.18	2.75
17	8.40	6.11	5.18	4.67	4.34	4.10	3.93	3.79	3.59	3.46	3.08	2.65
18	8.29	6.01	5.09	4.58	4.25	4.01	3.84	3.71	3.51	3.37	3.00	2.57
19	8.18	5.93	5.01	4.50	4.17	3.94	3.77	3.63	3.43	3.30	2.92	2.49
20	8.10	5.85	4.94	4.43	4.10	3.87	3.70	3.56	3.37	3.23	2.86	2.42
21	8.02	5.78	4.87	4.37	4.04	3.81	3.64	3.51	3.31	3.17	2.80	2.36
22	7.95	5.72	4.82	4.31	3.99	3.76	3.59	3.45	3.26	3.12	2.75	2.31
23	7.88	5.66	4.76	4.26	3.94	3.71	3.54	3.41	3.21	3.07	2.70	2.26
24	7.82	5.61	4.72	4.22	3.90	3.67	3.50	3.36	3.17	3.03	2.66	2.21
25	7.77	5.57	4.68	4.18	3.86	3.63	3.46	3.32	3.13	2.99	2.62	2.17
26	7.72	5.53	4.64	4.14	3.82	3.59	3.42	3.29	3.09	2.96	2.58	2.13
27	7.68	5.49	4.60	4.11	3.78	3.56	3.39	3.26	3.06	2.93	2.55	2.10
28	7.64	5.45	4.57	4.07	3.75	3.53	3.36	3.23	3.03	2.90	2.52	2.06
29	7.60	5.42	4.54	4.04	3.73	3.50	3.33	3.20	3.00	2.87	2.49	2.03
30	7.56	5.39	4.51	4.02	3.70	3.47	3.30	3.17	2.98	2.84	2.47	2.01
32	7.50	5.34	4.46	3.97	3.65	3.43	3.26	3.13	2.93	2.80	2.42	1.96
34	7.45	5.29	4.42	3.93	3.61	3.39	3.22	3.09	2.90	2.76	2.38	1.91
36	7.40	5.25	4.38	3.89	3.58	3.35	3.18	3.05	2.86	2.72	2.35	1.87
38	7.35	5.21	4.34	3.86	3.54	3.32	3.15	3.02	2.83	2.69	2.32	1.84
40	7.31	5.18	4.31	3.83	3.51	3.29	3.12	2.99	2.80	2.66	2.29	1.80
60	7.08	4.98	4.13	3.65	3.34	3.12	2.95	2.82	2.63	2.50	2.12	1.60
120	6.85	4.79	3.95	3.48	3.17	2.96	2.79	2.66	2.47	2.34	1.95	1.38
∞	6.63	4.61	3.78	3.32	3.02	2.80	2.64	2.51	2.32	2.18	1.79	1.00

Table A2.6 (contd) Critical values of F (ANOVAS) at various levels of probability. For your F value to be significant at a particular probability level, it should be equal to or larger than the critical values associated with v_1 and v_2 in your study. (Reproduced from Lindley DV, Scott WF (1995) New Cambridge Statistical Tables, 2nd edition. Cambridge University Press, with permission.)

d. Critical values of F at $p < 0.001$

v_2	v_1 1	2	3	4	5	6	7	8	10	12	24	∞
1	*4053	5000	5404	5625	5764	5859	5929	5981	6056	6107	6235	6366*
2	998.5	999.0	999.2	999.2	999.3	999.3	999.4	999.4	999.4	999.4	999.5	999.5
3	167.0	148.5	141.1	137.1	134.6	132.8	131.5	130.6	129.2	128.3	125.9	123.5
4	74.14	61.25	56.18	53.44	51.71	50.53	49.66	49.00	48.05	47.41	45.77	44.05
5	47.18	37.12	33.20	31.09	29.75	28.83	28.16	27.65	26.92	26.42	25.14	23.79
6	35.51	27.00	23.70	21.92	20.80	20.03	19.46	19.03	18.41	17.99	16.90	15.75
7	29.25	21.69	18.77	17.20	16.21	15.52	15.02	14.63	14.08	13.71	12.73	11.70
8	25.42	18.49	15.83	14.39	13.48	12.86	12.40	12.05	11.54	11.19	10.30	9.34
9	22.86	16.39	13.90	12.56	11.71	11.13	10.69	10.37	9.87	9.57	8.72	7.81
10	21.04	14.91	12.55	11.28	10.48	9.93	9.52	9.20	8.74	8.44	7.64	6.76
11	19.69	13.81	11.56	10.35	9.58	9.05	8.66	8.35	7.92	7.63	6.85	6.00
12	18.64	12.97	10.80	9.63	8.89	8.38	8.00	7.71	7.29	7.00	6.25	5.42
13	17.82	12.31	10.21	9.07	8.35	7.86	7.49	7.21	6.80	6.52	5.78	4.97
14	17.14	11.78	9.73	8.62	7.92	7.44	7.08	6.80	6.40	6.13	5.41	4.60
15	16.59	11.34	9.34	8.25	7.57	7.09	6.74	6.47	6.08	5.81	5.10	4.31
16	16.12	10.97	9.01	7.94	7.27	6.80	6.46	6.19	5.81	5.55	4.85	4.06
17	15.72	10.66	8.73	7.68	7.02	6.56	6.22	5.96	5.58	5.32	4.63	3.85
18	15.38	10.39	8.49	7.46	6.81	6.35	6.02	5.76	5.39	5.13	4.45	3.67
19	15.08	10.16	8.28	7.27	6.62	6.18	5.85	5.59	5.22	4.97	4.29	3.51
20	14.82	9.95	8.10	7.10	6.46	6.02	5.69	5.44	5.08	4.82	4.15	3.38
21	14.59	9.77	7.94	6.95	6.32	5.88	5.56	5.31	4.95	4.70	4.03	3.26
22	14.38	9.61	7.80	6.81	6.19	5.76	5.44	5.19	4.83	4.58	3.92	3.15
23	14.19	9.47	7.67	6.70	6.08	5.65	5.33	5.09	4.73	4.48	3.82	3.05
24	14.03	9.34	7.55	6.59	5.98	5.55	5.23	4.99	4.64	4.39	3.74	2.97
25	13.88	9.22	7.45	6.49	5.89	5.46	5.15	4.91	4.56	4.31	3.66	2.89
26	13.74	9.12	7.36	6.41	5.80	5.38	5.07	4.83	4.48	4.24	3.59	2.82
27	13.61	9.02	7.27	6.33	5.73	5.31	5.00	4.76	4.41	4.17	3.52	2.75
28	13.50	8.93	7.19	6.25	5.66	5.24	4.93	4.69	4.35	4.11	3.46	2.69
29	13.39	8.85	7.12	6.19	5.59	5.18	4.87	4.64	4.29	4.05	3.41	2.64
30	13.29	8.77	7.05	6.12	5.53	5.12	4.82	4.58	4.24	4.00	3.36	2.59
32	13.12	8.64	6.94	6.01	5.43	5.02	4.72	4.48	4.14	3.91	3.27	2.50
34	12.97	8.52	6.83	5.92	5.34	4.93	4.63	4.40	4.06	3.83	3.19	2.42
36	12.83	8.42	6.74	5.84	5.26	4.86	4.56	4.33	3.99	3.76	3.12	2.35
38	12.71	8.33	6.66	5.76	5.19	4.79	4.49	4.26	3.93	3.70	3.06	2.29
40	12.61	8.25	6.59	5.70	5.13	4.73	4.44	4.21	3.87	3.64	3.01	2.23
60	11.97	7.77	6.17	5.31	4.76	4.37	4.09	3.86	3.54	3.32	2.69	1.89
120	11.38	7.32	5.78	4.95	4.42	4.04	3.77	3.55	3.24	3.02	2.40	1.54
∞	10.83	6.91	5.42	4.62	4.10	3.74	3.47	3.27	2.96	2.74	2.13	1.00

*Critical values to the right of $v_2 = 1$ should all be multiplied by 100, i.e. 4053 should be 40 5300.

NB   When there is no exact number for the df, use the next lowest number. For very large dfs (i.e. well over 120) you should use the row for infinity, marked ∞.

These values are all for a two-tailed test only.

Table A2.7   Critical values of U (Mann–Whitney U test) at various levels of probability. For your U value to be significant at a particular probability level, it should be equal to or less than the critical value associated with n_1 and n_2 in your study. (Reproduced from Runyon R, Haber A (1991) Fundamentals of Behavioral Statistics, 7th edn. with permission of McGraw-Hill Inc.)

a. Critical values of U for a one-tailed test at 0.005; two-tailed test at 0.01

n_2	1	2	3	4	5	6	7	8	9	10	11	12	13	14	15	16	17	18	19	20
1	–	–	–	–	–	–	–	–	–	–	–	–	–	–	–	–	–	–	–	–
2	–	–	–	–	–	–	–	–	–	–	–	–	–	–	–	–	–	–	0	0
3	–	–	–	–	–	–	–	–	0	0	0	1	1	1	2	2	2	2	3	3
4	–	–	–	–	–	0	0	1	1	2	2	3	3	4	5	5	6	6	7	8
5	–	–	–	–	0	1	1	2	3	4	5	6	7	7	8	9	10	11	12	13
6	–	–	–	0	1	2	3	4	5	6	7	9	10	11	12	13	15	16	17	18
7	–	–	–	0	1	3	4	6	7	9	10	12	13	15	16	18	19	21	22	24
8	–	–	–	1	2	4	6	7	9	11	13	15	17	18	20	22	24	26	28	30
9	–	–	0	1	3	5	7	9	11	13	16	18	20	22	24	27	29	31	33	36
10	–	–	0	2	4	6	9	11	13	16	18	21	24	26	29	31	34	37	39	42
11	–	–	0	2	5	7	10	13	16	18	21	24	27	30	33	36	39	42	45	48
12	–	–	1	3	6	9	12	15	18	21	24	27	31	34	37	41	44	47	51	54
13	–	–	1	3	7	10	13	17	20	24	27	31	34	38	42	45	49	53	56	60
14	–	–	1	4	7	11	15	18	22	26	30	34	38	42	46	50	54	58	63	67
15	–	–	2	5	8	12	16	20	24	29	33	37	42	46	51	55	60	64	69	73
16	–	–	2	5	9	13	18	22	27	31	36	41	45	50	55	60	65	70	74	79
17	–	–	2	6	10	15	19	24	29	34	39	44	49	54	60	65	70	75	81	86
18	–	–	2	6	11	16	21	26	31	37	42	47	53	58	64	70	75	81	87	92
19	–	0	3	7	12	17	22	28	33	39	45	51	56	63	69	74	81	87	93	99
20	–	0	3	8	13	18	24	30	36	42	48	54	60	67	73	79	86	92	99	105

b. Critical values of U for a one-tailed test at 0.01; two-tailed test at 0.02

n_2	1	2	3	4	5	6	7	8	9	10	11	12	13	14	15	16	17	18	19	20
1	–	–	–	–	–	–	–	–	–	–	–	–	–	–	–	–	–	–	–	–
2	–	–	–	–	–	–	–	–	–	–	–	0	0	0	0	0	0	0	1	1
3	–	–	–	–	–	–	0	0	1	1	1	2	2	2	3	3	4	4	4	5
4	–	–	–	–	0	1	1	2	3	3	4	5	5	6	7	7	8	9	9	10
5	–	–	–	0	1	2	3	4	5	6	7	8	9	10	11	12	13	14	15	16
6	–	–	–	1	2	3	4	6	7	8	9	11	12	13	15	16	18	19	20	22
7	–	–	0	1	3	4	6	7	9	11	12	14	16	17	19	21	23	24	26	28
8	–	–	0	2	4	6	7	9	11	13	15	17	20	22	24	26	28	30	32	34
9	–	–	1	3	5	7	9	11	14	16	18	21	23	26	28	31	33	36	38	40
10	–	–	1	3	6	8	11	13	16	19	22	24	27	30	33	36	38	41	44	47
11	–	–	1	4	7	9	12	15	18	22	25	28	31	34	37	41	44	47	50	53
12	–	–	2	5	8	11	14	17	21	24	28	31	35	38	42	46	49	53	56	60
13	–	0	2	5	9	12	16	20	23	27	31	35	39	43	47	51	55	59	63	67
14	–	0	2	6	10	13	17	22	26	30	34	38	43	47	51	56	60	65	69	73
15	–	0	3	7	11	15	19	24	28	33	37	42	47	51	56	61	66	70	75	80
16	–	0	3	7	12	16	21	26	31	36	41	46	51	56	61	66	71	76	82	87
17	–	0	4	8	13	18	23	28	33	38	44	49	55	60	66	71	77	82	88	93
18	–	0	4	9	14	19	24	30	36	41	47	53	59	65	70	76	82	88	94	100
19	–	1	4	9	15	20	26	32	38	44	50	56	63	69	75	82	88	94	101	107
20	–	1	5	10	16	22	28	34	40	47	53	60	67	73	80	87	93	100	107	114

Table A2.7 (contd) Critical values of U (Mann–Whitney U test) at various levels of probability. For your U value to be significant at a particular probability level, it should be equal to or less than the critical value associated with n_1 and n_2 in your study. (Reproduced from Runyon R, Haber A (1991) Fundamentals of Behavioral Statistics, 7th edn. with permission of McGraw-Hill Inc.)

c. Critical values of U for a one-tailed test at 0.025; two-tailed test at 0.05

n_2	1	2	3	4	5	6	7	8	9	10	11	12	13	14	15	16	17	18	19	20
1	–	–	–	–	–	–	–	–	–	–	–	–	–	–	–	–	–	–	–	–
2	–	–	–	–	–	–	0	0	0	0	1	1	1	1	1	1	2	2	2	2
3	–	–	–	–	0	1	1	2	2	3	3	4	4	5	5	6	6	7	7	8
4	–	–	–	0	1	2	3	4	4	5	6	7	8	9	10	11	11	12	13	13
5	–	–	0	1	2	3	5	6	7	8	9	11	12	13	14	15	17	18	19	20
6	–	–	1	2	3	5	6	8	10	11	13	14	16	17	19	21	22	24	25	27
7	–	–	1	3	5	6	8	10	12	14	16	18	20	22	24	26	28	30	32	34
8	–	0	2	4	6	8	10	13	15	17	19	22	24	26	29	31	34	36	38	41
9	–	0	2	4	7	10	12	15	17	20	23	26	28	31	34	37	39	42	45	48
10	–	0	3	5	8	11	14	17	20	23	26	29	33	36	39	42	45	48	52	55
11	–	0	3	6	9	13	16	19	23	26	30	33	37	40	44	47	51	55	58	62
12	–	1	4	7	11	14	18	22	26	29	33	37	41	45	49	53	57	61	65	69
13	–	1	4	8	12	16	20	24	28	33	37	41	45	50	54	59	63	67	72	76
14	–	1	5	9	13	17	22	26	31	36	40	45	50	55	59	64	67	74	78	83
15	–	1	5	10	14	19	24	29	34	39	44	49	54	59	64	70	75	80	85	90
16	–	1	6	11	15	21	26	31	37	42	47	53	59	64	70	75	81	86	92	98
17	–	2	6	11	17	22	28	34	39	45	51	57	63	67	75	81	87	93	99	105
18	–	2	7	12	18	24	30	36	42	48	55	61	67	74	80	86	93	99	106	112
19	–	2	7	13	19	25	32	38	45	52	58	65	72	78	85	92	99	106	113	119
20	–	2	8	13	20	27	34	41	48	55	62	69	76	83	90	98	105	112	119	127

d. Critical values of U for a one-tailed test at 0.05; two-tailed test at 0.10

n_2	1	2	3	4	5	6	7	8	9	10	11	12	13	14	15	16	17	18	19	20
1	–	–	–	–	–	–	–	–	–	–	–	–	–	–	–	–	–	–	0	0
2	–	–	–	–	0	0	0	1	1	1	1	2	2	2	3	3	3	4	4	4
3	–	–	0	0	1	2	2	3	3	4	5	5	6	7	7	8	9	9	10	11
4	–	–	0	1	2	3	4	5	6	7	8	9	10	11	12	14	15	16	17	18
5	–	0	1	2	4	5	6	8	9	11	12	13	15	16	18	19	20	22	23	25
6	–	0	2	3	5	7	8	10	12	14	16	17	19	21	23	25	26	28	30	32
7	–	0	2	4	6	8	11	13	15	17	19	21	24	26	28	30	33	35	37	39
8	–	1	3	5	8	10	13	15	18	20	23	26	28	31	33	36	39	41	44	47
9	–	1	3	6	9	12	15	18	21	24	27	30	33	36	39	42	45	48	51	54
10	–	1	4	7	11	14	17	20	24	27	31	34	37	41	44	48	51	55	58	62
11	–	1	5	8	12	16	19	23	27	31	34	38	42	46	50	54	57	61	65	69
12	–	2	5	9	13	17	21	26	30	34	38	42	47	51	55	60	64	68	72	77
13	–	2	6	10	15	19	24	28	33	37	42	47	51	56	61	65	70	75	80	84
14	–	2	7	11	16	21	26	31	36	41	46	51	56	61	66	71	77	82	87	92
15	–	3	7	12	18	23	28	33	39	44	50	55	61	66	72	77	83	88	94	100
16	–	3	8	14	19	25	30	36	42	48	54	60	65	71	77	83	89	95	101	107
17	–	3	9	15	20	26	33	39	45	51	57	64	70	77	83	89	96	102	109	115
18	–	4	9	16	22	28	35	41	48	55	61	68	75	82	88	95	102	109	116	123
19	0	4	10	17	23	30	37	44	51	58	65	72	80	87	94	101	109	116	123	130
20	0	4	11	18	25	32	39	47	54	62	69	77	84	92	100	107	115	123	130	138

Dashes in the table mean that no decision is possible for those n values at the given level of significance.

Table A2.8 Critical values of H (Kruskal–Wallis test) at various levels of probability. (For your H value to be significant at a particular probability level, it should be equal to or larger than the critical values associated with the ns in your study.) (Reproduced from Kruskal WH, Wallis WA (1952). The use of ranks in one-criterion variance analysis. Reprinted with permission from The Journal of the American Statistical Association. Copyright (1952) by the American Statistical Association. All rights reserved.)

| Size of groups | | | | | Size of groups | | | | |
n_1	n_2	n_3	H	p	n_1	n_2	n_3	H	p
2	1	1	2.7000	0.500	4	3	2	6.4444	0.008
2	2	1	3.6000	0.200				6.3000	0.011
2	2	2	4.5714	0.067				5.4444	0.046
			3.7143	0.200				5.4000	0.051
3	1	1	3.2000	0.300				4.5111	0.098
3	2	1	4.2857	0.100				4.4444	0.102
			3.8571	0.133	4	3	3	6.7455	0.010
3	2	2	5.3572	0.029				6.7091	0.013
			4.7143	0.048				5.7909	0.046
			4.5000	0.067				5.7273	0.050
			4.4643	0.105				4.7091	0.092
3	3	1	5.1429	0.043				4.7000	0.101
			4.5714	0.100	4	4	1	6.6667	0.010
			4.0000	0.129				6.1667	0.022
3	3	2	6.2500	0.011				4.9667	0.048
			5.3611	0.032				4.8667	0.054
			5.1389	0.061				4.1667	0.082
			4.5556	0.100				4.0667	0.102
			4.2500	0.121	4	4	2	7.0364	0.006
3	3	3	7.2000	0.004				6.8727	0.011
			6.4889	0.011				5.4545	0.046
			5.6889	0.029				5.2364	0.052
			5.6000	0.050				4.5545	0.098
			5.0667	0.086				4.4455	0.103
			4.6222	0.100	4	4	3	7.1439	0.010
4	1	1	3.5714	0.200				7.1364	0.011
4	2	1	4.8214	0.057				5.5985	0.049
			4.5000	0.076				5.5758	0.051
			4.0179	0.114				4.5455	0.099
4	2	2	6.0000	0.014				4.4773	0.102
			5.3333	0.033	4	4	4	7.6538	0.008
			5.1250	0.052				7.5385	0.011
			4.4583	0.100				5.6923	0.049
			4.1667	0.105				5.6538	0.054
4	3	1	5.8333	0.021				4.6539	0.097
			5.2083	0.050				4.5001	0.104
			5.0000	0.057	5	1	1	3.8571	0.143
4	3	1	4.0556	0.093	5	2	1	5.2500	0.036
			3.8889	0.129				5.0000	0.048

Table A2.8 (contd) Critical values of H (Kruskal–Wallis test) at various levels of probability. (For your H value to be significant at a particular probability level, it should be equal to or larger than the critical values associated with the ns in your study.) (Reproduced from Kruskal WH, Wallis WA (1952) The use of ranks in one-criterion variance analysis. Reprinted with permission from The Journal of the American Statistical Association. Copyright (1952) by the American Statistical Association. All rights reserved.)

Size of groups					Size of groups				
n_1	n_2	n_3	H	p	n_1	n_2	n_3	H	p
			4.4500	0.071				5.6564	0.049
			4.2000	0.095				5.6308	0.050
			4.0500	0.119				4.5487	0.099
5	2	2	6.5333	0.008				4.5231	0.103
			6.1333	0.013	5	4	4	7.7604	0.009
			5.1600	0.034				7.7440	0.011
			5.0400	0.056				5.6571	0.049
			4.3733	0.090				5.6176	0.050
			4.2933	0.122				4.6187	0.100
5	3	1	6.4000	0.012				4.5527	0.102
			4.9600	0.048	5	5	1	7.3091	0.009
			4.8711	0.052				6.8364	0.011
			4.0178	0.095				5.1273	0.046
			3.8400	0.123				4.9091	0.053
5	3	2	6.9091	0.009				4.1091	0.086
			6.8218	0.010				4.0364	0.105
			5.2509	0.049	5	5	2	7.3385	0.010
			5.1055	0.052				7.2692	0.010
			4.6509	0.091				5.3385	0.047
			4.4945	0.101				5.2462	0.051
5	3	3	7.0788	0.009				4.6231	0.097
			6.9818	0.011				4.5077	0.100
			5.6485	0.049	5	5	3	7.5780	0.010
			5.5152	0.051				7.5429	0.010
			4.5333	0.097				5.7055	0.046
			4.4121	0.109				5.6264	0.051
5	4	1	6.9545	0.008				4.5451	0.100
			6.8400	0.011				4.5363	0.102
			4.9855	0.044	5	5	4	7.8229	0.010
			4.8600	0.056				7.7914	0.010
			3.9873	0.098				5.6657	0.049
			3.9600	0.102				5.6429	0.050
5	4	2	7.2045	0.009				4.5229	0.099
			7.1182	0.010				4.5200	0.101
			5.2727	0.049	5	5	5	8.0000	0.009
			5.2682	0.050				7.9800	0.010
			4.5409	0.098				7.7800	0.049
			4.5182	0.101				5.6600	0.051
5	4	3	7.4449	0.010				4.5600	0.100
			7.3949	0.011				4.5000	0.102

NB   These values are all for a two-tailed test only.

Table A2.9   Critical values of S (Jonckheere trend test) at various levels of probability. (For your S value to be significant at a particular probability level, it should be equal to or larger than the critical values associated with C and n in your study.)

a. Significance level $p < 0.05$

C	2	3	4	5	6	7	8	9	10
3	10	17	24	33	42	53	64	76	88
4	14	26	38	51	66	82	100	118	138
5	20	34	51	71	92	115	140	166	194
6	26	44	67	93	121	151	184	219	256

b. Significance level $p < 0.01$

C	2	3	4	5	6	7	8	9	10
3	–	23	32	45	59	74	90	106	124
4	20	34	50	71	92	115	140	167	195
5	26	48	72	99	129	162	197	234	274
6	34	62	94	130	170	213	260	309	361

NB   These values are all for a one-tailed test only.

Table A2.10   Critical values of r_s (Spearman test) at various levels of probability. (For your r_s value to be significant at a particular probability level, it should be equal to or larger than the critical values associated with N in your study.) (Reproduced with permission from Olds EG (1949) The 5% significance levels for sums of squares of rank differences and a correction. Annals of Mathematical Statistics 20:1.)

	Level of significance for one-tailed test			
	0.05	0.025	0.01	0.005
	Level of significance for two-tailed test			
N (number of subjects)	0.10	0.05	0.02	0.01
5	0.900	1.000	1.000	–
6	0.829	0.886	0.943	1.000
7	0.714	0.786	0.893	0.929
8	0.643	0.738	0.833	0.881
9	0.600	0.683	0.783	0.833
10	0.564	0.648	0.746	0.794
12	0.506	0.591	0.712	0.777
14	0.456	0.544	0.645	0.715
16	0.425	0.506	0.601	0.665
18	0.399	0.475	0.564	0.625
20	0.377	0.450	0.534	0.591
22	0.359	0.428	0.508	0.562
24	0.343	0.409	0.485	0.537
26	0.329	0.392	0.465	0.515
28	0.317	0.377	0.448	0.496
30	0.306	0.364	0.432	0.478

NB   When there is no exact number of subjects use the next lowest number.

Table A2.11   Critical values of r (Pearson test) at various levels of probability. (For your r value to be significant at a particular probability level, it should be equal to or larger than the critical values associated with the df in your study. (Reproduced with kind permission of Longman Group Limited.)

	Level of significance for one-tailed test				
	0.05	0.025	0.01	0.005	0.0005
	Level of significance for two-tailed test				
df = N − 2	0.01	0.05	0.02	0.01	0.001
1	0.9877	0.9969	0.9995	0.9999	1.0000
2	0.9000	0.9500	0.9800	0.9900	0.9990
3	0.8054	0.8783	0.9343	0.9587	0.9912
4	0.7293	0.8114	0.8822	0.9172	0.9741
5	0.6694	0.7545	0.8329	0.8745	0.9507
6	0.6215	0.7067	0.7887	0.8343	0.9249
7	0.5822	0.6664	0.7498	0.7977	0.8982
8	0.5494	0.6319	0.7155	0.7646	0.8721
9	0.5214	0.6021	0.6851	0.7348	0.8471
10	0.4973	0.5760	0.6581	0.7079	0.8233
11	0.4762	0.5529	0.6339	0.6835	0.8010
12	0.4575	0.5324	0.6120	0.6614	0.7800
13	0.4409	0.5139	0.5923	0.6411	0.7603
14	0.4259	0.4973	0.5742	0.6226	0.7420
15	0.4124	0.4821	0.5577	0.6055	0.7246
16	0.4000	0.4683	0.5425	0.5897	0.7084
17	0.3887	0.4555	0.5285	0.5751	0.6932
18	0.3783	0.4438	0.5155	0.5614	0.6787
19	0.3687	0.4329	0.5034	0.5487	0.6652
20	0.3598	0.4227	0.4921	0.5368	0.6524
25	0.3233	0.3809	0.4451	0.4869	0.5974
30	0.2960	0.3494	0.4093	0.4487	0.5541
35	0.2746	0.3246	0.3810	0.4182	0.5189
40	0.2573	0.3044	0.3578	0.3932	0.4896
45	0.2428	0.2875	0.3384	0.3721	0.4648
50	0.2306	0.2732	0.3218	0.3541	0.4433
60	0.2108	0.2500	0.2948	0.3248	0.4078
70	0.1954	0.2319	0.2737	0.3017	0.3799
80	0.1829	0.2172	0.2565	0.2830	0.3568
90	0.1726	0.2050	0.2422	0.2673	0.3375
100	0.1638	0.1946	0.2301	0.2540	0.3211

NB When there is no exact df use the next lowest number.

Table A2.12   Critical values of *s* (Kendall's coefficient of concordance) at various levels of probability. (For your *s* value to be significant at a particular probability level, it should be equal to or larger than the critical values associated with n and N in your study.) (Adapted from Friedman M (1940) A comparison of alternative tests of significance for the problem of M rankings. Annals of Mathematical Statistics 11 : 1. (With permission of The Institute of Mathematical Statistics.))

a. Critical values of s at $p = 0.05$

n	$N = 3$	$N = 4$	$N = 5$	$N = 6$	$N = 7$
3	–	–	64.4	103.9	157.3
4	–	49.5	88.4	143.3	217.0
5	–	62.6	112.3	182.4	276.2
6	–	75.7	136.1	221.4	335.2
8	48.1	101.7	183.7	299.0	453.1
10	60.0	127.8	231.2	376.7	571.0
15	89.8	192.9	349.8	570.5	864.9
20	119.7	258.0	468.5	764.4	1158.7

b. Critical values of s at $p = 0.01$

n	$N = 3$	$N = 4$	$N = 5$	$N = 6$	$N = 7$
3	–	–	75.6	122.8	185.6
4	–	61.4	109.3	176.2	265.0
5	–	80.5	142.8	229.4	343.8
6	–	99.5	176.1	282.4	422.6
8	66.8	137.4	242.7	388.3	579.9
10	85.1	175.3	309.1	494.0	737.0
15	131.0	269.8	475.2	758.2	1129.5
20	177.0	364.2	641.2	1022.2	1521.9

NB The values are all for a one-tailed test only.

A dash in the table means that no decision can be made at this level.

Appendix 3

Answers to activities

Chapter 1

Activity 1.1

1. 46
2. −2
3. 43
4. 253
5. 9
6. 49
7. 54
8. 19
9. 104
10. 47
11. −6
12. −8
13. −48
14. −44
15. −42
16. −48
17. 45
18. −13
19. 7
20. −240

Chapter 4

Activity 4.1

The following are examples of nominal levels of measurement. Any variation on these which still involves allocating patients to a category is acceptable.

1. You might measure improvement in lumbar movement by asking the patient: Did you experience any improvement following physiotherapy? Yes/No
2. This might be measured by asking patients if they have had a reduction in chest infections and requiring them to answer 'Yes' or 'No'.
3. You assess whether or not a patient experienced an increased range of movement following manipulation by allocating him/her to either an 'Increase in movement' category or 'No increase in movement' category.
4. Patients could be classified as those who kept appointments and those who did not.
5. This might be assessed by asking patients to answer the following question: Did you find the treatment in the osteopathy treatment to be:

Acceptable ☐   Not acceptable ☐

Activity 4.2

Again, any variation on the answers suggested below is acceptable, as long as you are rank ordering your data according to the dimension you're interested in.

1. Improvement in lumbar movement might be measured by asking the patients to answer the following question: To what

extent did your movement improve following therapy?

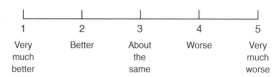

Alternatively, you could rank order your subjects according to how much they improved.

2. This might be measured by assessing the patients along a scale of incidence of chest infection thus:

The incidence of chest infection following breathing exercises was:

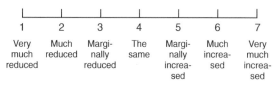

Similarly, you could rank order the patients according to their incidence of chest infections.

3. Range of movement could be assessed by either rank ordering the subjects from the greatest increase in movement to the smallest increase, or alternatively you could use a point scale thus:

The increase in range of movement in the leg following manipulation was:

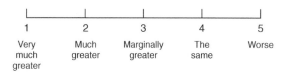

4. Likelihood of keeping appointments could be assessed by a point scale thus:

How likely is this patient to keep an appointment at the chiropractic clinic?

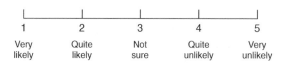

5. Assessing the quality of osteopathy treatment could be conducted along similar lines:

How would you rate the quality of the osteopathy treatment you received?

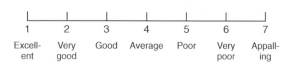

Activity 4.3

1. You could measure lumbar movement on an interval/ratio scale simply by assessing range of movement in degrees.
2. Incidence of chest infection could be assessed by noting the number of times each patient suffered a chest problem following breathing exercises.
3. Range of movement could be measured in degrees.
4. The number or percentage of appointments kept and missed could be monitored for each patient.
5. You could ask the patients to rate the quality of osteopathy by giving it marks out of 20 or 100.
6.   (i) Accuracy of shooting an arrow at a target could be measured:
   - on a nominal scale by counting up the number of hits and the number of misses.
   - on an ordinal scale by rank ordering each arrow's proximity to the target, giving a rank of 1 to the nearest, etc.
   - on an interval/ratio scale by measuring the distance of each arrow from the target, in centimetres or inches.
     (ii) Improvement in mobility after a hip replacement operation could be measured:
   - on a nominal scale by classifying the patients according to whether they:
     a. experienced an improvement in mobility or
     b. experienced no improvement in mobility
   - on an ordinal scale using a point scale thus:
   - What degree of improvement in mobility did this patient experience?

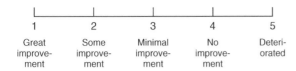

– on an interval/ratio scale by measuring the distance walked.

(iii) Relief of neck and arm pain following the use of remedial massage could be measured:

– on a nominal scale by classifying patients according to whether they experienced pain relief, or did not experience pain relief.

– on an ordinal scale by using a point scale thus:

How much pain relief did you experience after remedial massage?

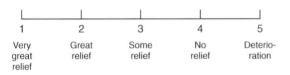

– on an interval/ratio scale by asking the patient the percentage of pain relief felt, e.g. was the pain about 50%/30%/25% less than it was prior to having remedial massage?

7. (i) Nominal
(ii) Ordinal (or interval if equal distances between points are assumed)
(iii) Interval/ratio
(iv) Interval/ratio
(v) Interval/ratio

Chapter 5

Activity 5.1

1. (a) Histogram (Fig. A3.1).
   (b) Frequency polygon (Fig. A3.2)
2. Frequency polygon with reduced number of units along the horizontal axis (Fig. A3.3)

Activity 5.2

1. (i) Mean: 73.091
   Median: 76
   Mode: 76

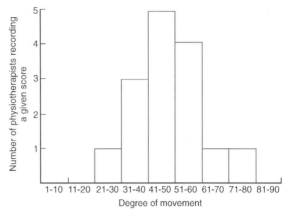

Figure A3.1 Histogram.

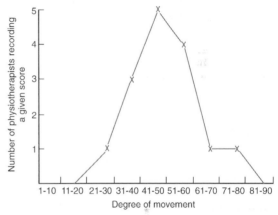

Figure A3.2 Frequency polygon.

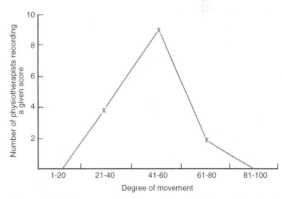

Figure A3.3 Frequency polygon with reduced number of units along the horizontal axis.

(ii) Mean: 28.667
Median: 27
Mode: 17
(iii) Mean: 50.1
Median: 47.5
Mode: 43

2. Set of data (i) has the largest range of scores while (ii) has the smallest.

Activity 5.3

1. (i) Range: 24

    Deviation: $14 - 19.444 = -5.444$
    $9 - 19.444 = -10.444$
    $21 - 19.444 = +1.556$
    $23 - 19.444 = +3.556$
    $18 - 19.444 = -1.444$
    $17 - 19.444 = -2.444$
    $33 - 19.444 = +13.556$
    $28 - 19.444 = +8.556$
    $12 - 19.444 = -7.444$

    Variance: 52.691
    Standard deviation: 7.259

    (ii) Range: 33

    Deviation: $71 - 67.571 = +3.429$
    $50 - 67.571 = -17.571$
    $48 - 67.571 = -19.571$
    $64 - 67.571 = -3.571$
    $80 - 67.571 = +12.429$
    $81 - 67.571 = -13.429$
    $79 - 67.571 = +11.429$

    Variance: 168.816
    Standard deviation: 12.993

2. You might assess the reliability of the weighing scales by taking several readings (e.g. 10) of the same piece of equipment to establish a constant, known weight and then repeat this on, say, four further occasions. For each set of 10 readings you might calculate the mean and the median to assess the homogeneity or similarity of the scores. You might also wish to calculate the range and the standard deviation to find out how disparate the readings are.

Activity 5.4

Cumulative frequencies for each class interval:

3
13
21
30
42
57
70
90

106
117
127
135
138
140

10th percentile = 66.375
20th percentile = 77.939
30th percentile = 86.5
40th percentile = 93.031
50th percentile = 100.5
60th percentile = 105.4
70th percentile = 111.0
80th percentile = 118.315
90th percentile = 127.8

Activity 5.5

63 words = 7th percentile (rounded up to the nearest whole number)
77 words = 19th percentile (rounded up to the nearest whole number)
138 words = 97th percentile (rounded up to the nearest whole number)

Activity 5.6

Child A (24.25 months) z score = 3.751
Child B (22.5 months) z score = 2.571
Child C (19.25 months) z score = 0.714

Activity 5.7

1. 95% of patients will have heart rates of between 66 and 98 during weeks 10–20 of pregnancy.
2. 2.36% of patients will have heart rates of between 99 and 106.
3. This patient comes in 0.135% of the population in terms of heart rate.

Chapter 6

Activity 6.1

The two variables in each hypothesis are:

1. Age of patient (child or adolescent) and compliance with exercise regime.
2. Sex (male or female) and responsiveness to remedial massage.

3. Sex (male or female) and progress on therapy.
4. Type of treatment centre (outpatients or sports injuries) and recovery rate for leg fractures.
5. Type of training (degree vs. diploma) and professional competence.

Activity 6.2

The null hypotheses for these experimental hypotheses are:

1. There is no relationship between age of patient with scoliosis and compliance with an exercise regime.
2. There is no relationship between the sex of arthritis patients and responsiveness to remedial massage.
3. There is no relationship between sex of patient with torticollis and progress on therapy programmes.
4. There is no relationship between the type of treatment centre and recovery rates for leg fractures.
5. There is no relationship between type of training and professional competence in clinical therapists.

Activity 6.3

1. IV = sex of patient.
   DV = tendency to complain about pain.
   IV manipulated by selecting one group of male patients and one group of female patients.
2. IV = type of walking aid.
   DV = mobility.
   IV manipulated by selecting a number of patients and deciding which walking aid each should receive.
3. IV = type of hospital.
   DV = absenteeism.
   IV manipulated by selecting one group of occupational therapists working in a psychiatric hospital and another group working in a general hospital.
4. IV = sex of patient.
   DV = degree of rapport.
   IV manipulated by selecting one group of male patients and one group of female patients.

5. IV = podiatry schools' entry requirements.
   DV = pass rate on final exam.
   IV manipulated by selecting a number of schools requiring 'A'-level physics and a number of schools not requiring 'A'-level physics.

Activity 6.4

Other possible explanations for improved communication amongst these chiropractors might be:

1. Simply the fact that they were a bit older and therefore a bit more experienced and socially skilled.
2. Experiencing a period of illness themselves which made them more aware of the patient's need for communication.
3. Reading a book on counselling and communication skills.
4. Attending another sort of course.

   Plus, of course, many other possible reasons.

Activity 6.5

Designs for hypotheses on page 74.

1.	Pre-test measure of DV	Condition	Post-test measure of DV
Control group	Compliance	No information	Compliance
Experimental group	Compliance	Information	Compliance

2.	Pre-test measure of DV	Condition	Post-test measure of DV
Experimental group	Sympathy	Experience as hospital patient	Sympathy
Control group	Sympathy	No experience as hospital patient	Sympathy

3.		Condition	Measure of DV
Experimental group 1		<5 years	Motivation
Experimental group 2		>10 years	Motivation

Activity 6.6

See Fig. A3.4.

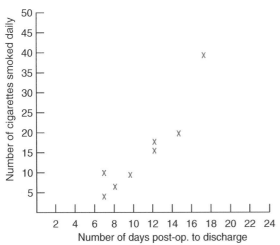

Figure A3.4 Frequency polygon with reduced number of units along the horizontal axis.

Activity 6.7

1. (i) A positive correlation is predicted, with high scores on age being associated with high scores on rehabilitation time. This would be represented by a general upward slope on a scattergram and a correlation coefficient of around +1.0.
    (ii) A negative correlation is predicted with high scores on distance being associated with low scores on attendance. This would be represented by a general downward slope on a scattergram and a correlation coefficient of around −1.0.
    (iii) A positive correlation is predicted with low scores on 'A'-levels being associated with low final exam scores. An upward slope and a correlation coefficient of around +1.0 would be anticipated.
    (iv) A negative correlation is predicted with high scores on occupational stress being associated with low scores on job satisfaction. A general downward slope and a correlation coefficient of around −1.0 would be predicted.
2. From strongest to weakest, the coefficients are:

    $$-0.73 + 0.61 - 0.42 + 0.21 - 0.17 + 0.09$$

Chapter 8

Activity 8.1

Some of the constant and random errors involved in these experiments are outlined in Tables A3.1 and A3.2. You may have thought of many more.

Activity 8.2

From greatest support to least:
$p = 0.01\%$ $p = 3\%$ $p = 5\%$ $p = 7\%$ $p = 15\%$ $p = 19\%$

Table A3.1 Hypothesis: men are more likely to suffer respiratory complications following cardiothoracic surgery

Constant error	Solution	Random error	Solution
1. Age of patient	Ensure both groups are of comparable age	1. Personality	
2. Nature of illness	Ensure both groups are being treated for the same complaint	2. Attitude	
3. Previous health	Establish comparability of previous health in both groups	3. Supportive family	
4. Previous relevant illnesses	Ensure both groups have had similar number/types of relevant illness	4. Biochemical make-up	Random selection of patients in each group
5. Smoker/non-smoker	Ensure that no S in either group smokes	5. Inherent and undetected lung defects	
6. Vital capacity	Ensure that both groups have comparable vital capacity		

Table A3.2   Hypothesis: chiropractic achieves recovery rates for lumbar spine injury that are different from those of physiotherapy

Constant error	Solution	Random error	Solution
1. Age of patient	Ensure both groups of patients are of comparable age	1. Motivation of patient and therapist	
2. Nature of injury	Ensure the type of injury is the same in each case	2. Personality of patient and therapist	
3. Fitness of patient	Ensure comparability of previous fitness in both groups	3. Attitude of patient and therapist	Randomly select patients from each situation to take part in the experiment
4. Sex of patient	Ensure both groups comprise either all males, all females, or an equal number of each sex	4. Biochemical make-up	
5. Amount of time spent in treatment	Ensure that the amount of treatment is standardised in each case	5. Inherent and undetected bone defects	
6. Quality of treatment	Ensure that the type and quality of treatment is standardised in each case		

Table A3.3

	Probability that the results are due to chance (%)
$p = 0.01$	1
$p = 0.07$	7
$p = 0.03$	3
$p = 0.05$	5
$p = 0.50$	50

Converted to a decimal:

$p = 0.0001$ $p = 0.03$ $p = 0.05$ $p = 0.07$
$p = 0.15$ $p = 0.19$

Activity 8.3

See Table A3.3

Chapter 9

Activity 9.1

1. Chi-squared test (data are nominal).
2. Wilcoxon or related t test.
3. Spearman (data are ordinal for seniority of chiropractor).
4. Mann–Whitney U test (data are ordinal).
5. Friedman or one-way ANOVA for related samples.
6. Kruskal–Wallis (data are ordinal).

Activity 9.2

1. One-tailed (more effective).
2. Two-tailed (differentially effective).
3. One-tailed (less pain).
4. Two-tailed (difference in strength).
5. One-tailed (more effective in diminishing primary hypertension).

Converting the one-tailed hypotheses to two-tailed:

1. There is a difference in the effectiveness of praise as a motivator when used in a group or a one-to-one situation.
2. There is a difference in the reported pain of patients who attend for chiropractic or conventional traction treatment.
3. The elimination of lactose in the diet and pharmacological intervention are differentially effective in diminishing primary hypertension.

Converting the two-tailed hypotheses to one-tailed:

1. Social modelling is more (less) effective than social skills training in developing interaction skills of head injury patients.
2. Strength of muscle contraction in a selected muscle group is reduced (increased) more by 2 minutes of infrared radiation than by 2 minutes of specific warm-up.

Chapter 13

Activity 13.1

1. (i) $p < 0.025$ significant
   (ii) $p < 0.005$ significant
   (iii) $p = 0.02$ significant
   (iv) p is greater than 0.05, and is therefore not significant
   (v) $p < 0.001$ significant
   (vi) $p < 0.05$ significant
2. $\chi^2 = 9.6$; $p < 0.01$

   Using the McNemar test ($\chi^2 = 9.6$) the results were significant ($p < 0.01$ two-tailed). These results suggest that providing information about the reasons for changing on-call duty hours significantly alters clinical therapists' views in favour of the change.

Activity 13.2

1. See Table A3.4.
2. (i) $p < 0.05$ significant
   (ii) $p < 0.01$ significant
   (iii) $p < 0.025$ significant
   (iv) $p < 0.01$ significant
   (v) $p < 0.1$ not significant
   (vi) $p < 0.05$ significant
   (vii) $p < 0.01$ significant
   (viii) $p < 0.01$ significant
3. $T = 0$
   $N = 9$
   $p < 0.005$, one-tailed
   Using a Wilcoxon on the data ($T = 0$, $N = 9$)

Table A3.4

Subject	Condition A	Condition B	d	Rank
1	10	9	+1	3.5
2	8	9	−1	3.5
3	9	7	+2	7
4	6	7	−1	3.5
5	5	4	+1	3.5
6	8	3	+5	11
7	7	6	+1	3.5
8	9	9	0	Omit
9	9	6	+3	8
10	5	6	−1	3.5
11	7	3	+4	9.5
12	8	4	+4	9.5

the results were found to be significant at $p < 0.005$ (one-tailed). These results support the hypothesis that traction is significantly more effective than surgical collars in the treatment of cervical spondylosis.

Activity 13.3

1. (i) $p = 0.033$ significant
   (ii) $p < 0.02$ significant
   (iii) $p < 0.072$ not significant
   (iv) $p < 0.001$ significant
   (v) $p < 0.008$ significant
   (If you got any of these wrong, or are confused about the answers, do check that you were using the correct table.)
2. $\chi_r^2 = 2.658$, $p < 0.305$; not significant

   Using a Friedman test to analyse the data, the results were not significant ($\chi^2 = 2.658$, $p < 0.305$). This suggests that there is no significant difference in the tone of the quadriceps muscle between Asian, Caucasian and African–Caribbean children. The null hypothesis can therefore be accepted.

Activity 13.4

1. (i) $p < 0.01$ significant
   (ii) $p = 0.05$ significant
   (iii) $p < 0.05$ significant
   (iv) $p < 0.001$ significant
   (v) p is greater than 0.05 and is therefore not significant
2. $L = 105$, $p < 0.05$

   Using the Page's L trend test to analyse the data, the results were significant ($L = 105$, $p < 0.05$). These results support the experimental hypothesis that hydrotherapy is more effective than exercise, which in turn is more effective than massage in the mobilisation of lower limbs paralysed following a stroke.

Chapter 14

Activity 14.1

1. (i) $p < 0.025$ significant
   (ii) $p < 0.1$ not significant
   (iii) $p < 0.01$ significant
   (iv) $p < 0.01$ significant
   (v) $p < 0.02$ significant

2. $t = 2.362$; df = 11; $p < 0.025$

Using a related t-test to analyse the data, the results were found to be significant at $p < 0.025$ ($t = 2.362$, df = 11). This suggests that student chiropractors with 'A'-level physics do better in their first-year theory exam marks than students without 'A'-level physics. The null hypothesis can therefore be rejected in favour of the experimental hypothesis.

Activity 14.2

1. (i) $p < 0.05$ significant
    (ii) $p < 0.01$ significant
    (iii) p is greater than 0.05 and is therefore not significant
    (iv) $p < 0.025$ significant
    (v) $p < 0.05$ significant
    (vi) $p < 0.025$ significant
2. See Table A3.5
    F ratio = 3.529; df_{bet} = 2; df_{error} = 10; p is not significant.
    F ratio$_{subj}$ = 3.424; df_{subj} = 5; df_{error} = 10; $p < 0.05$; significant.

    These results suggest that there is no significant effect from the different types of therapy used, but that the sets of matched subjects were significantly different from one another, and were therefore an atypical sample. These results can be expressed in the following way:

    Using a one-way ANOVA for related samples, no significant differences were found between the three treatment conditions (F = 3.529, df_{bet} = 2, df_{error} = 10). This suggests that the type of therapy used on hip replacement patients has no significant effect on mobility after 1 week. However, significant differences were

Table A3.5

Source of variation in scores	SS	df	MS	F ratio
Variation in scores between conditions	31.445	2	15.723	3.529
Variation in scores between subjects	76.278	5	15.256	3.424
Variation in scores due to random error	44.555	10	4.456	
Total	152.278	17		

found between the sets of matched subjects, (F = 3.424. df_{subj} = 5, df_{error} = 10, p < 0.05). This indicates that the subject sample was an atypical group and may represent a flaw in the sampling procedure. The null hypothesis must therefore be accepted.

Activity 14.3

Comparisons:
a. Condition 1 (seminar) × Condition 2 (tutorial)

$$F' = (C - 1)3.29 = 9.87$$

$$F = 2.8, p > 0.05; \text{not significant}$$

This suggests that the tutorial method is not significantly more effective than seminars in promoting understanding among a group of clinical therapy students.

b. Condition 1 (seminar) × Condition 3 (lecture)

$$F' = (C - 1)3.29 = 9.87$$

$$F = 0.194; \text{not significant}$$

This suggests that there is no difference in the effectiveness of seminar or lecture methods in developing understanding among clinical therapy students.

c. Condition 1 (seminar) × Condition 4 (reading)

$$F' = (C - 1)3.29 = 9.87$$

$$F = 6.078, p > 0.05; \text{not significant}$$

This suggests that seminars are no more effective than reading for developing understanding in a group of clinical therapy students.

d. Condition 2 (tutorial) × Condition 3 (lecture)

$$F' = (C - 1)3.29 = 9.87$$

$$F = 4.465, p > 0.05; \text{not significant}$$

These results indicate that the tutorial is no more effective than lectures in developing student clinical therapists' understanding.

e. Condition 2 (tutorial) × Condition 4 (reading)

$$F' = (C - 1)5.42 = 16.26$$

$$F = 17.124, p < 0.01; \text{significant}$$

These results suggest that tutorials are significantly more effective than reading for developing understanding in a group of clinical therapy students.

f. Condition 3 (lecture) × Condition 4 (reading)

$$F^1 = (C-1)3.29 = 9.87$$

$$F = 4.101, p > 0.05; \text{ not significant}$$

These results suggest that lectures are no more effective than reading in promoting clinical therapy students' understanding.

Chapter 15

Activity 15.1

1. (i) $p < 0.025$ significant
    (ii) $p < 0.02$ significant
    (iii) $p < 0.05$ significant
    (iv) p is greater than 0.10 and is therefore not significant
    (v) $p < 0.005$ significant
2. $\chi^2 = 8.377$ df = 1, $p < 0.005$

    Using a χ^2 to analyse the data ($\chi^2 = 8.377$, df = 1) the results were significant ($p < 0.005$, one-tailed). This means that the null hypothesis can be rejected and that teachers of clinical therapy are more likely to study for Open University degree courses than clinically based therapists.

Activity 15.2

1. (i) $p < 0.05$ significant
    (ii) $p < 0.05$ significant
    (iii) $p < 0.01$ significant
    (iv) $p < 0.005$ significant
    (v) $p < 0.05$ significant
    (vi) p is larger than 0.10 and is therefore not significant
2. $U = 45$, p < 0.01, one-tailed test

    Using a Mann–Whitney U test on the data ($U = 45, N_1 = 14, N_2 = 14$) the results were found to be significant at $p < 0.01$ for a one-tailed hypothesis. This suggests that the experimental hypothesis has been supported and that paraffin wax is more effective than a hot soak as a preparation for mobilising exercises with post-fracture patients.

Activity 15.3

1. (i) $p < 0.046$ significant
    (ii) $p = 0.049$ significant
    (iii) $p < 0.05$ significant
    (iv) $p < 0.011$ significant
    (v) $p < 0.01$ significant
    (vi) p is larger than 0.05 and is therefore not significant
2. $H = 6.26, N_1 = 5, N_2 = 5, N_3 = 5, p < 0.049$

    Using a Kruskal–Wallis test on the data ($H = 6.26, N_1 = 5, N_2 = 5, N_3 = 5$), the results were found to be significant ($p < 0.049$ for a two-tailed test). This suggests that the three methods of giving lumbar mobility exercise instructions are differentially effective. This means the null hypothesis can be rejected and the experimental hypothesis supported.

Activity 15.4

1. (i) $p < 0.01$ significant
    (ii) p is greater than 0.05 and so the results are not significant
    (iii) $p < 0.05$ significant
    (iv) $p < 0.01$ significant
    (v) $p < 0.05$ significant
    (vi) p is greater than 0.05 and therefore the results are not significant
2. $A = 128, B = 192, S = 64, C = 3, n = 8, p < 0.05$

    Using a Jonckheere trend test to analyse the results ($S = 64, C = 3, n = 8$), the results were found to be significant ($p < 0.05$, one-tailed). This suggests that there is a significant trend in the probability of keeping outpatients' appointments, according to social class, with social class 3 being the most likely to keep them, followed by social class 2, and finally class 4. The null hypothesis can be rejected.

Activity 15.5

1. (i) p is greater than 10% and so the results are not significant
    (ii) $p < 0.05$ significant
    (iii) $p < 0.05$ significant
    (iv) p is greater than 5%, and so the results are not significant
    (v) $p < 0.02$ significant
2. $\chi^2 = 5.095$, df = 2, p is greater than 5% and so is not significant.

Using an extended χ^2 on the data ($\chi^2 = 5.095$, df = 2), the results were found to be not significant (p is greater than 5%). Therefore the null hypothesis is accepted; there is no significant relationship between keeping an outpatient appointment and ease of journey, using public transport.

Chapter 16

Activity 16.1

1. (i) $p < 0.05$ significant
    (ii) $p < 0.02$ significant
    (iii) $p = 0.01$ significant
    (iv) p is larger than 5% and so the results are not significant
    (v) $p < 0.01$ significant
2. $t = 2.43$; df = 25; $p < 0.025$.

Using an unrelated t-test on the data ($t = 2.43$, df = 25), the results were significant ($p < 0.025$ for a one-tailed test). The null hypothesis can be rejected. This suggests that absenteeism is significantly greater among basic-grade clinical therapists than among senior clinical therapists.

Activity 16.2

1. (i) $p < 0.01$ significant
    (ii) $p < 0.001$ significant
    (iii) $p < 0.05$ significant
    (iv) $p < 0.01$ significant
2. $F = 2.171$, p is greater than 5% and is therefore not significant.

Using a one-way ANOVA for unrelated subject designs on the data (F = 2.171, $df_{bet} = 2$, $df_{error} = 18$), the results were found to be not significant (p is greater than 5%). This means that the null hypothesis must be accepted and that there is no relationship between the type of therapy given to traumatic brain injury patients and their neuropsychological progress.

Activity 16.3

1. a. Comparison of 1992 and 1997
        $F = 4.982$
        p is not significant
        i.e. 'A'-level results were not significantly higher in 1997 than in 1992.
   b. Comparison of 1992 and 2002
        $F = 35.124$
        $p < 0.001$
        i.e. 'A'-level results were significantly higher in 2002 than in 1992.
   c. Comparison of 1997 and 2002
        $F = 13.649$
        $p < 0.01$
        i.e. 'A'-level results were significantly higher in 2002 than in 1997.

Chapter 17

Activity 17.1

H_1 There is a relationship between the age of the patient and vital capacity.

a. Correlational design
   You would select one group of subjects who represented a whole range of ages (e.g. 15–65). You would then measure their vital capacities to see if there was any correlation between age and vital capacity.

b. Experimental design
   You have two possible options here. First, you might select two groups of subjects one being at the youngish end of the age range and the other being at the older end.

   Group 1   15–30 years (for example)
   Group 2   50–65 years (for example)

   You would measure their vital capacities to see if there was any difference between the groups.
   Alternatively, you might select a third group who represented a mid-age range thus:

   Group 1   15–25 years (for example)
   Group 2   35–45 years (for example)
   Group 3   55–65 years (for example)

Table A3.6

Source of variation	SS	df	MS	F ratio
Variation due to treatment, i.e. between conditions	180.952	2	90.476	2.171
Variation due to random error	750	18		41.667
Total	930.952	20		

Again you would compare their vital capacities for differences between the groups.

Activity 17.2

1. $p < 0.01$
   p = not significant
   $p = 0.02$
   p = not significant
   $p < 0.005$
2. Results of the calculation of the Spearman rho:
   $r_s = -0.827$
   $p = < 0.01$ (two-tailed)
   Using a Spearman test on the data, ($r_s = -0.827$, $N = 10$) the results were found to be significant ($p < 0.01$ for a two-tailed test). This suggests that there is a significant negative correlation between the length of lunch-break and clinical competence. The null hypothesis can, therefore, be rejected.

Activity 17.3

1. (i) $p < 0.05$
   (ii) p = not significant
   (iii) $p < 0.005$
   (iv) $p = 0.02$
   (v) $p < 0.001$
2. Results of the calculation of the Pearson product moment correlation:
   $r = +0.899$
   $p < 0.005$ (one-tailed)
   Using a Pearson product moment correlation test on the data ($r = +0.899$, df = 6), the results were found to be significant ($p < 0.005$, for a one-tailed test). This means that there is a significant positive correlation between students' marks on their first-year exam and their averaged continuous assessment mark through the year. The null hypothesis can therefore be rejected.

Activity 17.4

1. (i) $p < 0.05$
   (ii) p is greater than 5% and is therefore not significant

(iii) $p < 0.01$
(iv) $p < 0.01$
(v) p is greater than 5% and is therefore not significant.
2. Results of the calculation of the Kendall coefficient of concordance
   $s = 77$, $W = 0.616$
   $p < 0.05$
   Using the Kendall coefficient of concordance on the data ($s = 77$, $W = 6.61$, $n = 5$, $N = 4$), the results were found to be significant ($p < 0.05$ for a one-tailed test). This suggests that there is significant agreement on lumbar mobility when measured by the double inclinometer method. The null hypothesis can be rejected.

Activity 17.5

$a = 0.939$, $b = 0.47$

(i) This patient would be in labour for 11.175 hours.
(ii) This patient would be in labour for 8.459 hours.
(iii) This patient would be in labour for 14.569 hours.

Chapter 18

Activity 18.1

1. The proportion of non-attenders in the outpatient clinic will be somewhere between 0.3 and 0.46 (for 95% confidence level).
2. The average amount of clinical therapy time that learning disabled children will require will be between 2.25 and 4.15 hours, per child, per week (99% confidence level).
3. The average life-expectancy of your ultrasound machine is estimated, with 90% confidence, to fall within the interval 4.07–4.53 years.

Appendix 4

A sample critique of a published article

The article to be evaluated appeared in Manual Therapy in 2000. It was written by Amir Tal-Akabi and Alison Rushton, both of whom are physiotherapists. To critique the article, the questions put forward as a framework in Chapter 12 will be used, along with comments about how these relate to the article. The article itself will appear, in full, first, followed by the critique. If you want to use this Appendix as a self-assessment exercise, you can cover my suggested critique of the paper and then compare your comments and mine when you've finished. I would like to re-emphasise that I am not a physiotherapist and therefore some of my comments about the clinical aspects of the study may well seem naïve. Also, you may have other comments in addition to those presented here, or you may disagree with my evaluation. There is no absolute in critiquing research, and the framework and responses I suggest should therefore be taken as indicative, rather than definitive.

Manual Therapy (2000) **5(4)**, 214–222
© 2000 Harcourt Publishers Ltd
doi:10.1054/math.2000.0355, available online at http://www.idealibrary.com on **IDEAL**

Original article

An investigation to compare the effectiveness of carpal bone mobilisation and neurodynamic mobilisation as methods of treatment for carpal tunnel syndrome

A. Tal-Akabi*, A. Rushton[†]

Clinical Physiotherapist, Bern, Switzerland, [†]Senior Lecturer, Coventry University, Coventry, UK

SUMMARY. Carpal tunnel syndrome is the most common peripheral entrapment neuropathy. There is little literature available that addresses the management of this condition, which may partly explain why physiotherapy is often overlooked as a treatment approach in its management. This study investigated the effects of two manual therapy techniques in the treatment of patients experiencing carpal tunnel syndrome. An experimental different subject design compared three groups of subjects in three different conditions (two treatment interventions and one control group). Each group consisted of seven patients. The objectives of the study were: (1) to investigate differences between treated and untreated groups; (2) to investigate differences in the effectiveness of treatment I (median nerve mobilization) compared with treatment II (carpal bone mobilization). Measurements were taken applying several measurement tools, including active range of wrist movement (ROM flexion and extension), upper limb tension test with a median nerve bias (ULTT2a), three different scales to evaluate pain perception and function, and lastly numbers of patients continuing to surgery in each group were compared. In visual terms a clear trend was demonstrated between subjects who received treatment compared to those who were not treated, in particular the descriptive analysis of results for ULTT2a and numbers of patients continuing to surgery. When analysed statistically, less could be concluded. Only scores on a Pain Relief Scale ($P < 0.01$) demonstrated highly significant differences between the three groups when analyzed using Kruskal–Wallis Test. In exploring the results of the two intervention groups, no statistically significant difference in effectiveness of treatment was demonstrated between carpal bone mobilization and median nerve mobilization. © 2000 Harcourt Publishers Ltd.

INTRODUCTION AND LITERATURE REVIEW

Carpal tunnel syndrome (CTS) is the most common peripheral entrapment neuropathy and it affects women more than men (Phalen 1966; Cailliet 1994; Katz 1994). This condition has recently become a growing reason for workers' compensation claims due to absence from work (Dean & Louis 1992; Harter et al. 1993; Katz et al. 1998).

The literature regarding some aspects of treatments and their risks is enlightening. For example, surgery to release the pressure from the median nerve may be

Amir Tal-Akabi, MSc, Manipulative Therapy MCSP, MMACP, MSVOMP, MSAMT, Clinical Physiotherapist Bern, Switzerland, Alison Rushton, MSc, MCSP, Dip TP, MMACP, Senior Lecturer in Physiotherapy Coventry University and Course Leader for the MSc Manipulative Therapy course, Coventry, UK.
Correspondence to A.T.-A., Stapfeboden 332, 3625
Heiligenschwendi, Switzerland, Tel: + +41 33 243 49 52;
E-mail: amir_tal@hotmail.com

helpful but it can have a 15–20% failure rate (Katz 1994). Complications can and do occur with both known procedures (Palmer & Toivonen 1999) but, various conservative methods are also available and might provide relief. Harter et al. (1993) reported satisfactory results after treating 188 patients with different conservative methods such as resting splints, anti-inflammatory drugs, vitamin B6 and steroid injections. However, there are also some risks involved in some of the common conservative treatments for carpal tunnel syndrome such as vitamin B6 or steroid injections (Katz 1994; Murray et al. 1994; Tavares & Giddins 1996).

Some of the physiotherapy methods for treating CTS such as electrotherapy may offer some symptomatic relief. However, such methods do not address the pathological neurodynamics of the median nerve and its surrounding structures (Butler 1991). Anecdotal clinical evidence supports physiotherapeutic intervention with these patients as improvement has been seen in response to a variety of manual therapy treatment approaches. There is also some evidence of chiropractic or osteopathic manual intervention providing some relief of symptoms for patients experiencing CTS (Sucher 1993; Bonebrake 1994; Sucher 1994; Valenta & Gibson 1994; Davis et al. 1998). However, there were some methodological problems with these studies that therefore limit generalization. For example inclusion/exclusion criteria do not consider factors contributing to the neuropathy such as double crush syndrome and, thoracic or cervical origin of symptoms. Questions are also raised regarding the reliability and accuracy of the palpation methods, the method of measuring ROM employed by Sucher (1994), and the lack of statistical analysis of the results. In some studies (Bonebrake 1994; Davis et al. 1998) it is also not possible to determine which conservative method of treatment was effective as many different methods were employed. Generalization is also limited in the single case study by Valenta and Gibson (1994) due to its poor design and subsequent lack of analysis.

Other research has explored the biomechanical changes of the transverse carpal ligament and the degenerative changes to the connective tissue and tenosynovium (Schuind et al. 1990; Allampallam et al. 1996), these degenerative changes could explain the common limitation of reduced active ROM of the wrist (Sucher 1994). Several authors have suggested treating CTS with manipulation of the carpal bones (Patterson 1998; Sucher & Hinrichs 1998) and Maitland (1991) suggested mobilizing the pisiform and stretching the flexor retinaculum. Literature concerning the effects of joint mobilisation as applied by manual therapists is however lacking and at present there is no specific literature exploring the treatment of CTS.

Some studies have investigated the effects of nervous system mobilization on nerve entrapment problems (Butler 1991; Elvey 1995; Shacklock 1995a). The rationale in treating patients with nervous system mobilization is an attempt to improve axonal transport and by this mechanism to improve nerve conduction (Butler & Gifford 1989; Shacklock 1995a,b). Mobilization of a nerve may reduce the pressure existing within the nerve and could therefore result in an improvement of blood flow to the nerve. Consequently, regeneration and healing of an injured nerve may also occur (Butler 1991). Rozmaryn et al. (1998) treated patients experiencing CTS with nerve gliding exercises and report in 70.2% of patients good or excellent results. A combined approach was illustrated by Exelby (1995) who investigated lateral glide of the proximal row of carpal bones (as described by Mulligan 1992) while maintaining tension on the median nerve.

From the existing literature it is therefore considered that different manual therapy techniques may help

those patients who are interested in treatment other than surgery. However, due to the lack of literature within this area it seems that there is an urgent need for structured research to inform patient management.

METHODOLOGY

The aims of this study were firstly to investigate the effectiveness of manual therapy intervention in patients experiencing CTS when compared to a control group, and secondly to investigate the difference in effectiveness between two approaches to manual therapy treatment for CTS, carpal bone mobilization and mobilization of the nervous system. The subsequent research null hypothesis was that there will be no significant differences in the recovery of patients experiencing CTS according to whether they have been treated with neurodynamic mobilization, carpal bone mobilization or received no treatment at all.

An experimental different subject design enabled comparison between the two interventions and a control group as follows:

Group I 7 CTS patients	received	Condition 1 Neurodynamic mobilization
Group II 7 CTS patients	received	Condition 2 Carpal bone mobilizations
Group III 7 CTS patients	received	Condition 3 Control group (no treatment)

Incidental sampling from a waiting list for surgery provided a sample population of 21 patients experiencing CTS. The ratio of male to female was 1:2. Their ages ranged from 29 to 85 years with the mean age of 47.1 (S.D. 14.8). In looking at the presentation of symptoms, 12 right hands and 9 left hands were presented with 9 patients presenting with bilateral symptoms. The mean duration of symptoms for the subjects was 2.3 years (S.D. = 2.5) with a range of 1 to 3 years. After selection, the subjects were randomly allocated to one of the three groups by pulling names out of a hat.

Inclusion criteria included a positive electrodiagnostic test, positive clinical tests (Phalen/Tinel's), positive upper limb tension test 2a with a median nerve bias (ULTT2a), with positive diagnosis of CTS by a surgeon indicating that the patient was a candidate for decompression surgery. Exclusion criteria included known psycho-social problems, diabetes mellitus, herpes zoster, rheumatoid arthritis, pregnancy, hyperthyroidism, known congenital abnormality of the nervous system, and cervical or thoracic spine origin of symptoms on assessment.

Several measurement tools were selected for use in this study in order to reflect the multidimensional presentation of CTS that encompasses its characteristic presentation of pain, daily pattern, and limitation of range of movement and function. Initially it was planned that electrodiagnostic tests would be utilized but the reliability and validity of their results of these tests have been questioned (Redmond & Rivner 1988; Glowacki et al. 1996). A pilot study explored issues of reliability for the measurement tools that had not been previously investigated.

Symptom diary

The subjects were requested to complete a 24 h daily symptom diary as used by Elton et al. (1979) (see Fig. 1). The Visual Analogue Scale (VAS) component provided information regarding severity of symptoms and the diary provided information on duration and frequency of the symptoms. The reliability and sensitivity of VAS has already been established (Huskisson 1974; Huskisson et al. 1976). Furthermore, it was concluded by Levine et al. (1993) that measurement of severity of symptoms and functional scales in patients experiencing CTS are reproducible, internally consistent and responsive to clinical change.

Functional box scale

Huskisson et al. (1976) developed a functional scale and tested it on patients with rheumatoid arthritis. For the purpose of this study the most limited function was discussed with the patients and a slightly modified scale, the functional box scale (FBS) (Waterfield & Sim 1996) combined with a simple descriptive scale was used (Fig. 2).

Pain Relief Scale

When assessing the effects of treatment, the Pain Relief Scale (PRS) was found to be more effective and more sensitive, compared to other scales (Huskisson, 1974). Fig. 3 shows the modified PRS used in this study.

Measurement of Active range of movement – wrist flexion and extension

Measurements of Range of movement (ROM) were taken by an independent examiner as described by Daniels & Worthingham (1986) using a standard goniometer. The same goniometer was used for all measurements.

Upper limb tension test 2a, the median nerve biased test

Being a specific tension test that has been developed to bias the median nerve (Butler 1991), it was performed in this study to reproduce symptoms or identify changes in existing symptoms. For the purpose of this study the test measured positive/negative responses only. Butler's definition (1991, p 162–163)

Please mark below level of severity of your symptoms. Record ONLY waking hours.
Use one chart for each day and please record at least four different times a day.
Please record also times at night that your symptoms woke you up.
Please chose one of the following scores:

0   No symptoms (you are able to do every kind of your daily activity)
1   Low level of symptoms (you are aware of it only when you direct attention to it).
2   Symptoms which could be ignored at times.
3   Constant symptoms but you are able to continue working.
4   Very severe level of your symptoms which makes concentration difficult, but undemanding tasks can be coped with.
5   Intense incapacitating symptoms.

Date .... Day ....

	5	6	7	8	9	10	11	12	1	2	3	4	5	6	7	8	9	10	11	12	1	2	3	4
5																								
4																								
3																								
2																								
1																								
0																								

Fig. 1—Weekly symptoms chart (incorporating Visual Analogue Scale).

© *2000 Harcourt Publishers Ltd*

Effectiveness of carpal bone and neurodynamic mobilization as treatments for carpal tunnel syndrome   217

Please mark on the scale below your present ability/disability to button/unbutton a shirt or to grip. Please choose one of the following scores:

0   Able to do alone without any problem
1   Able to do alone with slight ability problem
2   Able to do alone with some difficulties
3   Able to do alone but with a lot of difficulties
4   Not able to do alone

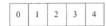

Fig. 2—The Functional Box scale (modified box scale of pain and simple descriptive scale).

definition was applied concerning positivity of the test:

- It reproduces the patient's symptoms.
- The test responses can be altered by movement of distant body parts
- There are differences in the test from the left side to the right side and from what is known to be normal.

The order of the ULTT2a was standardized in a pilot study as is described in Butler (1991, p 153) as slight glenohumeral abduction, shoulder girdle depression, elbow extension, lateral rotation of the whole arm, wrist, thumb & finger extension and finally glenohumeral abduction. All movements were taken to the end of available range (R2) or to the point where first symptoms were produced (P1).

Subjects continuing to surgery

Each subject was followed up after intervention to see if they proceeded to surgery.

Procedures

All measurements except the PRS measurement were undertaken by an independent examiner pre treatment intervention to obtain baseline readings. All the measurement tools were then utilized post intervention by the same independent examiners.

Please mark on the scale below your experience of symptom relief following the treatment you have received. Please choose one of the following scores:

0   I have **not** experienced any relief of my symptoms
1   The symptoms relief can be described as poor
2   Moderate symptom relief
3   I have a good amount of symptom relief
4   I have excellent symptom relief but still not complete
5   I have complete symptom relief

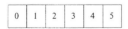

Fig. 3—The modified pain relief scale.

The procedure for treatment was as follows: subjects in group I were treated with ULTT2a mobilization (Butler 1991, p 154); group II were treated by carpal bone mobilization (posterior-anterior and/or anterior-posterior mobilization techniques) and flexor retinaculum stretch (Maitland 1991, p 205). Grade of treatment, amplitude of mobilization, and the progression of treatment was decided on an individual patient basis depending upon the irritability and severity of the individual patient's symptoms (Butler 1991; Maitland 1991). Group III received no intervention.

All data were analyzed using the SPSS computer package for Windows release 6.0, employed with a critical value of P set by convention at 0.05 (Hicks, 1995). The reliability studies were analyzed using Kendall's coefficient of concordance as recommended by Hicks (1995) for repeated measurements. The related t test was applied for within group pre and post test analysis (VAS and ROM), and the ANOVA between conditions was utilized for the analysis of ROM. The Kruskal–Wallis test (Hicks, 1995) was employed to analyze the PRS, FBS and VAS, while data obtained from the ULTT2a and numbers continuing to surgery were analyzed descriptively. All tests utilized were two tailed.

No change in the original surgical treatment plan for the patients was expected. The subjects were selected from the surgical waiting list and the surgical option remained available during and at the end of the study. Every subject participating in the study was asked to give informed consent and had the opportunity to withdraw at any time during the study without affecting their right for surgery. The study was granted the approval of the involved hospital's Research Ethics Committee and their Research & Development Committee.

RESULTS

Results from the VAS

Table 1 illustrates the results of the VAS. Using a Kruskal–Wallis test on the data ($H = 6.406$, $n = 21$) the results were found to be significant at $P < 0.05$. This suggests that there is a significant difference in the VAS scores post treatment intervention of three different interventions.

The results for each group pre and post treatment intervention were analyzed using the related t-test looking for differences within the groups. For group III the results were not significant ($P > 0.05$) but for groups I and II the results were highly significant ($P < 0.02$, $P < 0.001$ respectively), suggesting that there was a difference pre and post treatment intervention in both treated groups.

© 2000 Harcourt Publishers Ltd

Table 1. Results of Visual Analogue Scale Measurement pre and post treatment (RX) intervention

n	Group I pre RX intervention	Group I post RX intervention	Group II pre RX intervention	Group II post RX intervention	Group III pre RX intervention	Group III post RX intervention
1	0	0	2	1	2	3
2	1	0	2	1	1	2
3	3	1	4	1	4	2
4	4	2	1	0	2	2
5	3	2	2	0	0	1
6	4	4	2	0	3	3
7	2	2	3	2	2	2
Total	17	11	16	5	14	15
Mean	2.42	1.57	2.2857	0.71	2	2.14
related		$t = 2.52$		$t = 5.28$		$t = -0.35$
t-test		Significant $P<0.02$		Significant $P<0.001$		Not significant
analysis						

Results of the functional box scale measurements

A correlation study was conducted in order to find the correlation of this tool with the VAS and to inform regarding its reliability. Using a Spearman test on the data (rs $= +0.804$, $n = 18$) the results were found to be significant ($P<0.05$ for a one tailed test).

Table 2 illustrates the results of the FBS. Using a Kruskal–Wallis test on the data post treatment intervention (H $= 5.27$, $n = 21$) the results were found to be not significant at $P<0.05$. This suggests that there is no significant difference in the FBS scores post treatment intervention for the three different interventions.

Results of the pain relief scale (PRS)

Table 3 illustrates the results of the PRS post treatment intervention. Using a Kruskal–Wallis test on the data (H $= 13.58$, $n = 21$) the results were found to be significant at $P<0.05$. This suggests that there was a significant difference in the PRS scores post treatment intervention for the three different interventions.

Results of ROM measurements of wrist flexion/extension

A pilot study was conducted initially to establish the intra-tester reliability for the measurement of ROM

flexion/extension (F/E), using Kendall's coefficient of concordance (Hicks 1995) the results were found to be significant ($P<0.05$) for a one tailed test, establishing satisfactory reliability. Table 4 illustrates the results of wrist ROM flexion between subjects. Using a related t test the results of pre and post intervention measurements were found to be significant for group I.

Table 5 illustrates the results of ROM measurement for wrist extension between subjects. Using a related t test the results were found to be significant for groups I and II.

In further exploring the results of wrist ROM F/E between conditions, a one way ANOVA for unrelated designs demonstrated F $= 0.99$, df$_{bet} = 2$, df$_{error} = 18$ for flexion ROM, and F $= 1.243$, df$_{bet} = 2$, df$_{error} = 18$ for extension ROM, the results therefore were not significant. This suggests that there is no relationship between the type of treatment given to the subjects and the subsequent measurement of ROM of the wrist.

Results of the ULTT2a

Intra tester reliability was established within the pilot study, with Kendall's coefficient of concordance (Hicks, 1995) being significant ($P<0.05$) for a one tailed test. Figure 4 illustrates the results of the ULTT2a post treatment intervention between

Table 2. Results of the Functional Box Scale Measurements Treatment scores pre and post treatment (RX) intervention

n	FBS Group I pre RX intervention	FBS Group I post RX intervention	FBS Group II pre RX intervention	FBS Group II post RX intervention	FBS Group III pre RX intervention	FBS Group III post RX intervention
1	0	0	1	1	0	0
2	1	0	2	0	3	3
3	4	1	4	1	4	4
4	1	0	1	0	2	2
5	2	1	0	0	3	3
6	3	3	3	1	3	3
7	3	3	3	2	2	2
Total	14	8	14	5	17	17
Mean	2	1.14	2	0.71	2.42	2.42

© *2000 Harcourt Publishers Ltd*

Table 3. Results of the Pain Relief Scale Measurement post Treatment intervention

n	PRS Group I	PRS Group II	PRS group III
1	5	3	0
2	4	3	0
3	3	4	0
4	4	5	0
5	3	3	0
6	1	5	0
7	2	3	0
Mean	3.14	3.71	0
Total	22	26	0

groups. Visual analysis suggests that the manual therapy interventions are associated with the improvements seen in the ULTT2a.

Number of subjects continuing to surgery

An important indication for effectiveness of the treatment in this study was the number of subjects who returned to their originally planned surgery. Only two patients from group I and one patient from group II chose to continue to surgery, while six patients from group III (control) continued with their planned surgery (Fig. 5).

SUMMARY OF RESULTS

Table 6 summarizes the results of the statistically significant findings to aid clarity for consideration in the discussion. As the Table 6 illustrates, two of the between condition analyses were statistically significant, the Kruskal–Wallis (PRS and VAS) suggesting differences between the three groups. Beyond this the three between subject analyses of related t tests (VAS and ROM F/E) suggest differences within groups I (VAS, ROM F/E) and II (VAS, ROM ext).

DISCUSSION

This study set out to investigate the effectiveness of two methods of mobilization in the management of

(CTS) compared to a control group. It was found that the differences in scores for the VAS were statistically significant between the three conditions ($P < 0.05$). Furthermore, a visual improvement is suggested by the VAS for groups I and II, supported by a statistically significant related t test pre and post intervention for groups I and II, suggesting some improvement.

Although the results on the FBS were not statistically significant, most subjects from both treated groups scored their inability to perform certain activities lower after 3 weeks of treatment. This suggests that improvement in function was achieved in the treated groups. The results post treatment intervention for the FBS although visually different were not statistically significant ($P > 0.05$). Development of the methodology and in particular utilizing a larger sample size would be useful in exploring this effect further.

The results of the PRS were highly significant ($P < 0.01$) and demonstrated that there were differences between the three groups. The differences in the results can be seen from the visual analysis and it is apparent that group II did slightly better than the other groups. However, a small sample size and a placebo effect may have contributed to the positive results.

In analyzing the results between subjects of ROM flexion, group I was significantly better and group II was visually better although the results were not statistically significant. Comparison of the results for ROM extension indicate that both groups I & II showed significant improvement whereas group III did not. This highlights a clear difference in favour of the treated groups. Had the sample size been larger, the results from ROM flexion group II may also have reached significance.

When analyzing the results of ROM between conditions visually it can be seen that for ROM flexion and extension groups I & II both demonstrated improvement whereas group III did not. Despite these trends, statistical analysis employing an ANOVA demonstrated that the visual differences were not statistically significant. However, it might be

Table 4. The results of measurement of active ROM wrist flexion (ROMF) pre and post treatment intervention

n	ROMF group I pre RX (degrees)	ROMF group I post RX (degrees)	ROMF group II pre RX (degrees)	ROMF group II post RX (degrees)	ROMF group III pre RX (degrees)	ROMF Group III post RX (degrees)
1	60	70	52	46	53	52
2	55	61	63	76	41	50
3	57	74	56	60	62	61
4	35	52	48	45	55	56
5	55	65	60	69	62	62
6	46	42	51	65	32	35
7	55	62	24	59	58	59
Total	363	426	354	420	363	375
Mean	51.85	60.85	50.57	60	51.85	53.57
Related	$t = 3.302$		$t = 1.834$		$t = 1.29$	
t-test analysis	Significant <0.05		Not significant		Not significant	

© 2000 Harcourt Publishers Ltd

Table 5. The results of active wrist ROM extension (ROME) pre and post treatment intervention

n	ROME group I pre RX (degrees)	ROME group I post RX (degrees)	ROME group II pre RX (degrees)	ROME group II post RX (degrees)	ROME group III pre RX (degrees)	ROME group III post RX (degrees)
1	45	74	39	58	47	48
2	67	69	59	69	65	66
3	70	71	66	72	61	63
4	38	60	66	74	59	60
5	55	82	70	71	60	75
6	45	52	54	71	50	48
7	59	64	46	63	74	70
Total	379	472	400	478	416	430
Mean	54.14	67.42	57.14	68.28	59.42	61.42
Related *t*-test analysis	$t = 2.87$ Significant <0.05		$t = 4.38$ Significant < 0.05		$t = 0.86$ Not significant	

that in a study with a larger sample the differences between the conditions would have reached significance.

Although good intra-tester reliability for measuring wrist ROM was found, difficulties were encountered while performing the active movement measurements on some subjects. It was found that in some cases symptoms of pain or paraesthesia were the limiting factor and not the actual physiological range of the wrist as found on healthy subjects in the pilot study. However, it can be argued that the same factor that caused the limitation of active ROM in the main study was responsible for the dysfunction of the patients, making this a useful test and in practice an indication of the subjects' willingness to perform the movement. Improvement of symptoms subsequently resulted in improvement of ROM (see results). These findings justify the measurement of active rather than passive physiological ROM.

Visual analysis of the results of the ULTT2a illustrated differences in the improvement between the three groups post treatment. All subjects in the non intervention group III still had positive tests post treatment but the results of groups I & II demonstrated improvement. It can also be seen that group I who received nerve mobilization did slightly better than group II who received carpal bone mobilization. This can perhaps be explained by the nature of the technique chosen for group I which treated directly the pathomechanics of the median nerve i.e. vascular and mechanical factors of the nerve (Sunderland 1978; Lundborg 1988; Mackinnon & Dellon 1988). Group II, who received treatment for the nerve interfacing, also achieved improvement of the pathomechanics of the median nerve. However, it might be that problems along the course of the median nerve proximal to the wrist contributed to the incomplete recovery of the neurodynamics of some patients from group II, i.e. the double crush syndrome (Upton & McComas 1973). It was initially intended to use the extended Chi square on the ULTT2a data, but due to the limited number of subjects it was not possible to fulfil the requirements of minimum numbers in the contingency table for this test. It was therefore not possible to explore the above visually observed differences through statistical analysis.

Perhaps the most important indication for effectiveness of the treatment in this study was the number of treated subjects who returned to their originally planned surgery, where both treatment intervention groups illustrated a considerable change in results compared to the control group. This decision was left completely to the patients considering their experience of symptom relief, improvement of function

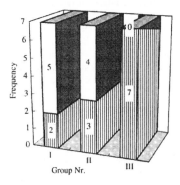

Fig. 4—Bar graph demonstrating the results of the ULTT2a post RX intervention in terms of a positive or negative test (all subjects tested positive prior to intervention) ▦ positive; □ negative.

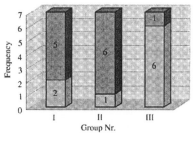

Fig. 5—Bar graph demonstrating the number of subjects continuing to surgery post intervention (all subjects were intending to undergo surgery prior to intervention) ▦ no operation; ▦ operation.

© *2000 Harcourt Publishers Ltd*

Table 6. Summary of the statistically significant results

Statistical analysis	Measurement tool	Statistically significant group
Kruskal–Wallis	PRS and VAS	between I II and III
Related *t* test	ROM flex	I
Related *t* test	ROM ext	I and II
Related *t* test	VAS	I and II

and the change in the nocturnal behaviour of the symptoms. The same limitation to this analysis applies as to the ULTT2a where statistical analysis was not possible due to the spread of subjects across the contingency table for an extended Chi square test.

As discussed in the literature review, several measures were chosen to reflect the multidimensional nature of CTS. It was not a surprise to therefore see the differences in results gained from the different measurement tools. One of the reasons for these differences could be the different nature of the scales. For example, the PRS measured the relief of symptoms post intervention and compared one group of no scores against two groups of scores on this scale. The use of electro-diagnostic testing would strengthen the results of this study, but the reliability and validity of these tests would need to be improved.

The results of this study suggest that differences existed between the recovery of patients experiencing CTS who received specific manual treatment intervention and those who were not treated. These results also support Butler (1991) who describes the peripheral nervous system as having considerable regenerative powers. These results are also in agreement with Harter et al. (1993) and Rozmaryn et al. (1998) who used other conservative methods of treatment and with the chiropractic and osteopathic researchers who used different manipulation techniques on CTS and claim good results (Sucher 1993; Bonebrake 1994; Sucher 1994; Valenta & Gibson 1994).

Butler (1991) suggests a few hypotheses that may explain the improvement seen after treating the patients with different methods of manual therapy. Mobilization of the carpus may result in alteration of the pressure in the nervous system and subsequently to a dispersion of any existing intra-neural oedema. The carpal tunnel with the flexor retinaculum is part of the interface of the median nerve, and mobilization of the interface could therefore have an effect on any extraneural component which is the cause of the problem (Butler 1991). Treatment of the interface may assist in normalizing the pressure gradients in the carpal tunnel and consequently normalize the blood supply and the axonal transport system (Butler 1991). Against this, any other existing factors such as congenital abnormalities in the nervous system could predispose the subject to the development of carpal tunnel syndrome. Such abnormalities may have lessened the patient's potential for recovery.

Although some statistically significant results were obtained from this experimental study, no conclusion can be drawn regarding the longer term effects. Some studies have addressed longer time scales (Sucher 1994; Kluge et al. 1996; Rozmaryn et al. 1998). Unfortunately the time restrictions of this study did not permit further follow up. Had the study continued for a longer period of time, the different treatments could be monitored for the longevity of their effects.

Generalization of the results of this study is limited due to several factors, some of which have been discussed above. Because of the interesting results obtained, this study would be worthwhile repeating with a larger sample size and randomly selected subjects recruited from more than one site.

CONCLUSION

This study has investigated the effects of two manual therapy techniques as treatment for patients experiencing CTS. Several measurement tools were utilised to evaluate effectiveness of treatment. The results were not always statistically significant, but in visual terms a clear trend was demonstrated between subjects who received treatment compared to those who were not treated.

The results of this study are encouraging to manual therapists. However, as discussed it has several limitations and the results therefore cannot be generalised to all patients experiencing CTS. The study has failed to show significant differences in the effectiveness between mobilization of the median nerve and carpal bone mobilization in the treatment of patients presenting with carpal tunnel syndrome. However, the results indicate that even after such a short period of time, some patients with no other contributing factors (see exclusion criteria), might benefit from a specific treatment with neurodynamic techniques, or with mobilization of carpal bones. This research has therefore demonstrated that patients experiencing CTS can improve after manual therapy, and therefore provides support for the use of manual therapy in the conservative management methods of treating patients with this condition with satisfactory results. However, more research needs to be carried out to further support these findings.

References

Allampallam K, Chakraborty J, Bose KK, Robinson J (1996) Explant Culture, Immunofluorescence and Electron-Microscopic Study of Flexor Retinaculum in Carpal Tunnel Syndrome. Journal of Occupational & Environmental Medicine 38(3): 264–271

Bonebrake AR (1994) A Treatment for Carpal Tunnel Syndrome: results of follow-up study (letter; comment). Journal of Manipulative & Physiological Therapeutics 17(8): 565–567

© 2000 Harcourt Publishers Ltd

Butler D (1991) Mobilization of the Nervous system, 1st edn, Churchill Livingstone, Melbourne

Butler D, Gifford L (1989) The Concept of Adverse Mechanical Tension in the Nervous System, Part 2: Examination and Treatment. Physiotherapy 75(11): 629–636

Cailliet R (1994) Hand Pain and Impairment, 4th edn., FA Davis, Philadelphia

Daniels L, Worthingham C (1986) Muscle Testing: Techniques of Manual Examination. 5th edn. W.B. Saunders, Philadelphia

Davis PT, Hulbert JR, Kassak KM, Meyer JJ (1998) Comparative Efficacy of Conservative Medical and Chiropractic Treatment for Carpal Tunnel Syndrome: a randomized clinical trial. Journal of Manipulative & Physiological Therapeutics 21(5): 317–326

Dean S, Louis MD (1992) The Carpal Tunnel Syndrome in the Work Place, in: Millender LH, Louise DS, Simmons BP. Occupational Disorders of the Upper Extremity. Chapter 12. Churchill Livingstone

Elton D, Burrows GD, Stanley GV (1979) A Multidimensional Approach to the Assessment of Pain. Australian Journal of Physiotherapy 25(1): 33–37

Elvey RL (1995) Peripheral Neuropathic Disorders and Neuromusculoskeletal pain, in: Shacklock MO (ed), Moving in on Pain. Butterworth-Heinemann, Oxford

Exelby L (1995) Mobilisation with Movement, A Personal View. Physiotherapy 81(12): 724–729

Glowacki KA, Breen CJ, Sacher K, Weiss AP (1996) Electrodiagnostic Testing and Carpal Tunnel Release Outcome. Journal of Hand Surgery 21A(1): 117–121

Harter BT Jr, McKiernan JE Jr, Kirzinger SS, Archer FW, Peters CK, Harter KC (1993) Carpal Tunnel Syndrome: Surgical and Non-surgical Treatment. Journal of Hand Surgery 18A(4): 734–739

Hicks CM (1995) Research for Physiotherapists, Project design and analysis, 2nd edn, Churchill Livingstone, Edinburgh

Huskisson EC (1974) Measurement of Pain. The Lancet ii: 1127–1131

Huskisson EC, Jones J, Scott PJ (1976) Application of Visual-Analogue Scales to the Measurement of Functional Capacity. Rheumatology and Rehabilitation 15(3): 185–187

Katz RT (1994) Carpal Tunnel Syndrome: A practical review. American Family Physician 49(6): 1371–1379

Katz JN, Keller RB, Simmons BP, Rogers WD, Bessette L, Fossel AH, Mooney NA (1998) Maine Carpal Tunnel Study: outcomes of operative and nonoperative therapy for carpal tunnel syndrome in a community-based cohort. Journal of Hand Surgery (Am) 23(4): 697–710

Kluge W, Simpson RG, Nicol AC (1996) Late Complications After Open Carpal Tunnel Decompression. Journal of Hand Surgery 21B(2): 205–207

Levine DW, Simmons BP, Koris MJ, Daltory LH, Hohl GG, Fossel AH, Katz JN (1993) A Self-Administered Questionnaire for the Assessment of Severity of Symptoms and Functional Status in Carpal Tunnel Syndrome. Journal of Bone & Joint Surgery 75A(11): 1585–1592

Lundborg G (1988) Nerve Injury and Repair. Churchill Livingstone, Edinburgh

Mackinnon SE, Dellon AL (1988) Surgery of the Peripheral Nerve. Thieme, New-York

Maitland GD (1991) Peripheral Manipulation 3rd edn. Butterworth-Heinemann, Oxford

Mulligan BR (1992) Manual Therapy "NAGS", "SNAGS", "PRP'S" etc. 2nd edn. Plane View Services, New Zealand

Murray DP, Saccone PG, Rayan GM (1994) Complications After Subfascial Carpal Tunnel Release. Southern Medical Journal 87(3): 416–418

Palmer AK, Toivonen DA (1999) Complications of Endoscopic and Open Carpal Tunnel Release. Journal of Hand Surgery (Am) 24(3): 561–565

Patterson MM (1998) Manipulation can Stretch the Transverse Carpal Ligament. Journal of the American Osteopathic Association 98(12): 662

Phalen GS (1966) The Carpal Tunnel Syndrome, Seventeen Years' Experience in Diagnosis and Treatment of Six Hundred Fifty-Four Hands. The Journal of Bone and Joint Surgery 48A(2): 211–228

Redmond MD, Rivner MH (1988) False Positive Electrodiagnostic Tests in Carpal Tunnel Syndrome. Muscle & Nerve 11: 511–517

Rozmaryn LM, Dovelle S, Rothman K, Olvey KM, Bartko JJ (1998) Nerve and Tendon Gliding Exercises and the Conservative Management of Carpal Tunnel syndrome. Journal of Hand Therapy 11(3): 171–179

Schuind F, Ventura M, Pasteels JL (1990) Idiopathic Carpal Tunnel Syndrome: Histologic Study of Flexor Tendon Synovium. Journal of Hand Surgery 15A(3): 497–503

Shacklock MO (1995a) Neurodynamics. Physiotherapy 81(1): 9–15

Shacklock MO (1995b) Clinical Application of Neurodynamics, in: Shacklock MO, Moving in on Pain. Butterworth-Heinmann, Oxford

Sucher BM (1993) Myofascial Manipulative Release of Carpal Tunnel Syndrome: Documentation with Magnetic Resonance Imaging. Journal of American Osteopathic Association 93(12): 1273–1278

Sucher BM (1994) Palpatory Diagnosis and Manipulative Management of Carpal Tunnel Syndrome. Journal of the American Osteopathic Association 94(8): 647–663

Sucher BM, Hinrichs RN (1998) Manipulative Treatment of Carpal Tunnel Syndrome: biomechanical and osteopathic intervention to increase the length of the transverse carpal ligament. Journal of the American Osteopathic Association 98(12): 679–686

Sunderland S (1978) Nerves and Nerve Injuries. 2nd edn. Churchill Livingstone, Edinburgh

Tavares SP, Giddins GEB (1996) Nerve Injury Following Steroid Injection for Carpal Tunnel Syndrome. Journal of Hand Surgery 21B(2): 208–209

Upton ARM, McComas AJ (1973) The Double Crush in Nerve-Entrapment Syndromes. The Lancet ii: 359–362

Valenta R, Gibson H (1994) Chiropractic Manipulation in Carpal Tunnel Syndrome. Journal of Manipulative & Physiological Therapeutics 17(4): 246–249

Waterfield J, Sim J (1996) Clinical Assessment of Pain by a Visual Analogue Scale. British Journal of Therapy and Rehabilitation 3(2): 94–97

© *2000 Harcourt Publishers Ltd*

ABSTRACT OR SUMMARY

1. Is the title a clear and succinct statement of the research study?

The title provides a clear and unambiguous message that the study will be a comparison of the effectiveness of two treatment techniques (carpal bone mobilisation and neurodynamic mobilisation) for a specified clinical problem (carpal tunnel syndrome). The title, therefore, is entirely unambiguous in its aims and any reader interested in the topic of treatments for carpal tunnel syndrome would be able to make an immediate assessment about the article's relevance.

2. Does the Abstract provide a clear statement of the aims, methods, results and conclusions/implications of the study?

The first two lines of the Summary/Abstract provide a clear contextual background and justification for the study, in that the prevalence of carpal tunnel syndrome is highlighted, together with a statement about the lack of research on the physiotherapeutic management of the problem. The case for the study is clearly and simply made. The authors continue with the aim (sentence 3), which is a comparison of the effectiveness of two physiotherapy techniques in the management of carpal tunnel syndrome. The research design they used is clearly stated (experimental, different subject, two treatment interventions and a control group), and the group size for each of the three conditions is reported (7 per group). The authors go on to refine their aims into specific outcome objectives (line 6, the comparison of treatment with no treatment and the comparison of intervention 1 with intervention 2). Four types of outcome measures (data collected) were noted: range of wrist movement, upper limb tension, three pain scales and subsequent need for surgery. The analysis of the results included both an 'eyeballing' of the data, which suggested at first glance that both treatments were more effective than no treatment, as well as formal analysis using inferential statistics. The Summary indicated that the results were not statistically significant between the treatment and non-treatment groups, and neither was there a statistically significant difference between the two types of treatment. The only exception was a pain relief scale, which the authors note 'demonstrated highly significant differences between the three groups when analysed by the Kruskal –Wallis test'. While the probability value is clearly stated, there is no statement as to which of the three groups experienced least pain and nor are the actual values for the test results recorded. Therefore, from the Summary, the data appear to have been analysed appropriately. The conclusions of the study have been stated in the last sentence and directly answer the research question implicit in the title

3. After reading the Abstract, are you clear in your mind about the nature of the study?

Overall, this is a lucid and succinct account of a small-scale research study, which addresses most of the key

issues. As a non-physiotherapist and with no knowledge of the clinical area, I feel quite happy about what was done and why. The design and method of the study are entirely suitable for its aims and fully address the research questions.

INTRODUCTION

4. Is there an adequate description of the general context of the study?

The first paragraph of the Introduction makes a clear statement about the extent of the problem, as well as the knock-on effect for absenteeism and compensation claims. Therefore, the gravity of the problem and the practical real-life implications provide not only the context for the study, but also begin to make the case for carrying it out. The study has both clinical and practical relevance.

5. Is the literature review thorough, relevant, recent and properly used to provide a structured argument leading to the reason for conducting the reported piece of research?

The authors start the literature review (second paragraph) by reporting the results of surgical interventions for carpal tunnel syndrome, noting that, overall, the outcomes from these are less than totally successful, with a number of associated risks. The second paragraph, in essence, highlights the deficiencies with surgery and conservative medical interventions and begins to build the argument for a consideration of alternative (i.e. physiotherapy) treatments.

The next paragraph reviews some conventional physiotherapy interventions and points out their limitations (second sentence); it also refers to alternative chiropractic and osteopathic techniques, critiquing the available literature with reference to the methodological inadequacies of the studies. This paragraph therefore continues to develop the case against existing non-surgical treatment options, again implicitly suggesting that other interventions need to be evaluated.

Paragraph 4 is concerned with a theoretical physiological/anatomical account of the implications of carpal tunnel syndrome. In particular, it focuses on the impact of the condition for wrist movement and the interventions that have been used to improve joint mobility. The authors emphasise the fact that these interventions have not been properly evaluated. This paragraph, then, focuses down onto two specific issues that were central to Tal-Akabi and Rushton's study: namely, the problems of wrist movement (one of their outcome measures) and the lack of scientific evidence for joint mobilisation (one of their treatment interventions). This rather more theoretical section adds more weight to the case for their study.

The next paragraph addresses another anatomical/ physiological aspect of carpal tunnel syndrome, that of nervous system mobilisation. The theory underpinning this is succinctly covered and the research that has evaluated this approach is summarised. Together with the preceding paragraph, it is clear to the reader that there are two possible management techniques for carpal tunnel syndrome, which have been neither compared nor fully investigated for their effectiveness. The final paragraph in the Introduction explicitly makes this point and at the same time concludes the case for carrying out the current study. The structure of the Introduction, which goes from the general (prevalence and real-world implications of carpal tunnel syndrome), through to more specific treatment issues (lack of evidence for, and limitations of, surgical, as well as some physiotherapeutic, chiropractic and osteopathic interventions) and finally to a very focused theoretical and research-based account of two management approaches that form the basis of the authors' study, makes a clear and succinct case for the experiment. It follows clearly the inverted triangle format (Fig. 11.1) outlined on page 150, allowing the reader to progress from an understanding of the general clinical and practical issues to an informed position of the limitations of existing treatment techniques and the reasons for conducting this evaluation study. As the journal restricts the length of an article to 4000 words maximum, the coverage of the existing literature within these parameters is thorough and directly relevant to the problem. Moreover, with regard to the contemporaneous nature of the review, the vast majority of the citations are dated within the 1990s. Given that the article itself appeared in 2000, was probably submitted for publication a year before that and conducted 2–3 years before its appearance (around 1997–78), it might reasonably be concluded that the literature was up-to-date at the time of going to press. Without specialist knowledge of the topic area or undertaking a thorough search of journals and CD-ROMs, this is a useful yardstick for a reader to use when assessing the quality of a literature review. The Introduction to this article, then, satisfies all the requirements contained in question 5 of the critique guidelines. Overall, the clarity and comprehensiveness of the Introduction demonstrate the researchers' grasp of the clinical and theoretical aspects of the syndrome; also the clear case made for undertaking the study demonstrates the practical relevance and value of the project.

6. Is the hypothesis (if appropriate) clearly stated and the predicted relationship between the variables apparent?
Because the authors have clearly stated that this is an experimental, different-subject design (Summary/Abstract, lines 4–5), an hypothesis is essential. While some journals require this to be specified at the conclusion of the Introduction, here the authors have stated the hypotheses as the aims of the study in the Methodology section; this is quite acceptable. The first hypothesis clearly predicts a relationship between intervention (IV) and effectiveness (DV). The second hypothesis predicts a difference in effectiveness (DV) between the two treatment types used, i.e. carpal bone mobilisation and neurodynamic mobilisation (IV). The direction of the hypotheses (both of which are two-tailed) is implicit. The fact that no trend or

direction is predicted for the results is entirely appropriate in the light of the available research evidence, which does not indicate that one of the treatment techniques is any better than the other. Since it is important for a one-tailed prediction to be justified by a clear directional picture provided by the existing literature, a one-tailed prediction would not have been suitable here. The null hypotheses are also properly stated. The precisely cited aims of the study enable the reader to make a subsequent assessment of the suitability of the design as a test of the hypotheses.

7. If the research does not test the hypothesis, are the aims of the study clear?
See question 6 above.

8. Are the aims or hypothesis useful to clinical therapy?
As the focus of the study is a comparison of two treatment techniques in an important area of physiotherapy which had hitherto been under-researched, the topic is of great relevance.

9. Is the project likely to be of value to clinical therapy?
As carpal tunnel syndrome is 'the most common peripheral entrapment neuropathy' (Tal-Akabi and Rushton, p. 214), it must, by definition, constitute a significant clinical problem for the health care professions. Moreover, because there is limited evidence about suitable interventions, this piece of research had the capacity to inform physiotherapy management of a frequently occurring patient condition. Therefore, whatever the findings, they should be able to guide physiotherapy provision for carpal tunnel patients; consequently, the project was a relevant and valuable one.

METHOD

10. Has the design of the study been properly described?
The researchers not only state that a different-subject experimental design was used, they also provide a model of the study, showing which patient group received which intervention. This illustration greatly clarifies the design used and accords perfectly with the model provided on Table 9.3 outlined on page 150 of this text.

11. Has the researcher made it clear why this design was chosen?
The researchers state clearly in the second paragraph of the Methodology that this design 'enabled comparison between the two interventions and a control group' (p. 215); the chosen design has therefore been fully justified in the light of the study's aims.

12. Is the design appropriate for the aims/hypothesis stated in the Introduction?
The different-subject design is absolutely correct for the stated hypothesis. It would be entirely inappropriate to use

a same-subject design here, because it would be impossible to isolate the results of a given intervention if all the patients received both treatment types. In other words, there would be no way of disentangling which technique was having the effect, since any improvements for the patient might be the cumulative effect of both interventions. Re-read pp. 93–96 if you're not clear about this. Consequently, the best way of testing the stated hypotheses is by using separate (or different) groups of subjects, each of which receives one treatment, and then comparing the clinical outcomes of each. The design, then, is entirely right.

13. Are sources of error acknowledged and controlled?
These are dealt with explicitly in response to questions 23 and 28, as well as implicitly in various parts of the article. This critique refers to the sources of error addressed in:

- questions 14 and 16: re: incidental sampling methods
- question 14: re: issues of co-morbidities
- question 15: re: age of participants, length of time with syndrome
- question 20/21: re: procedures adopted in the study, especially order of assessments taken, individual nature of clinical treatment interventions, reliability of measurements
- question 22: re: instructions to patients.

The critique in regard to these points highlights some aspects of the design that could potentially have biased the results. Where the researchers have addressed these, it has been noted. To avoid repetition, these points will not be reiterated in response to this question.

14. Is the sample suitable? Of an appropriate size? Fully described? Properly selected?
The sample comprised 21 carpal tunnel syndrome patients selected from a waiting list for surgery. Therefore, given that the focus of the study was carpal tunnel syndrome, these patients, at face value, were self-evidently suitable in terms of their clinical problem. Clear inclusion/exclusion criteria were specified in paragraph 4 of the Methodology and in this sense describe the participants adequately, although it is often clearer to tabulate the sample's relevant details. The exclusion criteria reflect some of the constant errors that might have distorted the results. For example, patients with rheumatoid arthritis and diabetes were eliminated from the study, presumably because their co-morbidities would counteract and obscure the effects of treatment for carpal tunnel syndrome. The patients were selected using a non-probability method of incidental sampling, which, strictly speaking, is not appropriate for experimental designs and inferential statistical analysis, although it is frequently used in practice as a base for inferential analysis (see pp. 29–30). Furthermore, at 7 patients per group, the sample was very small. Later, in the Discussion, the authors fully acknowledge the implications for the results that their sampling process and participant numbers might have. I shall deal with these points in the next question.

15. Were any sources of bias or error evident in the sample and/or in the process by which they were chosen?
The sample was a small non-probability sample, which would mean that there may be some potential for bias (see questions 14 and 16). However, the authors acknowledge this in the Discussion and the limitations it would impose on generalising from the results. They have clearly stipulated the exclusion/inclusion criteria used and the way in which the subjects were randomised to conditions. Given the small-scale exploratory nature of the study, the approach adopted was reasonable. A more detailed response to these points can be found in questions 14 and 16.

16. Would this impact upon the study's outcomes?
The patients selected, although clinically fairly similar at baseline, were heterogeneous in some regards, in that their age range was 29–85 years and the length of time they had experienced the problem ranged from 1 to 3 years. It is conceivable that older patients and those who had had the problem for longer might be more resistant to, or profit less from, treatment. I fully accept, though, that, as I am not a physiotherapist, these comments may be invalid and that neither age nor length of time with the condition may be relevant to the outcomes. It is also important to emphasise that homogeneity of the sample is difficult to achieve in an applied study, and, moreover, is not necessarily desirable because it limits the generalisability of the results (see p. 99). Usually, the implications of these individual differences would normally be acknowledged in the discussion of the results, and taken into account when drawing conclusions. Moreover, how representative the sample was of the parent population would also need to be addressed in the discussion, especially since the sampling technique was not random (see later in this section). It must, though, be emphasised that applied clinical research cannot be perfect and therefore, while the above comments about the sample are valid in research terms, it must always be fully acknowledged that, in real-world research, ideal samples cannot be obtained.

The sample was a small one (7 per group) and this will compromise the generalisability of the results, a point addressed clearly by the authors later in the Discussion. While it is recognised that this is a piece of applied research, the numbers are very small and my own feeling is that the study would have been better classified as a pilot study, preparatory to informing a later larger-scale project. As one aim of a pilot study is to explore the feasibility of undertaking a bigger investigation, smaller numbers can be used.

In addition, the authors use incidental sampling, which is a non-probability method of selecting participants, frequently used but not strictly appropriate for inferential statistics (see pp. 29–30). As inferential statistics rest on the assumption that the results from a small sample can be generalised to the population from which it was drawn, it is important that a sample is representative of its parent population. If the participants are a convenient incidental sample, then they are less likely to reflect the population characteristics; consequently, the results are likely to be less applicable to other carpal tunnel syndrome patients. The authors do acknowledge this in the discussion and conclusion of their study, and their interpretation of the results and recommendations for practice are made in the light of the sample's shortcomings. The nature of the sampling procedure also serves to support the recommendation that this study might have been better construed as a pilot study, since the same level of methodological rigour is not as essential for a pilot project as for a full-scale one, because the purposes of each are somewhat different.

The method of randomising patients to treatments was a simple, but acceptable, one, although the authors do not mention who conducted the randomisation process. While this study was not classified as an RCT (randomised controlled trial), the randomisation process is intended to minimise bias, so it would have been useful for the researchers to clarify whether either of them had been involved in the allocation process and, if so, what steps they took to ensure that experimenter involvement at this stage did not influence the procedure, and hence the results.

17. Was any mechanical apparatus used in the study and, if so, was it properly described? Was it suitable for the project?

Under the subheading 'Measurement of active range of movement – wrist flexion and extension' it is reported that a standard goniometer was used. Since the universal goniometer is widely used, this does not require further explanation. However, in the following section, which describes the upper limb tension test (ULTT2a), no apparatus was mentioned, although photographic recording of movement can be used. As practitioner judgement is an accepted clinical method of assessing upper limb tension, and because the authors presumably anticipated that the results of this study would be implemented in clinical practice, it would be highly unlikely that photographic techniques would be used in everyday practice to monitor the effects of treatment. Therefore, because of the applied nature of this study, it is perfectly acceptable to use the evaluation measures that practitioners would routinely use in clinical situations. Both the goniometer and ULTT2a are standard clinical procedures used for assessing these functions and so these measurement techniques are entirely suitable.

18. Were any other materials used, such as questionnaires, score sheets, attitude scales, etc.?

The authors used a number of other materials in their outcome measurements, namely a symptom diary, a functional box scale and a pain relief scale (referred to in the Summary/Abstract as 'three different scales to evaluate pain perception and function' (p. 214). They also used the median nerve biased test to measure upper limb tension.

19. Were these described fully and/or included in the Appendix, if appropriate?

20. Were any questionnaires or scales which were used properly constructed and adequately tested before using them in the study? Were they suitable for their purpose?

In order to avoid repetition, questions 19 and 20 will be taken together. The first non-mechanical measurement reported is a symptom diary (referred to as the Visual Analogue Scale or VAS), which is described both verbally and diagrammatically (Figure 1). While this diary is clearly and cogently justified, I had difficulty in fully understanding Figure 1, because the horizontal and vertical numbers are not labelled. However, as I am not a physiotherapist, I am prepared to accept that Figure 1 would have more meaning to the profession. Nonetheless, it would be important for the authors to emphasise how they instructed the patients to complete this task, so that the participants were fully and clearly informed. It should be noted, too, that although the text immediately above the figure describes the meaning of the 0–5 vertical scale, this measure is not a conventional visual analogue scale (see pp. 42–43).

The authors also used the 'functional box scale' (FBS), which was a modification of an established procedure for measuring hand/wrist function. Adaptation of standard procedures is both acceptable and appropriate if nothing precisely suitable is available, although it would be useful to identify the alterations that were made. The article suggests that the measure was discussed, and therefore effectively tried out with the actual sample, as a means of pretesting the feasibility of the measure. This stage was essentially a mini-pilot and would have been useful for highlighting any difficulties experienced by the participants. The authors present an illustrative example of this scale, but, to the non-expert, it is unclear whether the FBS only focuses on doing up/undoing shirts/buttons and on gripping, or whether there are other functional tests incorporated in the measure. As any article might be read by a wide-ranging audience, it might have been better to clarify this.

The authors also use a pain relief scale (PRS) that is a modification of an established scale. The same comments regarding the nature of the changes made and the exact content of the measurement scale also apply here. The final assessment was whether or not the patients proceeded to surgery following treatment. This is a straightforward, real-life test of whether or not the interventions had been clinically effective for the participants.

To conclude, then, the measures appear to be absolutely suitable for their purpose, but it might have been useful to specify the nature of the modifications made and the precise details of the measuring instruments. However, it should always be recognised that the word limit imposed on any article means that some information must be omitted. This paper presents a lot of detail, and in this respect is a good model; a couple of sentences addressing the points noted above would have made it even more lucid.

21. Is the description of what was done absolutely clear?

22. Does it state the order in which things were done?

Again, for the purpose of brevity, questions 21 and 22 will be taken together. The procedure is clearly stated as involving independent pre-and post-treatment assessments of the stipulated DVs. The only exception is the pain relief scale, which logically can only be used after treatment to assess the degree to which pain was relieved by the intervention. The use of independent people to collect the data is a good design consideration, since it minimises the potential for bias. However, it would have been useful to note the number of independent data collectors involved and the way in which they were involved. For example, did one person do all the pre-and post-tests for one group? Or did three or four people take the same measurement for each patient, in order to check the reliability of the readings?

Each of the experimental groups received their allocated intervention (either median nerve mobilisation or carpal bone mobilisation), while the control remained as a non-intervention group. A clear statement of the length of the individual treatment sessions and the overall intervention period would be a valuable piece of information for researchers wishing to replicate this study. However, at the end of the second paragraph of Procedures, the authors do make it clear that the nature of the treatment was not standardised within an intervention group, but, rather, was tailored to individual need. This is an interesting point that illustrates the difference between an applied and a controlled lab-based study. While pure experimental research should endeavour to ensure that any intervention is undertaken in the same way for all participants, responding to patient need and reflecting standard clinical practice is more appropriate for applied research. Therefore, the procedure adopted by the authors was entirely appropriate for a real-life study and was probably essential to obtaining ethical approval and patient consent.

The description of the analyses states which software package and which tests were used to analyse the data. The issue of reliability studies is introduced here for the first time and therefore raises some questions. Reliability studies of the three pain symptom/function tests or the measures taken by the independent assessors? Certainly, the evaluation of measurement reliability against other scales is a very valid and desirable design consideration, but a few more details would have made the nature of these completely clear. The appropriate 5% significance level was used, although this point will be referred to later in response to question 33.

The use of parametric vs. non-parametric tests for the types of data collected was appropriate, with the possible exception of the related t-test used to analyse the 0–5 symptom scale on the symptom diary. This has been described by the authors as a visual analogue scale and the data have been treated as interval/ratio (as indicated by the use of the parametric related t-test). However, a visual

analogue scale is by convention an unmarked 10 cm line and the scores are the distance between the 0 end and the mark placed by the respondent (see pp. 42–43). These data can be treated as interval/ratio and analysed by parametric tests. However, the authors use a 0–5 scale, which is neither a conventional visual analogue scale and nor is it interval/ratio data. It is true to say, though, that in practice many researchers assume equal intervals in such scales, thereby enabling them to use parametric tests. Where variations to conventional analytical methods are used, they should be justified. The authors correctly state that the tests were all two-tailed, which is consistent with the stated hypotheses.

The issue of ethics was properly addressed, in that subjects were asked to give informed consent and the whole proposal was approved by the relevant ethics committees. These stages are essential in studies involving human participants.

The general order of the assessments (i.e. before/after) is made clear, although the specific order of which outcome was measured when, is not reported. This could have been important, in that it is conceivable that feedback from one assessment might have influenced the patient's reportage of other outcomes. For example, if the range of wrist movement was measured first by the goniometer and was found to have increased following treatment, this might impact upon the patient's subsequent interpretation of the pain levels experienced or their reported functional ability. The problem of order effects is covered in Chapter 8 and should be addressed where multiple measures of a single-subject sample are being taken.

23. Does it provide a verbatim report of any instructions given to the subjects? Were the instructions clear?

The symptom diary presumably required patients to complete the form at home, which meant that these were self-completing measures. Any tool (e.g. survey questionnaire) that requires the subject to respond independently, away from the researcher/data collector, must be absolutely unambiguous in its requirements and instructions (see Chapter 3), otherwise misunderstanding can result. As was noted in the response to question 20, the method of completing the symptom diary could have been made more explicit in the article.

24. Were the sources of error dealt with appropriately?

There are many sources of error that can bias the outcomes of a research study (see Chapter 8) and these need to be acknowledged. The authors refer, in the Discussion, to two potential sources of error in the study: sample size and the sampling process. They also specify appropriate exclusion/inclusion criteria for the sample (see below). With any applied study, a perfect research design is impossible to obtain, and it is important for researchers to acknowledge the compromises made. The authors have done this here, which is a good index of their awareness of the implications of their design decisions.

However, order effects of testing could have influenced the results (see answer to question 23) and, while the researchers may have dealt with this in the conduct of their study, it would have been useful to mention this in the report. Experimenter bias was also a possible source of distortion and, in response to this, the authors use an independent person to collect the before/after data. The inclusion/exclusion criteria deal with some sources of constant error, but there are other individual differences (such as age, length of time with condition; see responses to questions 14 and 15) which might have been relevant to include.

25. Was the method of data collection clearly described and appropriate?

The researchers were interested to assess the impact of different forms of treatment on various clinical and functional outcomes, and so the methods they used to evaluate these outcomes are appropriate.

26. Were the data suitable measures of the dependent variable (if the study tested an hypothesis) or of the information required by the survey's aims?

The authors were concerned to assess the effectiveness of two different treatments with a control group on a number of mobility, functional and pain measures. They therefore used relevant data to assess these outcomes (symptom diary, functional box scale, pain relief scale, range of wrist movement and ULTT2a). They also justify the use of these over other available techniques, which is a very good feature.

27. Were the subjects treated well, their rights and confidentiality protected?

The authors make it clear that the patients could withdraw at any point without compromising their treatment. This is entirely consistent with ethical recommendations (see pp. 86–89). The fact that the participants gave informed consent prior to the start of the study implies that they were cognisant of what would be involved (final paragraph of the Methodology). Nothing is said about the confidentiality of results, nor how the data were stored.

28. Was the study ethical?

The use of a control group always raises ethical questions, since this, by definition, is a non-treatment group. When selecting participants, however, the researchers would have had to make it clear that there would be a chance of being allocated to the control group; therefore, consenting to these terms meant that the patients were also agreeing to this possibility.

29. Could you repeat this study to the letter if it was considered necessary?

The description of the study thus far has been quite detailed, to the point that I would estimate that it could be fairly accurately replicated. More precise details of the order of testing and the modifications to the materials would have enabled absolute replication of these aspects. Overall, the Methodology section is clear, detailed and concise and would afford general replication.

RESULTS

30. Are the graphs (if provided) clear, self-explanatory and useful?

Two bar graphs are presented, one for the ULTT2a test and one for continuation to surgery. Both are clearly labelled, with a useful legend, which makes them self-explanatory.

31. Are the tables (if used) clearly labelled and constructed, with an obvious relevance to the study?

Six tables are presented, one for each of the data sets for the five outcome measures used, and one summarising the significant findings. The tables are clearly labelled and relate directly to the measures of the DV. The tables are unusual in that they report the raw data, made possible, presumably, by the small subject numbers involved. This, of course, makes it possible for the reader to check the analyses, if so wished. It would have been sufficient, though (unless it is journal policy to produce the raw data), simply to tabulate the results of the different analyses.

32. Are the statistical tests used the correct ones for the project's design?

The researchers have analysed the data from each of the outcome measures by making two separate sets of comparisons. First, they have compared the treatment outcomes at post test, for each of the three groups, using either a one-way ANOVA for unrelated designs, or its non-parametric equivalent, the Kruskal–Wallis. This between-group comparison was intended to establish whether one treatment was more effective than the others. Second, in order to see whether each intervention had any effect on a specified DV, they have used a related t-test on the before/after data for each group. This within-group comparison was intended to ascertain whether there were any before/after differences for each treatment intervention; in other words, did the treatment have any effect on baseline symptoms/functions? The researchers, therefore, have treated the results as though they have emerged from two separate designs – a between-group design to compare the three interventions and a within-group design to assess the before/after effects – and they have analysed the results from each design separately. Therefore, if we take, for example, the VAS, they have used four analyses: a non-parametric Kruskal–Wallis, plus three related t-tests.

However, this mixture of between-and within-group design is classified as a mixed design, because three independent groups have been used (two types of treatment and a control), each of which is measured on each outcome on two occasions (before and after treatment), and the results must be analysed as a single data set. Therefore, the researchers have a mixture of a different-subject design (treatment types + control) and a same-subject design (before and after measures) within the same study (see Fig. A4.1).

This design is one we haven't covered in the book, because of its complexity, but its analysis requires a form of ANOVA called mixed between-within group analysis of

Between-group comparison (i.e. comparison of different interventions)

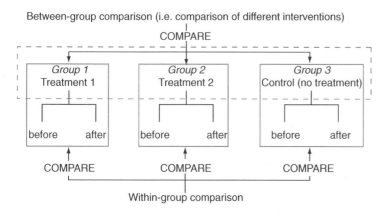

Figure A4.1 Mixed between-/within-group design used by authors in the critiqued article.

variance or a split-plot analysis of variance (ANOVA). This analysis simultaneously makes every possible comparison between sets of results (e.g. Control group before vs. Treatment group 1 after, Treatment group 2 before vs. Treatment group 2 after, Treatment group 1 after vs Treatment group 2 after, etc.). This ANOVA would be very difficult to compute by hand and the results it generates can be very hard to interpret, even though post-hoc comparisons of means would reveal where the differences in the results lay (see section on Scheffe, pp. 230–233). However, it is the correct test to use with the interval/ratio data here, as it would enable the researchers to analyse each outcome measure for each group, before and after, simultaneously. There is no non-parametric equivalent of the mixed design ANOVA for use with ordinal data (analysed here by the Kruskal–Wallis). What the researchers have done instead is to use either parametric or non-parametric one-way ANOVA for independent samples to compare the between-group findings and then to re-analyse the data using the related t-test to see if there were any before/after differences within each group. While this appears to be entirely logical, it is not really correct. Repeated analysis of the data set in this way can lead to Type I errors (i.e. concluding that the hypothesis has been supported when, in fact, it hasn't). The analyses used by the authors could possibly have been justified if they had made the (strong) case that there is no non-parametric equivalent of the split-plot ANOVA, and that they were not interested in all the comparisons the correct ANOVA would have computed; to compensate for the chance of Type I errors, they could have reduced the significance level for the t-tests to 0.01 (see p. 110). Also, had the study been set up as a pilot, the use of the current statistical techniques might have been acceptable as an exploratory process (simply because a pilot can be used to see if there are any findings worth pursuing further in a large-scale study). However, pilot studies can also use less stringent significance levels (i.e. 10%). So the authors could possibly have made a case for their choice of analysis, had they used either a more stringent significance level, or classified the study as a pilot. In addition, they would also have had to emphasise the lack of an appropriate non-parametric test and that

they were only interested in selected comparisons, rather than all the possible ones that the split-plot ANOVA would have yielded. It should, though, be noted that the version of SPSS that the authors used did not have the correct split-plot ANOVA available; this may explain the use of alternative analyses.

The authors also use a parametric related t-test for pre-and post-analysis of the VAS (symptom diary). Because the reported scale goes from 0 to 5, the data are not interval/ratio, making the use of the non-parametric Wilcoxon more appropriate. It should be emphasised that some researchers make the assumption that the intervals on an ordinal scale are equivalent and consequently use parametric tests to analyse the data. While this debate is beyond the scope of this text, it is still probably safer to follow the maxim 'when in doubt, use a non-parametric test'.

In conclusion, therefore, while the general principles of selecting statistical analysis based on unrelated vs. related designs were correct, because this study used a mixture of both in a split-plot design, the results must be treated as a single data set and analysed by a split-plot (or mixed design) ANOVA. However, it should not be assumed that the correct mixed-design ANOVA would necessarily yield different results. The raw data have been re-analysed using the correct tests and the findings are reported under question 34.

33. Is the selected level of significance appropriate for the topic area?
This question is partly addressed by the response to the above question. Insofar as the study was not expected to have adverse consequences in the event of the hypothesis not being supported, a 5% significance level was appropriate (see p. 110). However, the authors have analysed the data in a way that increases the possibility of a Type I error occurring; to counteract this, a lower significance level (e.g. 1% or 0.1%) would be more suitable. Conversely, had the authors presented this as a small-scale pilot study to establish whether or not a larger study was worth conducting, a less stringent significance

level (e.g. 10%) could have been adopted. So the answer to the question is not clear-cut.

34. Is the *p* value clearly stated and correct for the hypothesis as stated (i.e. one- or two-tailed)?

The Results section is subheaded, which makes it particularly easy to follow. The authors clearly state that the results of the Kruskal–Wallis test on the visual analogue scores from the symptom diary were significant at <0.05 and the implications of this are also highlighted. The results of the pre/post tests for each group's symptom diary scores are also succinctly reported, with obtained p values of >0.05, <0.02 and <0.001. The meaning of these results is noted. Rather than as an H value. It is not specified whether the hypothesis was one-or two-tailed. The results and raw data are presented in Table 1. With the caveats noted in the previous answer, this is a very clear section.

There are two sets of results from the FBS measurements; the first introduces a concept tangentially referred to in the text, that of correlation (see Question 23, above). The authors have very usefully and legitimately investigated the degree of association between the symptom diary scores and the functional box scores, to ascertain whether they are reliable measures (see page 243 for reliability issues). The results of the Spearman are presented as p < 0.05, rho = +0.804, N = 18. However, it is not clear which sets of results have been correlated (before/after, by treatment group/overall, etc.); it is therefore difficult to ascertain where the N value comes from.

The results of the Kruskal–Wallis test for the FBS measures are clearly presented (although, as noted above, for these sample sizes, the value of χ^2 rather than H should really have been recorded). The authors, however, do note the meaning of their calculations and the results and raw data are shown in Table 2. Similarly, the results of the pain relief scale are clearly presented and interpreted. Again, with the above provision in Question 32, these are lucid sections.

The results of the range of movement (ROM) tests are presented both as a test of its reliability as well as comparisons between the three treatment groups and within-group before/after comparisons. With regard to the reliability test, it is stated that a Kendall coefficient of concordance was calculated and found to be significant. While this test is an appropriate assessment of the level of agreement between a number of ratings, it is not clear what exactly the Kendall was calculated on (how many sets of readings or raters). The second analysis reported in this section was the within-group before/after measures, using a related t-test. The raw data and findings for the ROM flexion measures are clearly presented in Table 4 and suggest that only group 1 demonstrated any significant difference in movement following treatment. The results are stated as being significant at p < 0.05. Similar analyses were undertaken for the ROM extension results (Table 5), with p values of <0.05 being reported for each of the two treatment groups.

The third analysis reported is a one-way ANOVA to compare the outcomes for ROM flexion and extension for all three groups; this accurately notes that the F values are not significant (although, again, this should be interpreted with caution, since this ANOVA was not really the correct test). Re-analysis of the data using a mixed between-within-group ANOVA revealed non-significant p values in each case, with F values of 0.225 for the flexion results and 0.133 for the extension results, confirming the authors' findings. This means that the appropriate statistical test did not generate different results.

The next set of analyses deals with the ULTT2a assessments, again testing for inter-tester reliability using a Kendall coefficient of concordance, as well as graphing the results (see question 30 for comments on this). The final analysis related to the need for subsequent surgery. The authors present the raw data here, without any significance testing. Because of the design and the small numbers involved, this is quite appropriate.

The authors provide a summary of significant results in Table 6, which is useful, and, in my view, is a model which should be more widely adopted in articles. It should, though, be said that non-significant results can be as valuable as significant ones and, therefore, should not be overlooked.

My computer re-analysis of all the raw data revealed exact p values. SPSS analysis provides precise probability values for each calculation and it is usual to record these. It should also be noted that I used a different version of SPSS to that used by the researchers, and this might have generated slightly different information.

DISCUSSION

35. Are the results and conclusions clearly stated?

The authors reiterate their findings for each outcome measure used; they also provide a succinct conclusion, which takes account of some of the study's limitations. The conclusion does not make extravagant claims, but, rather, tentatively provides a general recommendation for therapists dealing with carpal tunnel syndrome patients. The conclusions (given the caveat above) are entirely appropriate.

36. Are they related to other studies in the area, thereby putting them into a broader research framework?

While the results from the symptom diary, FBS, PRS and both ROM measures are discussed independently of other research, those from the ULTT2a are presented and explained with reference to four other pieces of published work, which contextualise the study. The overall findings (paragraphs 10, 11 and 12) are discussed in relation to other work on carpal tunnel syndrome, and relevant research is cited by way of explanation of the current findings

37. Is a cogent theoretical explanation for the findings provided?

The authors provide a useful theoretical interpretation of the ULTT2a results, especially with reference to the observed differences in outcome between the two treatment groups (paragraph 7, Discussion). In addition, the general findings are explained in terms of other research work, most notably the work on the nervous system by Butler (1991). The authors also, quite rightly, observe that their results are compromised by some methodological issues, such as the measuring instruments used (paragraph 9) and the implications of the small sample size.

38. Are the results interpreted fully and correctly, or selectively and/or extravagantly?

The authors cover all their outcome measures properly, identifying their implications and limitations. No results are omitted from the discussion, nor are wild claims made for the interventions used. They use due caution in their recommendations.

39. Are any flaws in the study's design highlighted, together with recommendations for improvement?

The authors correctly refer several times to the limitations imposed by the small sample size (e.g. end of paragraph 2, final paragraph). They also refer to the restrictions on data analysis that this created, noting, rightly, which tests could have been used had a larger sample been involved (e.g. the use of the extended c^2 to analyse the ULTT2a results). They identify the difficulties encountered when taking measurements on wrist ROM (paragraph 6), but neatly justify its use, in preference to alternatives. The issue of longer-term effects of treatment are discussed in the penultimate paragraph, together with the implicit suggestion that a longer-term project would have answered some of these questions. The final sentence of the discussion suggests the use of a random, as opposed to an incidental, sample in a future study, thereby implicitly recognising the shortcomings of the sampling approach adopted here.

40. Are the results interpreted with these in mind?

The impact of sample size on the results is referred to several times, and the inability to draw conclusions about long-term effects of treatment is also mentioned. The fact that generalisability of the results is limited is identified as a problem of the small sample. Problems with ROM measurement techniques (see above and paragraph 6) are discussed thoroughly with regard to outcome data, but the technique is also well-justified. See also the response to question 38.

41. Are any practical ramifications of the results discussed?

The authors make appropriately tentative recommendations that manual therapy might be a useful conservative treatment for carpal tunnel syndrome patients with no other co-morbidities. This paper could therefore inform the physiotherapeutic management of this patient group.

42. Do any ideas for further projects emerge?

The authors identify the need for longer-term studies which might ascertain the degree to which patient benefits could

be maintained, the replication of the study with a larger, randomly selected sample, and the possibility of a multi-site project.

REFERENCES

43. Is every article, study, research report and book quoted in the reference section?

Yes.

44. Do these references give all the required information?

Yes, with the exception of the Dean and Louis reference, which omits the place of publication, and the Upton and McComas reference, which omits the volume and part number of the Lancet.

OVERALL CONSIDERATIONS

45. Was the project a worthwhile one, contributing to the knowledge base of physiotherapy?

Given the prevalence of carpal tunnel syndrome, its salience and the lack of established management guidelines of the condition, this study was a very valuable one.

46. Was it clearly written, so that the content was easily accessible to the reader?

Although there were one or two queries (see above), this article was sufficiently clearly written that I, as a non-physiotherapist, could easily understand the problem area, its implications and the ramifications of the findings; moreover, I could also assess the suitability of the design for the study of this clinical problem. The writing style is an excellent academic one, combining clarity with objectivity and succinctness. Therefore, my assessment is that the article is well written, clearly structured and, where specialist terms have been used, they have been defined at the point of introduction.

47. Is the report scientific and objective both in the way in which it was conducted as well as the way in which it was analysed and written up?

The study used a number of techniques that ensured scientific objectivity, e.g. the way in which the patients were randomised to conditions, the use of independent data collectors, the control condition, etc. While the use of a convenient incidental sample selected from a waiting list has the potential to introduce bias, the authors acknowledge this. Overall, the report was written objectively and scientifically.

48. Is the report devoid of jargon?

The authors use a number of technical/specialist terms. However, their usage constitutes a valid form of shorthand

and is therefore not unnecessary. Moreover, where abbreviations have been used, they have been defined at the point of introduction. The article is sufficiently clear that a non-physiotherapist could make sense of it.

49. Has the research project advanced clinical therapy in any way?

Insofar as the project highlights a highly relevant clinical problem, cautiously suggests some conservative management techniques and points the way to further relevant studies, the answer is undoubtedly 'yes'. The authors, though, are properly careful not to make any sweeping statements about treatment for carpal tunnel syndrome, but, rather, offer their research as a source of information for physiotherapists.

Overall, the study was neat, valuable, well-designed and competent, with a clear focus on a highly relevant clinical issue. It might have been better to present it as a pilot trial, which would mean that many of the foregoing comments would have been less relevant, since a pilot study is typically used to assess the feasibility of a larger-scale investigation and therefore does not need to adopt the same rigour.

Glossary

abstract (also called a summary) a résumé, usually found at the beginning of journal articles, which summarises the key features of the study.

action research a practical problem-driven approach to research that involves collaboration between practitioner and researcher. The process is cyclical, in that interventions are implemented and evaluated, modifications are made to the interventions, the modifications are then evaluated, changes made and so on.

analysis of variance (ANOVA) a statistical technique that allows the simultaneous comparison of three or more sets of data derived from experimental designs. There are a number of variants on this technique which allow the researcher to analyse data from different-, same/matched-subject designs, or a mixture of both. While there are non-parametric analysis of variance tests, the term ANOVA is commonly taken to mean the parametric variety, while the non-parametric tests are referred to by specific names (e.g. Kruskal–Wallis test).

apparatus any equipment used in a research project.

attitude scale a technique of measuring attitudes in a quantifiable and relatively scientific way. It involves several stages, each of which is intended to ensure that the tool is valid and reliable.

bar graph a graph used to show the frequency of a given event by the height of vertically arranged bars or columns. These bars have spaces between them.

baseline a stage in a research project (usually before the study has started) when the subjects receive no treatment or intervention.

bias any distortion in results due to flaws in the design of the study. (See also experimenter bias.)

Bland and Altman Agreement test a graphical technique used in reliability studies which involves plotting measurement error against two standard deviations either side of the mean.

central tendency a description of a set of results which typically makes use of the average score, the most commonly occurring score and the mid-score of that set of data.

characteristic some feature of a population for which the researcher wishes to make an estimate from a sample of that population.

chi-squared (χ^2) test a non-parametric statistical test used to analyse two sets of nominal data from different subject designs which employ two groups of subjects only. (See also extended χ^2 test).

clinical significance the degree to which a set of results has some clinical meaning or relevance. Sometimes results can be statistically significant but clinically meaningless.

closed-response question   any question that is framed in such a way that only a limited number of answers are possible.

confidence interval   a range in a set of scores derived from a sample, in which the population characteristic is confidently expected to fall.

confidence level   the degree of confidence which can be placed in an estimate of a population characteristic. It is expressed as a percentage; the most commonly used levels are 90%, 95% and 99%.

confidence limits   the upper and lower figures of the confidence interval.

constant error   any source of bias and error in a research project that will influence the results in a constant and predictable way. They must be controlled or eliminated; if they are not then the conclusions may be wrong, misleading and possibly dangerous.

control group   a group of subjects in an experimental design which does not receive any treatment or intervention. This group can then be compared with the experimental group which does receive some intervention, in order to establish the effects of the independent variable.

correlation coefficient   a numerical value somewhere between −1.0 and +1.0 which indicates the degree and nature of the association between sets of data derived from a correlation design.

correlational design   design that tests an experimental hypothesis by collecting data on both the variables in the hypothesis to see if the data are related in some way. The two relationships that are of interest are positive correlations and negative correlations (see entries under these headings).

counterbalancing   a technique used in research design to overcome the bias caused by order effects. It involves ensuring that the order of testing a group of subjects is alternated so that any results will not be influenced by the sequence of testing.

data   the facts and figures collected during a research project.

decile   equivalent to 10 percentile points in that it is the point in a data base below which 10% (or multiples of 10%) of the scores lie;

e.g. the 3rd decile indicates the point below which the bottom 30% of the scores lie.

degrees of freedom   a complex concept involved in some statistical tests which refers to the extent to which data have the capacity to vary once certain limits have been imposed. It is abbreviated to 'df' and is very easy to calculate.

Delphi technique   a method of obtaining consensus agreement from a panel of experts on a topic for which there is either inconsistent empirical evidence or very little evidence.

dependent variable   the variable in an experimental hypothesis which changes as a result of manipulating the independent variable. The changes in the dependent variable constitute the data in a study and can be thought of as the effects of the manipulation of the independent variable.

descriptive statistics   methods of describing a set of results in terms of their most interesting characteristics.

different-subject design   experimental design that uses two or more separate or different groups of subjects each of which is tested once. The groups are then compared for any differences between them. Sometimes known as a between-or unrelated-subjects design.

discussion   a section of a research report that discusses the findings of that research.

double-blind technique   an aspect of research design whose aim is to minimise the biasing effect that subjects and experimenters may have on the results by knowing what the aims of the study are. The double-blind procedure involves keeping the subjects ignorant of the project's aims until after the data have been collected, as well as using someone other than the main researcher to collect the data. This person will also be unaware of the purpose of the research project.

effect size   the size of the clinical significance or effect of the independent variable on the dependent variable; this is distinct from statistical significance.

estimation   a form of scientific 'best guessing' where estimates of a population characteristic are made on the basis of knowledge of the sample characteristic. It is a useful tool in planning.

ethics   a set of guidelines imposed on a study to ensure that the project will not compromise or upset the subjects in any way.

experimental condition   a group of subjects in an experimental design who receive some form of intervention or level of the independent variable. This group may be compared with other experimental groups who receive a different form of intervention or with a control group who receive no intervention at all.

experimental design   a method of testing hypotheses which involves manipulating the independent variable(s) in the experimental hypothesis and monitoring what impact this has on the dependent variable. By doing this, cause and effect can be established.

experimental hypothesis   a prediction of a consistent and reliable relationship between two or more variables. The experimental hypothesis is the starting point of any piece of experimental research and is often referred to in the literature as H_1.

experimenter bias effects   a source of bias to the results which results from the experimenter (usually unwittingly) influencing subjects' responses so that they fulfil the experimenter's aims. It can be counteracted to some extent by using a naive data collector.

extended chi-squared (χ^2) test   a non-parametric statistical test for use with nominal data and different subject designs. It is used with more than two nominal categories and/or more than two groups of subjects.

false positive   an incorrect decision in diagnosis or screening tests, which classifies a patient as having a disease/condition, when in fact they don't have it.

false negative   an incorrect decision in diagnosis or screening tests, which classifies a patient as not having a disease/condition, when in fact they do have it.

fatigue effects   an aspect of order problems where subjects do worse on the second or subsequent testing because of fatigue. This can mask the real effects of the independent variable.

frequency distribution graph   a graph which presents the frequency with which any given event occurs. These graphs can be bar graphs, histograms and frequency polygons (see separate entries).

frequency polygon   a frequency distribution graph which is characterised by the single continuous line drawn between the points on the graph.

Friedman test   a non-parametric analysis of variance for use with same- or matched-subject design, using more than two testing conditions. The data can be ordinal or interval/ratio, but this test is most likely to be used with ordinal data.

grounded theory   a research approach in which data are first systematically collected and then theories and hypotheses generated to explain the data.

histogram   a frequency distribution graph characterised by the use of adjacent vertical columns.

incidental sample   a method of selecting subjects for study that involves using the most readily available people.

independent variable   that variable in the experimental hypothesis which is manipulated so that the impact of this on the dependent variable can be observed. It can be thought of as the cause of something happening.

inferential statistics   a statistical technique whereby results derived from a sample of subjects are also inferred to apply to the population from which they come.

interclass correlation coefficient (ICC)   a statistical method used in reliability studies which assesses the degree of closeness between raters' measurements, when the data are interval/ratio.

inter-observer reliability   the degree to which two or more people agree in their observations of an event.

interval   level of measurement usually linked with the ratio level of measurement, this is a level of data which: (a) allows parametric statistical tests to be performed; (b) assumes equal intervals in measurement between the data; (c) has no absolute zero (i.e. a score of 0 does not mean the absence of that characteristic).

interview a conversation between the researcher and the subject which aims to elicit information relevant to the research topic. This interview may follow prescribed topics (structured interview) or may be entirely open (unstructured interview).

introduction (to a research report) the section of a research report which reviews the relevant literature and provides a rationale and the aims of the study in question.

Jonckheere trend test a non-parametric statistical analysis which is used with three or more separate groups of subjects (a different-subject design), ordinal or interval/ratio data and for which the results are expected to be in a specified trend.

Kappa also known as Cohen's Kappa, this measures the agreement between two raters, when nominal data are used.

Kendall's coefficient of concordance a non-parametric statistical test used with correlational designs and ordinal data which assesses the extent of agreement between three or more sets of data.

Kruskal–Wallis test a non-parametric analysis of variance test used with three or more separate groups of subjects (a different-subject design) and ordinal or interval/ratio data.

levels of measurement the data collected from a piece of research fall into one of four levels of measurement, which differ in their sophistication and the type of calculation that can be performed on them. These levels are (in order of sophistication from least to most): nominal (least) ordinal interval ratio (most).

linear regression a statistical technique used with sets of data known to be correlated, such that values on one variable can be calculated from knowledge of the values on the other.

literature review a survey of all the research relevant to the topic in question, which allows the researcher to establish what has already been carried out.

Mann–Whitney U-test a non-parametric statistical test used with two separate groups

of subjects (a different-subject design) and ordinal or interval/ratio data.

matched–subject designs types of experimental designs that involve matching subjects on all those factors which may affect the results. While these designs have the advantage of not being affected by individual differences and order effects, they are very difficult to carry out properly.

materials any non-mechanical items used in a piece of research, e.g. questionnaires, blood pressure sheets, etc.

McNemar test a non-parametric statistical test used with same- or matched-subject designs, two testing conditions and nominal data. It assesses the significance of any changes noted over the two testings.

mean the average score in a set of data, calculated by adding up all the scores and dividing the total by the number of scores in the set of data.

median the middle score in a set of data, such that there are as many scores above it as below. It is also the 50th percentile point and the 5th decile.

method the section of a research report which describes in detail what was done, how and with whom, in a piece of research. It should be sufficiently detailed that anyone who reads this section should be able to replicate the study exactly.

mode the most frequently occurring score in a set of data.

negative correlation the relationship between two sets of data derived from a correlational design, whereby high scores on one set of data are associated with low scores on the other.

negative skew a frequency distribution distorted to one side because too many subjects recorded high scores.

nominal level of measurement a very basic level of measurement (sometimes referred to as categorical data) which simply allocates subjects or their responses to named categories. It is characterised by the following: (a) only non-parametric statistical analyses can be performed on these data; (b) the categories are mutually exclusive;

(c) there is no commonly understood value attached to the category labels.

non-parametric tests   techniques of data analysis that are less sensitive and rather cruder than parametric tests. They can be used, in principle, with all levels of measurement, but are most commonly associated with the nominal and ordinal levels.

normal distribution   a symmetrical bell-shaped curve which has certain properties that are critical to statistical inference.

null hypothesis   the prediction which counters the claim made by the experimental hypothesis in a study. The null hypothesis predicts there is no relationship between the variables in the experimental hypothesis. It is often referred to in the literature as H_0.

observation   a technique of conducting research which involves the researcher simply observing what goes on in naturalistic settings.

one-tailed hypotheses or tests   these refer to hypotheses where a prediction is made that the results of the study will be in a specific direction.

open-ended questions   questions that allow the respondent to reply in a free and unstructured way to any given question.

order effects   a source of bias usually found in same-subject designs where the order in which the subjects were tested rather than the independent variable producing the results. This can be overcome by counterbalancing the order of testing.

ordinal level of measurement   a type of data which allows the researcher to rank order subjects along the dimension of interest (e.g. least improvement–most improvement). An important feature of this scale is that, while it allows the researcher to impose a numerical score on the subject's response, the differences between the points on the scale are not equal.

Page's L trend test   a non-parametric test used with same- or matched-subject designs which yields three or more sets of ordinal or interval/ratio data. A particular characteristic is that a trend in the results is specifically predicted.

parametric tests   techniques of statistical analysis which are said to be robust and sensitive. They require certain conditions or parameters to be fulfilled before they can be applied, the most important of which is that the data must be interval/ratio.

Pearson test   a parametric test for use with correlational designs and interval/ratio data.

percentile   indicates the percentage of scores that lie below a given score in a data base, e.g. the 15th percentile is the point in a data set below which 15% of the scores lie.

personal construct theory   a theory of personality developed by Kelly, which suggests that individuals constantly attempt to make sense of their own important experiences, life events and personal world. These salient features are called elements, and each is described by the individual using a limited set of bipolar descriptions called constructs. Together, the elements and constructs provide an insight into the individual, his/her values and perceptions. The method used to find out which elements and constructs are of relevance to a particular person is called 'repertory grid analysis'.

pilot study   a preliminary run of the main study to highlight any problems, which can then be corrected.

placebo effect   an interesting phenomenon whereby subjects show a significant degree of improvement even though their treatment is known to have no use.

point estimation   a statistical 'best guess' which provides a single figure estimate (usually an average or percentage figure) of a population characteristic based on information about the sample's characteristic.

population   a group of people all of whom have a characteristic in common which is of interest to the researcher, e.g. talipes. The sample for study in the research is drawn from this parent population.

population characteristic   see characteristic.

positive correlation   the degree of relationship between the data from two or more variables derived from a correlational design, such that high scores on one variable are associated with high scores from the other(s); similarly, low scores are associated with low scores.

positive skew   a frequency distribution where the data are distorted towards the lower scores, e.g. where students perform badly on an exam that is too difficult.

post-test   a measurement of the dependent variable which takes place after the intervention has occurred.

power level   the power of a statistical test to detect any impact of the independent variable on the dependent variable; the power of a test is partly dependent on the size of the sample involved.

practice effects   a variety of order effects whereby subjects perform better on second and subsequent testings and this improved performance masks the effects of the independent variable.

pretest   a measurement of the dependent variable which takes place before any intervention has occurred.

probability   the likelihood that random error is producing the results in a study. It is expressed as a percentage or decimal and is usually abbreviated to 'p'.

Q-methodology   a mixed qualitative/quantitative approach aimed at capturing subjective experiences; the technique clusters respondents according to the similarity of their reported experiences.

qualitative research   techniques of research investigation which collect non-numerical information from subjects.

quantitative research   techniques of research which collect non-numerical information from subjects.

questionnaire   a method of collecting information whereby subjects answer a set of questions usually predefined by the researcher.

quota sample   a process of selecting a sample to participate in a research study, such that preset quotas of subjects will be selected to represent categories deemed to be important.

random error   any source of bias or error in a piece of research which will affect the results in a random and unpredictable way. They include a variety of individual differences and cannot be eliminated completely.

random number tables   tables of randomly generated numbers which can be used to select a random sample of subjects for study.

random selection/sample   a method of selecting subjects to take part in a study, such that every member of the parent population has an equal chance of being chosen.

randomised controlled trials (RCTs)   these are considered to be the gold-standard research design in health care, because of their capacity to reduce bias; amongst other requirements, the design demands that control groups, strict randomisation procedures and blind procedures are used.

range   the difference between the lowest score and the highest score in a set of data.

ratio level of measurement   the 'highest' level of data which is characterised by equal intervals between the data points and an absolute zero which represents an absence of the quality in question.

references   a section in a research report that lists all the research articles referred to in the body of the report.

related t-test   a parametric statistical test for use with same- or matched-subject designs and two sets of interval/ratio data.

reliability   the degree to which a psychological test measures the same attribute each time it is used. It is an important feature of any psychological test.

repertory grid analysis   a technique deriving from personal construct theory that involves eliciting from an individual the most salient elements in his/her life; the individual is then asked to evaluate these elements using relevant bipolar constructs. The results provide a rich data bank of information about the way in which the individual makes sense of his/her personal world. The method can be adapted for many purposes and the results can be analysed in a variety of ways, both qualitatively and quantitatively.

representative sample   a sample that is typical or accurately reflects the population from which it comes.

research proposal   an outline of an anticipated piece of research covering background literature, aims, objectives, methodology, proposed analysis and a cost/benefit analysis. A research proposal is often required by ethical committees or when funding is applied for.

ROC (receiver operating characteristics)   a method used to assess the accuracy of diagnostic and screening tests in correctly identifying patients who either have or do not have a disease/risk factor.

same-subject design   a variant of experimental design which involves testing the same group of subjects on two or more occasions. They are typically used in before/after designs.

sample   a group of subjects selected from a parent population, who are used in a piece of research.

scattergram   a technique of plotting data, derived from correlational studies, in a graph. A general upward slope to the graph indicates a positive correlation; a general downward slope indicates a negative correlation.

Scheffé multiple range test   a statistical technique used in conjunction with parametric anovas which have yielded significant results. The Scheffé test allows the researcher to make an objective scrutiny of the data in order to establish which parts were responsible for the significant anova results.

sensitivity   a term used in diagnostic and screening tests to describe the ability of a test to correctly identify patients who have a disease/risk factor.

significance level   a cut-off point, usually of 5% or less, such that, if the results from a piece of research have a probability of 5% or less of being due to random error, then they are said to be significant. The null (no relationship) hypothesis can then be rejected in favour of the experimental hypothesis.

Spearman test   a non-parametric test for use with correlational designs and ordinal or interval/ratio data.

specificity   a term used in diagnostic and screening tests to describe the ability of a test to correctly identify patients who do not have a disease/risk factor.

standard deviation   a measure of the average amount that a set of scores varies or deviates from the mean.

standard score   see Z score.

stratified random sample   a method of selecting a sample from a population, so that subgroups of that population are represented in the sample.

subjects   the individual people who take part in a study.

survey   a method of collecting data which involves the researcher measuring relevant sample variables (often using a questionnaire) without any form of manipulation or systematic intervention.

systematic reviews   a rigorous, objective and comprehensive method of distilling all published and unpublished literature on a specified subject.

systematic sample   a method of selecting a sample for study by choosing every fourth, fifth, or whatever, member of the parent population.

Thurstone Paired Comparison Technique   a questionnaire-based method of eliciting rank-ordered preferences, using a system of forced-choice responses; it is particularly useful in identifying user priorities for service planning/modification.

true positive   a decision in diagnosis or screening tests, which correctly classifies a patient as having a disease/condition.

true negative   a decision in diagnosis or screening tests, which correctly classifies a patient as not having a disease/condition.

two-tailed hypothesis or test   an experimental hypothesis which simply predicts that the variables in the hypothesis are related, but does not specify the precise nature of that relationship.

Type I error   a conclusion that there is a relationship between the variables in the hypothesis, when in fact there is not.

Type II error   a conclusion that there is no relationship between the variables in the hypothesis when, in fact, there is.

unrelated t-test   a parametric statistical test used with two different groups of subjects and interval/ratio data.

validity   the degree to which a psychological test measures what it is intended to measure. There are four types of validity: construct validity refers to the degree to which a test measures the theoretical ideas underpinning a particular topic; content validity refers to the degree to which the test measures the overt manifestations of the theory; face validity refers to the degree to which the test looks as though it is measuring what it is supposed to measure; predictive validity refers to the degree to which responses to the test can predict future behaviour.

variable   any event or characteristic which has the capacity to vary (e.g. weight, age, etc.).

variance   the degree to which a set of scores vary or are dispersed.

weighted kappa   a statistical technique used in reliability testing, when two raters and ordinal data are used; the importance of any disagreements between the raters has to be decided in advance and factored into the calculation.

Wilcoxon test   a non-parametric statistical test used with same- or matched-subject designs, and two sets of ordinal or interval/ratio data.

Youden's index   a formula used in diagnostic and screening tests to determine a suitable threshold for classifying a patient as having or not having a disease or risk factor.

Z score   (also known as standard score) a measure of relative performance, in that it tells the researcher exactly how many standard deviations a given score is from the mean.

Index

WITHDRAWN
FROM STOCK
QMUL LIBRARY

WITHDRAWN
FROM STOCK
QMUL LIBRARY